Teaching the
Student with Spina Bifida

Teaching the Student with Spina Bifida

Edited by

Fern L. Rowley-Kelly, M.S.W., L.S.W.
Program Director
Spina Bifida Association of Western
 Pennsylvania
Pittsburgh, Pennsylvania

and

Donald H. Reigel, M.D.
Director
Pediatric Neurosurgery
Director
Spina Bifida Center
Allegheny General Hospital
Professor of Surgery (Neurosurgery)
Medical College of Pennsylvania
Pittsburgh, Pennsylvania

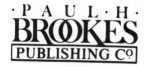

·P·A·U·L·H·
BROOKES
PUBLISHING Co.

Baltimore · London · Toronto · Sydney

Paul H. Brookes Publishing Co.
Post Office Box 10624
Baltimore, Maryland 21285-0624

Copyright © 1993 by Paul H. Brookes Publishing Co., Inc.
All rights reserved.

Typeset by Brushwood Graphics, Inc., Baltimore, Maryland.
Manufactured in the United States of America by
The Maple Press Company, York, Pennsylvania.

Permission to reprint the following quotations is gratefully acknowledged:

Pages 73–74:   Quotation from *School nurses working with handicapped children.*
Copyright © 1980, American Nurses' Association, Kansas City, MO, pp. 4–5.
Reprinted by permission.

Page 75:   Quotation from *Standards of school nursing practice.* Copyright ©
1983, American Nurses' Association, Kansas City, MO, pp.18–19. Reprinted by
permission.

Page 76:   Quotation from Grunfeld, C. (1984). *Physical disabilities.* Denver:
School Nurse Achievement Program at the University of Colorado School of Nursing, p. 32. Reprinted by permission.

Page 81:   Quotation from *School nurses working with handicapped children.*
Copyright © 1980, American Nurses' Association, Kansas City, MO, p. 5. Reprinted by permission. Also from Grunfeld, C. (1984). *Physical disabilities.* Denver: School Nurse Achievement Program at the University of Colorado School of
Nursing, p. vi. Reprinted by permission.

Pages 82–83:   Quotation from *Standards of school nursing practice.* Copyright
© 1983, American Nurses' Association, Kansas City, MO, pp. 3–5, 7–15. Reprinted by permission.

Library of Congress Cataloging-in-Publication Data
Teaching the student with spina bifida / [edited by] Fern L. Rowley-Kelly, Donald
H. Reigel.
      p.   cm.
   Includes bibliographical references and index.
   ISBN 1-55766-064-6 :
   1. Physically handicapped children—Education—United States. 2. Spina bi-
fida—United States. 3. Mainstreaming in education—United States. I.
Rowley-Kelly, Fern L., 1946–   II. Reigel, Donald H., 1937–
LC4231.T43   1992
371.91—dc20   92-15260
                                                                    CIP

British Library Cataloguing-in-Publication data are available from the British
Library.

Contents

The Editors

Fern L. Rowley-Kelly, M.S.W., L.S.W., Program Director, Spina Bifida Association of Western Pennsylvania, 320 East North Avenue, 7th Floor, South Tower, Pittsburgh, Pennsylvania 15212.

Fern L. Rowley-Kelly, M.S.W, L.S.W., has been an active participant in the Spina Bifida Association of Western Pennsylvania since 1978. She is presently the Program Director for the Association. She led the development of the national model camping program for children with spina bifida. She has also researched and developed the School Consultation and Personnel Training Program. Ms. Rowley-Kelly has conducted family research that resulted in the publication of *Behavioral Family Treatment for Families with an Adolescent with Spina Bifida: A Treatment Manual*. She has directed the development of the Gatehouse Program—a transition independence program for young adults with spina bifida. Her research of families with spina bifida has led to unique psychoeducational support for parents of children with spina bifida.

Donald H. Reigel, M.D., Director, Pediatric Neurosurgery, Tri-State Neurological Associates, and Director, Spina Bifida Center, Allegheny General Hospital, East Wing, 320 East North Avenue, Suite 302, Pittsburgh, Pennsylvania 15212

Donald H. Reigel, M.D., has been an important contributor in the development of support programs for people with spina bifida at The Woodlands—a $5 million, 32-acre facility that serves as the home of The Gatehouse, a residential, independent living, training program for young adults, a summer camping program for children and teens, and the development of model housing for adults. Dr. Reigel is the medical director of the Spina Bifida Center of Allegheny General Hospital, where more than 700 persons with spina bifida are treated. He is also Director of Pediatric Neurosurgery at Allegheny General Hospital and Professor of Surgery (Neurosurgery) at the Medical College of Pennsylvania. He is past president of the American Society of Pediatric Neurosurgeons and past Chairman of the Pediatric Section of the American Association of Neurological Surgeons. He is the Managing Editor of *Pediatric Neurosurgery*, an international journal dedicated to children's neurosurgery. He serves as Chairman of the Board of the Spina Bifida Association of Western Pennsylvania, which has been primarily responsible for developing programs of education and support for people with spina bifida.

Contributors

Suzanne Benintend Baker, P.T., M.Ed.
Spina Bifida Center
Allegheny General Hospital
7th Floor, South Tower
Pittsburgh, Pennsylvania 15212

William J. Casile, Ph.D.
Associate Professor
Department of Counseling,
    Psychology, and Special
    Education
Duquesne University
Pittsburgh, Pennsylvania 15282

Barbara Culatta, Ph.D.
Department of Communicative
    Disorders
Adams Hall
University of Rhode Island
Kingston, Rhode Island 02881

Nancy Hubley, Esq.
Education Law Center
1708 Law and Finance Building
429 4th Avenue
Pittsburgh, Pennsylvania 15219

Anne DesNoyers Hurley, Ph.D.
Massachusetts School of
    Professional Psychology
and Massachusetts Hospital
    School
322 Sprague Street
Dedham, Massachusetts 02026

Pamela Meyer Kunkle, B.A., B.S.
School Program Coordinator
Spina Bifida Association of
    Western Pennsylvania
320 East North Avenue
7th Floor, South Tower
Pittsburgh, Pennsylvania 15212

Ruth E. Leo, R.N.C., CRNP, M.Ed.
Assistant Professor of Nursing
Department of Nursing
Slippery Rock University
Slippery Rock, Pennsylvania
    16057-1326

Ellen Mancuso, B.A.
Education Law Center
Suite 610
801 Arch Street
Philadelphia, Pennsylvania 19107

Mary A. Rogosky-Grassi, O.T.R.
Spina Bifida Clinic
320 East North Avenue
7th Floor, South Tower
Pittsburgh, Pennsylvania 15212

Preface

The 1970s and 1980s saw many new questions and problems arising in the field of primary education as increasing numbers of children born with spina bifida entered public schools. This came about because of PL 94-142 and the fact that large numbers of children born with spina bifida were surviving in good health with the capacity to pursue a public education. Teachers and other school professionals with little experience in working with students with spina bifida were now facing new challenges. The parents of children with spina bifida were frightened and anxious about relinquishing daily care to educators. Students with spina bifida found themselves in a new and unfamiliar learning and social environment which produced a range of emotional, intellectual, and physical demands. Similarly, their classmates experienced discomfort because of the arrival of a new set of special students. *Teaching the Student with Spina Bifida* is written for all people concerned with the education of children with spina bifida.

The contributing authors of this book represent a variety of disciplines. They are intricately involved with efforts to enhance the lives of children with spina bifida. The authors, through their respective chapters, have made every effort to share their experience and work in order to produce confidence and security in the pursuit of education for students with spina bifida.

This book is divided into four sections. Section I, Health and Related Services in Educational Settings, addresses the health care needs of children with spina bifida. It indicates that health care and education of children with spina bifida may proceed in separate but integrated fashions, each contributing to the welfare of all students. Section II, Tailoring the Academic Program, discusses how careful neuropsychological testing and evaluation identify the learning skills of a student with spina bifida and may help to maximize his or her educational opportunity. In Section III, Beyond the Curriculum, the authors emphasize the fact that the education of students with spina bifida, as with all students, extends far beyond the classroom. This section discusses social and family issues that affect students with spina bifida and their rights and the resources available to ensure quality education. Section IV, Supporting Effective Education, concludes the book with a discussion of a school outreach program.

This book is dedicated to students with spina bifida. For the authors it has been a privilege to meet teachers and school professionals from many parts of the country who educate, assist, and inspire students with spina bifida. The authors discovered that, as in most educational settings, those who teach students with spina bifida often become learners as well.

The editors are grateful to Gay Simpson, Executive Director of the Spina Bifida Association of Western Pennsylvania, for her continuing support and encouragement. They are also thankful to all of the unnamed individuals who contributed silently and sincerely to the contents of this book.

Teaching the
Student with Spina Bifida

Health and
Related Services
in Educational Settings

Spina Bifida from Infancy through the School Years

Donald H. Reigel

Medical advances in the care of children born with spina bifida have enabled 90% or more of these children to survive through school age and enter classrooms throughout the United States. Thus, each year thousands of people working in the field of education experience the special challenges of providing maximal opportunity for the student with spina bifida. Although this birth defect is surprisingly common, many teachers will experience bewilderment and apprehension when they learn that a student with spina bifida will be in one of their classes or activity sessions. These feelings are often compounded by unfamiliarity and concern about the student with physical disability. Frequently, conversations with colleagues and friends will do little to alleviate the teacher's insecurity about his or her role in working with these pupils. Consultation with the school nurse and psychologist may be of help, but a search for current resource materials will lead to disappointment as the teacher attempts to prepare for the student with spina bifida. Since many of the student's past experiences with doctors and hospitals will provide important background for understanding and determining the student's future psychosocial and academic needs, this first chapter is devoted to the health care of the student with spina bifida.

Advances in medical care of people with spina bifida have led to the prediction that most may expect a nearly normal life span. In addition to the nervous system, spina bifida may be associated with abnormalities in other organ systems of the body. Therefore, quality health care requires the services of many specialists such as neurosurgeons (surgery of the brain and spinal cord), orthopedists (bracing, surgery of spine, hips, feet), urologists (surgical care of kidney and bladder), neurologists (seizure treatment), ophthalmologists (surgical treatment of problems of the eye), pediatricians, and a wide variety of other people working with these physicians. Most areas of the United States now have health care programs for spina bifida that include all of these medical specialists and also colleagues in psychology and the social sciences. These special programs are often regionalized and are called spina bifida centers or clinics. They are dedicated to the wellness of the person with spina bifida. This goal would be impossible without organized teamwork. Similarly, the educational goals for the student with spina bifida are best achieved by utilization of the team model (Figure 1.1). Ideally, the spina bifida health care program is only one part of the team that includes the parents, teacher, school nurse, special education teacher, psychologist, vocational rehabilitation counselor, and when available, special advocates for people with spina bifida. Review of Figure 1.1 will quickly show that the key team members are already in place in most school systems. This book provides the information required to enable this team to work together for benefit of the education of the student with spina bifida. Experience indicates that full, rewarding education is now possible for all students with spina bifida. Commitment to this goal will also lead to new reward and excitement for teachers and other school personnel.

WHAT IS SPINA BIFIDA?

Spina bifida is the most common crippler of children. In 1988 approximately 4 million children were born in the United States (Statistical Abstract of the United States, 1988). The incidence of spina bifida is thought to be 0.5–1.0 per thousand live births (Greenberg, James, & Oakley, 1983; Thompson & Rudd, 1976). Therefore, perhaps 4,000 children with spina bifida were born in 1988. Most people are surprised to learn that spina bifida is not a new disease and that archaeological discoveries have identified characteristic spinal changes in 7,000-year-old skeletons (Gool & Good, 1986). The incidence varies between countries and races. For instance, spina bifida occurs in 4–5 births per 1,000 in northern Ireland and less than 0.1 per 1,000 in Colombia, while appearing only rarely in blacks and Asians. There is a slightly higher occurrence among females than males (Reigel, 1989).

As with other complex diseases, there are gradations of severity of spina bifida. *Spina bifida occulta*, the most common and innocent form of spina bifida, occurs in one-third of the United States population. It is characterized by an absence of a small portion of the vertebrae (Figure 1.2) (Boone, Pansons, Lochman, & Sherwood, 1985). This abnormality is not detectable by physical examination and is most frequently discovered on an X ray obtained for routine purposes such as evaluation of

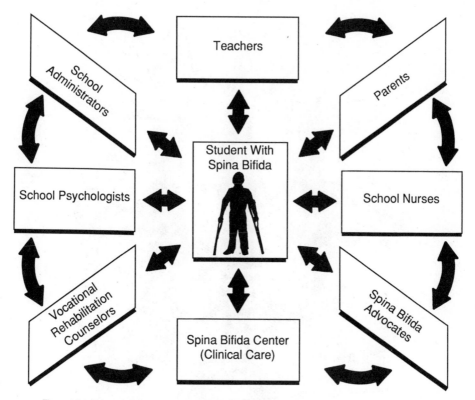

Figure 1.1. Team model for the education of the student with spina bifida.

back pain. Spina bifida occulta rarely affects the nervous system and is of little or no consequence to the person.

Meningocele is an abnormality present at birth and identified by a skin-covered mass (lump or swelling) located in the lumbar region (lower area of the spine). The mass or cyst contains cerebrospinal fluid and only rarely affects the spinal cord and nerves. Many people with meningocele have the lump surgically removed with no loss of neurologic function.

Myelomeningocele (spina bifida cystica) is the most severe form of spina bifida. It appears at birth as an open cyst or mass, usually located in the lumbar area, that may be leaking cerebrospinal fluid (see Figure 1.3). Myelomeningocele involves the lining of the spinal canal, the spinal cord, and nerves. Children born with this form of spina bifida have varying amounts of physical disability. Over 90% have some degree of weakness of their legs, inability to voluntarily control the bowel or bladder, and a variety of orthopedic abnormalities. Today, shortly after birth, almost all

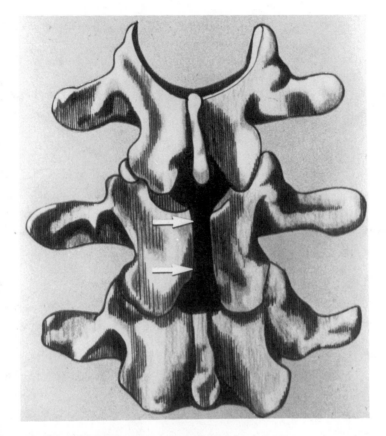

Figure 1.2. Spina bifida occulta. Arrows indicate missing spinous process.

children with myelomeningocele are treated with an operation to close the opening in the spine. Early surgery prevents infection of the central nervous system by removing the mass and closing the opening over the back. Also, closure of the opening with soft tissue and skin prevents additional injury to the nervous tissue. During surgery, a microscope is used to magnify the appearance of the spinal cord and thereby prevent injury to potentially functional tissue. The operation does *not* restore function of the abnormal nerve tissue. The operation takes 1–2 hours and if completed within the first few hours of life, the mother can begin holding and feeding the child within the first day. The most common complication of this surgery is infection and cerebrospinal fluid leakage. However, if promptly treated, these problems need not cause further disability. The goal of the early treatment program is for the child to leave the hospital at the time of the mother's discharge.

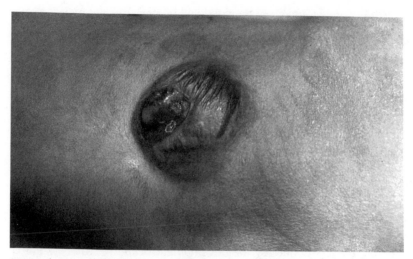

Figure 1.3.   Typical lumbar myelomeningocele. The head is to the left and the buttocks to the right.

The cause of spina bifida is unknown. Multiple factors seem to be related to its development such as race, malnutrition, and poverty; cluster-like occurrences point to possible environmental influences (Reigel, 1989). There also seems to be a family tendency or predisposition. For instance, if one sibling has spina bifida, the risk of a subsequent child having spina bifida increases to about 5%. If two previous children have spina bifida, the risk increases to approximately 12%–15% for a subsequent sibling to be born with spina bifida (Fraser, 1974). Studies of twins have failed to demonstrate a simple genetic inheritance (Thompson & Rudd, 1976).

Spina bifida develops during the first 26 days of intrauterine life of the fetus. Frequently the prospective parents have not yet become aware of the pregnancy (Warkany, 1977). It is important to understand that genetic inheritance has not been demonstrated; the parents or ancestors cannot be incriminated as a direct causal factor. Contrary to this fact, many parents harbor feelings of responsibility for the birth of a child with spina bifida. The lifelong guilt that follows becomes one of the origins of overprotection and relaxed parental demand that produces excessively dependent behavior in the child.

Although much of the developmental history of the pupil with spina bifida parallels that of peers, many differences will be found because of special health care that begins at birth and continues through life. During the preschool period and the early school years, required medical care profoundly affects the child, the family, and the educational process. Awareness of the medical events that occur during important stages of growth and development of the child will be of significant benefit to everyone concerned with the education of the student with spina bifida. Therefore, this chapter discusses the health care needs that occur during intrauterine life, the preschool years, ages 5–12, and from adolescence to adulthood. Each of these periods is associated with recurring and new experiences surrounding the acquisition of health care.

BEFORE BIRTH

The development of spina bifida begins during the first days of pregnancy. The human nervous system develops from a sheet of fetal cells known as neuroectoderm. With cell division and migration, this sheet of neural tissue rolls together to form a tube. From this neural tube, the nervous system (brain, spinal cord, and peripheral nerves) develop. Spina bifida occurs when, for unknown reasons, a portion of the neural tube fails to close. Subsequently the development of the nervous system is altered, resulting in an abnormal central nervous system (McLone, Suna, Collins, Poznanski, & Knepper, 1983). This failure of the neural tube to close properly occurs at 26–27 days of intrauterine life. Therefore, the events leading to the birth of a child with spina bifida have often occurred before most parents know that they are expecting a baby.

Today, prenatal diagnosis permits increasing numbers of expectant parents to prepare for a baby with spina bifida. However, despite the availability of prenatal testing, many newborns with spina bifida are not identified until birth. Whether an expectant couple learns that they are going to have a child with spina bifida during the fourth or fifth month of pregnancy or at the time of birth, they experience immense grief, precipitated by the loss of the dream of health and happiness for their new child. This grief is compounded by sadness about potential disability and suffering for their baby. Often during this period, misinformation is provided to the parents by well-meaning individuals that serves only to deepen their grief and subsequent depression and anger.

The prenatal diagnosis of a child with spina bifida is made by a combination of tests. First suspicion is often raised by a maternal blood test for the presence of a specific fetal protein (alpha-fetoprotein) (AFP) that leaks from the open spine of the fetus into amniotic fluid and subsequently enters the mother's bloodstream (Milunsky, 1979). If the blood serum alpha-fetoprotein is elevated, additional testing such as ultrasonographic imaging of the fetus and amniocentesis will be recommended. Amniocentesis is performed by aspirating a small amount of fluid from within the uterus. The fluid is then analyzed for alpha-fetoprotein and enzymes (Shurtleff, Lemire, & Warkany, 1986).

If these studies confirm the presence of spina bifida, the parents often face the agonizing decision whether to interrupt or continue with the pregnancy.

The obstetrician, pediatric neurosurgeon, and pediatrician attempt to provide each couple with factual information about the baby, the current outlook for children with spina bifida, and services available for health care and support of the family. If the parents elect to continue the pregnancy, the members of the spina bifida health care team work closely with them to prepare for the baby's arrival. Obviously prenatal preparation has many potential advantages for the parents. By the time of birth, they have already gone through the grief process and therefore are better prepared to concentrate on the care of the newborn child. By contrast, the parents who are shocked at the time of birth to learn that their child has spina bifida simultaneously have to learn about spina bifida, make treatment decisions, and struggle with grief and depression.

For most parents, pregnancy is a time of intense anticipation and dreams of the future. Often these dreams are for the anticipated child's activities, education, and intellect. The birth of a child with spina bifida turns these exciting thoughts to emotions of disappointment, grief, and depression. Therefore, the lifelong challenge of those concerned with this new child is to restore the parents' dreams of a joyful, rewarding, and meaningful life for their child. The provision of immediate comprehensive multidisciplinary care for the newborn enables the parents to concentrate on bonding with the baby. This form of total health care allows the infant to reach maximal developmental potential.

THE FIRST FIVE YEARS

Following birth, with the infant still in the delivery room, spina bifida is discovered by physical examination. The nurse or physician observes a cystic-like mass of variable size in the midline of the back, usually toward the bottom of the spine. Eighty-five percent will be located in the lumbar and sacral areas and the remainder will be scattered in the thoracic and cervical areas (see Chapter 2, Figure 2.1). This mass contains cerebrospinal fluid, the abnormal spinal cord, and other nervous tissue. With discovery of this form of spina bifida (myelomeningocele), the newborn is referred to a pediatric neurosurgeon for treatment. Often, medical care requires transfer of the baby to a hospital with a specialized treatment program for children with spina bifida. This type of transfer often separates the mother and infant. The baby goes to a children's unit and the mother remains in the community hospital, leaving the father to shuttle between family members and the two hospitals. With this separation, the mother may be excluded from active decisions and care of her newborn baby, a trauma that interferes with early bonding and increases the early grief and suffering of the parents. However, today, with prenatal diagnosis and preparation, many families choose to deliver their babies in medical centers where mother and child may be hospitalized together. If the baby with spina bifida was unanticipated, both the mother and baby can be transferred from the community hospital to a medical center where the baby can receive early surgical treatment and the mother can continue to receive her postpartum care. This move enables the parents to participate equally in medical decisions and take the important steps toward early bonding and care of the child.

Each newborn baby with spina bifida is promptly evaluated for associated health problems and degree of neurologic abnormality. The attending pediatric neurosurgeon and pediatrician then begin to teach the parents about the infant and the possible extent of the disability. The primary worries of the parents relate to the outlook for intellectual development, ambulation, and survival. They are given the current data that 95% or more of newborn children with myelomeningocele survive the newborn period. Eighty percent or more have normal intelligence and 85% learn to walk with or without some form of assistance such as crutches and braces (McLone & Naidich, 1989). Most parents are repeatedly instructed in the sad fact that the surgical treatment to close the opening of the back is done for the purpose of preventing infection and preserving existing function, but *not* to *restore* absent neurologic function. Often, despite repeated explanations, the parents cling to the hope that the primary operation will restore neurologic function that only heightens their emotional turmoil. In addition to acceptance of a child with weak legs, the parents learn that, because of abnormal nerve supply to the bladder and rectum, fewer than 5% of people with myelomeningocele develop voluntary control of these organs. The concept of artificially emptying the bladder and conditioning the bowel to prevent incontinence must be learned by parents and eventually the children.

Furthermore, the parents during the newborn period learn about **hydrocephalus**. This is a condition characterized by an excessive accumulation of cerebrospinal fluid within the brain (specifically the ventricles or caves of the brain) (Figure 1.4). Eighty to ninety percent of children born with myelomeningocele develop hydrocephalus (Reigel, 1989). Approximately 25% or more are born with hydrocephalus and an additional 60% develop it after the primary operation for closure of the opening on the back. Therefore, shortly after birth, most parents are forced to learn about a second condition requiring an additional operation—the placement of a cerebrospinal fluid shunt. The operative treatment of hydrocephalus consists of the insertion of a small silastic tube between the ventricles of the brain that detours the accumulating spinal fluid to an alternate site of absorption such as the abdomen or heart. This tube is

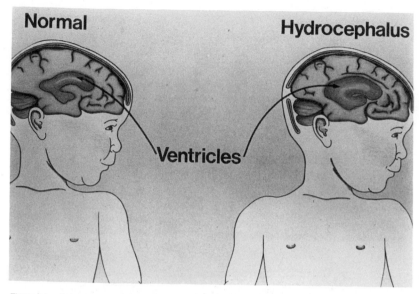

Figure 1.4.   Enlargement of the ventricular system characteristic of hydrocephalus.

located beneath the skin (Figure 1.5). Today, in a small percentage of patients, this operation is done just prior to the operation for closure of the back. Thus, within the first few hours of life, the child has two major operations. These procedures are done as soon as the neurosurgeon believes that the operations may be done without undue risk to the child and the parents are able to provide consent.

Following surgery, as soon as the baby is stable, the parents are permitted to hold and begin feeding the child. The purpose of the operation for hydrocephalus is to prevent excessive head growth and to permit normal brain growth. Since hydrocephalus persists throughout life, there is a continuous need for the cerebrospinal fluid shunt. Unavoidably, with growth and development, the complication of obstruction of cerebrospinal fluid flow through the shunt tubing is common. Therefore, many children have surgical revisions of their shunts. Infection may complicate operations to insert or revise shunts in 4%–10% of patients (Quigley, Reigel, & Kortyna, 1989). In the absence of infection, the parents are advised that they may expect intellectual development for their child that will match a peer group without spina bifida.

Immediately after birth, the clinical team begins intensive support and education of the parents. The staff continually assures the parents that their feelings of self-doubt, fears of inadequacy, and profound guilt are not unique to parents of children with spina bifida, but are common for all parents of children with health care problems. Staff members at-

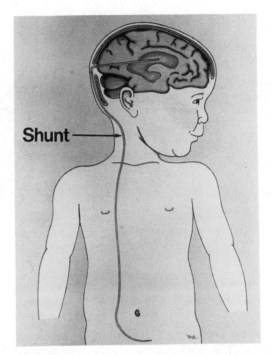

Figure 1.5.   Ventriculoperitoneal shunt. Excessive spinal fluid is diverted from the ventricles to the abdomen, where it is absorbed by a thin layer of tissue, the peritoneum, which lines the abdominal cavity.

tempt to demonstrate confidence in the parents' ability to care for and love their newborn while simultaneously establishing foundations for continuing care and compassion.

During the initial hospitalization, the baby is evaluated by an orthopedist in order to begin care of problems related to the skeletal system, such as leg and spine deformity. The most common problems of infancy requiring orthopedic management are **dislocated hip** and **club feet**. In the event of hip dislocation, the parents are instructed in nighttime positioning of the legs. Surgery to relocate the hips can be considered at about the age of 6 months. Club feet are treated with splints (Chapter 2) with the possibility of further casting or surgery. Early orthopedic management is highly successful and leads to improved potential for balance, sitting, and early ambulation (Mayfield, 1991; Menelaus, 1976).

From birth the parents will be taught the importance of emptying the child's bladder periodically. Because spina bifida damages the nerves to the bladder, the baby is not able to empty a full bladder completely. Retention of urine is also impaired because of the inability to relax the bladder outlet sphincters (the internal and external sphincters that function as outlet controls between the bladder and the urethra) (Figure 1.6). Initially, the parents are taught to compress the abdominal area over the bladder periodically in order to empty it (Crede maneuver). Failure to empty the bladder completely leaves residual urine that may cause bladder infection and subsequent kidney infection. However, for some children this manual method of emptying the bladder is inadequate and intermittent catheterization is required. For those children with poor sphincter control or a small bladder brought about by continuous abnormal contraction of the muscle wall of the bladder, medications may be prescribed that reduce bladder contraction such that dryness between catheterizations is achieved.

Today the goal of the early treatment program is to have the baby leave the hospital within the first week of life. When this day arrives, the parents are given a specific date for return to the spina bifida center for

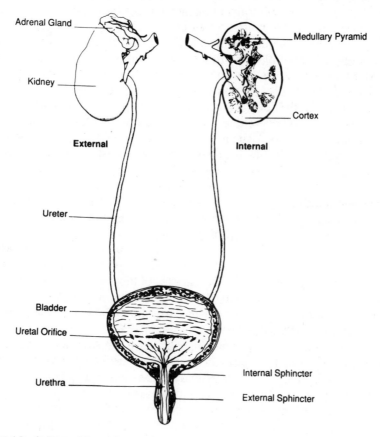

Figure 1.6. Anatomy of the urinary tract.

examination of the child and the beginning of continuing, comprehensive outpatient care and support. Detailed records will be maintained and copies will be forwarded to the family doctor or pediatrician.

Near the end of the first year of life, the orthopedist and physical and occupational therapists begin to develop plans for ambulation. The parents are taught to help the child use bracing designed to compensate for the level of lower extremity weakness (Chapter 2). Outpatient, community-based physical and occupational therapy programs work with the parents to teach the child to stand and walk with crutches between the age of 18 months and 2 years. Simultaneously, developmental patterns are evaluated and liaison with infant stimulation programs is established to achieve maximal developmental potential.

During the ensuing first 5 years of the child's life, there are repeated visits to the spina bifida center for examinations to identify and prevent potential health problems; assure function of the shunt; and detect skeletal changes, urinary tract infection, and seizure (epilepsy).

Thirty percent or more of children with spina bifida develop seizure, which is defined as an uncontrolled electrical discharge of the brain (Shurtleff & Dunne, 1986). During early childhood, seizure usually takes the form of petit mal, a brief staring episode of only a few seconds. Diagnosis is made by observation of characteristic episodes and an electroencephalogram (EEG). If untreated, seizure may lead to learning deficit. Seizure can be prevented with medications such as phenobarbital, Dilantin, and Tegretol. Usually by the time the child reaches preschool, seizure has been identified and successfully treated. These medications do not generally produce drowsiness or other side effects that interfere with education. Consultation with the school nurse helps to clarify questions about the child with spina bifida and a known seizure disorder. The appendix to this chapter provides answers to questions commonly asked by teachers of children with spina bifida.

Infants with spina bifida also show an increased incidence of **strabismus** (crossed eyes), necessitating yearly ophthalmologic examinations to identify weakness of the muscles of the eye. Correction may be achieved with medication and/or minor outpatient surgery. Persistent untreated strabismus occurring during early childhood may cause amblyopia (blindness) (Biglan, 1990).

All children with myelomeningocele have the **Arnold-Chiari malformation**, a variable displacement of the posterior part of the brain into the cervical spinal canal. It frequently causes easy gagging and difficult swallowing for the child. However, in the severest forms, it may cause breathing disorders and intermittent pneumonia. These severe problems usually appear within the first few weeks of life, but may appear at any time. The treatment of the mild forms of Arnold-Chiari malformation is usually supportive, whereas severe forms may require neurosurgical treatment. Routine and comprehensive visits to the spina bifida center facilitate prompt diagnosis.

Although periodic comprehensive medical evaluations are designed to prevent problems, they put the family and child at risk for excessive dependency on the health care team. Increasing dependency on and involvement with health care may also interfere with or cause neglect of traditional family relationships. Every effort is made by the spina bifida team to encourage and foster appropriate role definition. For instance, parents are frequently advised to concentrate on being the "parent" while permitting the doctor and nurse to provide health care. Emphasis is placed on a trusting, open relationship between the parents and the spina bifida center staff. Nonetheless, as the child proceeds through the first 5 years of life, medical evaluations and surgery cause fear, pain, and separation from family. It is natural that parental consolation, protection, and provision sow the seeds of dependency and social and emotional delay for the child. This sequence may also threaten important family dynamics as the child with spina bifida is propelled into dominant consideration in family decisions and activities.

AGE FIVE TO TWELVE

During the early school period, increased attention is placed on methods to overcome neurogenic bladder. This condition, caused by an abnormal nerve supply to the bladder, occurs even in children with minimal or no weakness of the legs. Most individuals (95%) with myelomeningocele do not have functioning nerves between the bladder and the brain. Therefore, they are unable to perceive a distended bladder. Equally, they cannot voluntarily relax the sphincter muscles and simultaneously contract the bladder wall to produce urination. This interference with innervation of the muscle wall of the bladder produces either a hypo- or hyperactive bladder.

With either form of bladder dysfunction, there is associated incontinence (involuntary release of urine). After the age of 2–3 years, incontinence causes increasing social problems such as strained peer interaction and withdrawal. Absence of skin sensation and conditioning to odor permit the incontinent child to seemingly ignore a situation that is embarrassing to peers and family members. Thus conflict, confusion, and self-depreciation are established and begin to alter psychological development. More importantly, neurogenic bladder may cause recurrent urinary tract infection and lead to subsequent kidney infection. Urinary tract infections arise most frequently because of inadequate emptying of the bladder and/or the backup of infected urine along the ureter (the tube that drains urine from the kidney to the bladder) (Figure 1.5). Recurrent kidney infections produce renal failure that may require dialysis and transplantation in order to prevent premature death. The goals of treatment of neurogenic bladder are:

1. Continence
2. Prevention of infection by providing a means of emptying the bladder
3. Preservation of kidney function

Today, for most students, all of these goals are achieved with clean intermittent catheterization (CIC) (Lapides, Prokno, Silber, & Lowe, 1972). A small tube or catheter that is clean, but not sterile, is inserted into the bladder through the urethra, the canal through which urine is released from the bladder. After the bladder is empty or urine stops flowing, the tube is withdrawn, cleansed with soap and water, and stored for future use. Clean intermittent catheterization is a safe and excellent method of emptying the bladder, proven to prevent infection, not to cause it (Ehrlich & Brem, 1982). This procedure is prescribed and taught under the direction of the urologist and thereafter is intermittently repeated by the student or an assistant. The risk of injury to the urethra or bladder is so small that children are frequently able to master the technique before the age of 6 years. Children with hyperactive bladders may be treated with a combination of CIC and medication to relax the bladder. For 80% or more of children with spina bifida, these methods lead to continence in the social setting. However, a small percentage require special surgical procedures to increase bladder capacity or prevent uncontrolled release of urine. Methods of controlling incontinence have become so reliable that when a student develops repeated incontinence, it should be reported to the school nurse and the parents. This change may signal urinary tract infection or neurologic change. An occasional accident may occur in the classroom and care should be taken to minimize embarrassment of the student and his or her classmates. Every effort should be made to permit and assist the student to practice his or her toilet habits privately and unobtrusively.

Just as the nerves to control urination are inadequate, so are the nerves that produce bowel control for the student with spina bifida. Therefore, voluntary bowel movements are impaired because the student cannot sense a full rectum or contract the external rectal sphincter (a circular muscle surrounding the rectum that in a contracted condition occludes the rectum). This impairment causes the child with spina bifida to have an occasional uncontrolled bowel movement (incontinence). An accidental bowel movement in the classroom is embarrassing for all, but may also lead to ridicule and isolation of the pupil. The goal of programs for bowel control is to develop a predictable time for bowel movements so that they may occur in private and in a socially accepted manner. In order to achieve this goal, training or conditioning of the bowel is required. The clinical staff works with the parents and the child to:

1. Choose a regular and private time for bowel movements.
2. Develop maximal dietary control to optimize consistency of the stool (generally, high-fiber).
3. Encourage exercise.
4. Develop postures that encourage evacuation.
5. Teach the use of suppositories and enemas.

Every effort is made to develop and habituate bowel movement activity to occur at a predictable time within the privacy of the home. Therefore, teachers need not actively participate in bowel continence programs. However, they do need to understand that occasional accidents may be unavoidable. An awareness of the helplessness the child may feel in this situation will help the teacher resist punitive measures and provide sensitive support. Since recurring episodes of stool incontinence may reflect intestinal or emotional problems, they should be reported to the school nurse and parents.

Urinary and bowel incontinence threaten the quality of life of the pupil just as distinctly as acute medical problems. Both have the potential to impair the educational experience and important social integration of the pupil significantly. An open and unemotional understanding of the origin and management of these problems permits the teacher to concentrate more effectively on the student's classroom activities. Although the school personnel first learn of these problems as the child begins attending school, the family has worked with the student to achieve continence since infancy. Therefore, the parents often are able to serve as a resource for the teacher and other staff members. A spirit of cooperation and respect among students, parents, and educators can only work to the benefit of the student.

Between the ages of 5–12 years, most children with or without spina bifida experience intermittent increases in height. For the student with spina bifida, these increases in growth may be associated with deterioration in strength of the legs, deformity of the lower extremities, spinal curvature (scoliosis), and change in control of urination. Although the cause of these changes may be complex and varied, one of the most common is the development of tethered spinal cord. This is a delayed complication of the first operation to close the opening of the back. With age the spinal cord adheres to surrounding tissues. Growth and activity cause stretching of the spinal cord with secondary injury and loss of function (Reigel, 1983). Tethered spinal cord is treated with a microsurgical operation and laser release of the spinal cord from the points of adhesion. The student with spina bifida is intermittently examined by staff at the spina bifida center who search for the onset of change related to tethered spinal cord. The overriding goal of the neurosurgeon and orthopedist is to help the child with spina bifida achieve and maintain maximal function of existing muscles and extremities.

Depending upon the level of spinal involvement, perhaps as many as 70% of children with spina bifida develop spinal curvature (**scoliosis**) requiring a surgical operation to fuse the spine (Shurtleff, Goiney, Gordon, & Livermore, 1976). Metallic rods and bone are placed beside the vertebral column and adhere to the spine, thereby strengthening the column and preventing progression of the curve. Steadily increasing spinal curve may cause life-threatening physical disability. Because the operation for scoliosis can also be life-threatening, many parents begin to worry about the onset of scoliosis. The treatment for curvature of the spine may result in prolonged periods of interruption of the student's education (6–12 months) and may require homebound tutoring or special adaptations in the classroom for the student with spinal orthoses (see Baker and Rogosky-Grassi, chap. 2, this volume). Successful completion of the treatment is associated with an improved outlook for student activities such as sitting and gait. Recent data suggest that treatment of tethered spinal cord decreases the incidence of scoliosis in some patients by as much as 40%–50% (Reigel, 1991). Details about orthopedic treatment of scoliosis can be obtained from the spina bifida center and the school nurse.

Thus, the important years between 5 and 12 are punctuated by health care demands upon the child and family. The student's school schedule is interrupted by intermittent visits to the spina bifida center. A variety of surgical operations may be required, some urgent and others anticipated and planned. In order not to disrupt the school years, students with spina bifida may sacrifice their free-spirited summer vacations in the pursuit of major health needs. Furthermore, intermittent health care crises are disruptive to the family's stability. Employment responsibilities and family budgets may be compromised. The anxiety produced by potentially life-threatening operations, irrespective of timing, produces insecurity. The early school years require parental support for the student that can only be tarnished by fright and uncertainty about the well-being of their children. The parents' and student's capacity to cope with the stress of intermittent acute health problems will be enhanced by an understanding and empathizing teacher. There is a certain normalcy and stability that comes to the family unit from school activities of the child with spina bifida that parallels that of pupils without spina bifida.

Finally, most children with spina bifida have siblings who attend school and who are equally threatened by stress and unsettling emotions that occur when their brother or sister with spina bifida faces a health care crisis. These children often suffer in silence and may be neglected because of parental focus on the child with spina bifida. The teacher's sensitivity to this group directly benefits the family unit and, therefore, indirectly, the student with spina bifida.

As the teachers reflect on this description of health care of the pupil with spina bifida, it should not be surprising if doubt and insecurity emerge. It may be helpful to realize that these feelings are not unique to the classroom, but are shared by all people involved with raising and loving the student with spina bifida. Just as the health care team has sought to assure the parents, so physicians and nurses seek to assure the education team. The responsibility of the teacher is to know the personality and behavior of the student with spina bifida and not to become a provider of health care within the school. Teachers should report change to the school nurse, parents, or members of the health care team. Most spina bifida centers provide continuous staff availability for questions arising within the school setting. If school attendance is a danger to the child, the parents are advised not to send the child to school. Trained to prevent crisis, most physicians and nurses err on the conservative side of this question. However, a sensitive understanding of the health care of a child with spina bifida will enhance not only the education, but also the health of the child. Despite this discussion, fear of an adverse medical crisis within the classroom will persist. In reality the incidence of crisis in the classroom for children with spina bifida is probably no different than for other students. Security comes from knowledge of basic first aid skills and the availability of a school nurse. Apprehensive regard for the student with spina bifida will produce an apprehensive education of the student. The future of the child with spina bifida is directly related to the team's ability to provide a full education side by side with good health care.

ADOLESCENCE TO ADULTHOOD

The hallmark of continuing medical care of the adolescent is recognition of chronic problems that may require ongoing treatment and may affect education. Many adolescents with spina bifida experience declining physical activity, rapid weight gain, and increasing social isolation that distinguishes them from the usual student. For many pupils with spina bifida, physical growth makes meaningful activity and exercise more difficult. Often they elect to use a wheelchair for ambulation in an attempt to match the increasing speed and intensity of activity of their peers. Occasionally a student perceives greater peer acceptance for a wheelchair rather than cumbersome and unsightly bracing. As fellow students begin the process of emancipation from parents, the students with spina bifida are often physically and psychologically unable to pursue activities leading to young adult freedom and identity. The chronic need for health care cements parental dependence and further inhibits student activity, producing even greater separation from peers. Special efforts to include the adolescent with spina bifida in all activities is helpful. Allotment of extra time for travel between classrooms and activities may also be of benefit.

Spina bifida not only interferes with the nerves that carry messages to muscles, but also those that send information from the skin to the brain. Therefore, students with spina bifida may not be able to perceive temperature, pain, and the location of their legs. Declining activity and exercise and increasing weight predisposes the student with spina bifida to unrecognized skin injury. These injuries often occur with prolonged periods of sitting and/or abnormalities of bracing that cause excessive pressure upon the skin of the buttocks and legs. The skin in these areas then breaks down, producing sores that are red and have the appearance of an ulcer. These sores are called decubiti (Figure 1.7). The development of decubiti on weight-bearing areas (soles of the feet and buttocks) further limits activity. Treatment often requires restriction of daily activities in order to eliminate excessive pressure and permit spontaneous healing. These limitations may alter classroom activity and even prevent school attendance. If spontaneous healing fails to occur, plastic surgery may be required, followed by prolonged hospitalization or homebound rest. If

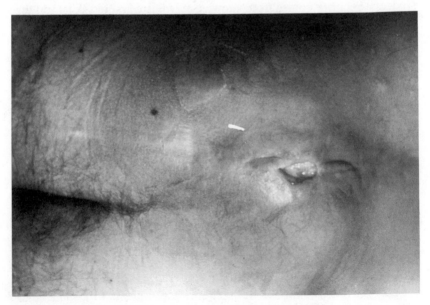

Figure 1.7.   A typical small pressure sore over the buttocks area (decubitus).

ever the axiom that "an ounce of prevention is worth a pound of cure" applies, it does to skin breakdown. Specific methods used to prevent skin breakdown (see Baker and Rogosky-Grassi, chap. 2, this volume) include:

1. The use of wheelchair cushions designed to relieve and equally distribute pressure on the buttocks
2. Teaching the child to shift his body weight within the wheelchair by doing pushups on the armrests of the wheelchair every 30–60 minutes while seated
3. The use of braces and crutches to avoid prolonged periods of sitting
4. Design of the child's work space to require movement, if possible
5. Evaluation of the fit of braces and provision by the spina bifida team of padding to prevent excessive skin pressure
6. Early recognition of areas of redness and swelling that may signal impending skin injury, and recommendation of corrective activity to prevent pressure sores

Prevention of skin injury requires continual vigilance on the part of the child, the family, and those observers working with the student. Suspicion of potential injury or existing skin injury should be reported to the school nurse.

Neurogenic bladder may lead to recurrent urinary tract infections. The use of clean intermittent catheterization (CIC) has decreased the incidence of infection. However, the occasional urinary tract infection is probably not preventable and may be associated with incontinence, headache, malaise, fever, vomiting, and loss of appetite. The recurrence of infections may be related to adolescent resistance to CIC, inadequate fluid intake, and obstruction to the flow of urine anywhere along the urinary tract. The spina bifida team carefully evaluates each student for change in kidney function and infection. Unexplained fever always raises the question of urinary tract infection. Urinary tract infections, particularly those confined to the bladder, may be treated with oral medication and usually do not disrupt school attendance. However, if the kidneys become infected and high fever develops, treatment may require hospitalization and intravenous antibiotic therapy. Obstruction to urine flow may require hospitalization and surgical treatment (Kass & Koff, 1983). Chronic urinary tract infections may cause high blood pressure (hypertension) that requires treatment with medications. Most physicians believe that chronic urinary tract infection leads to kidney failure and decreased life expectancy for the adult with spina bifida. For these reasons, symptoms of urinary tract infection should be reported to the school health nurse.

Uncontrolled seizure may interfere with classroom performance. With age, the form or type of seizure may change. Thus, in adolescence, instead of petit mal, seizure may be associated with loss of consciousness, abnormal respiration, repetitive flexion and extension of the extremities, and incontinence (grand mal). Medication that has been effective for control of seizure may fail as the adolescent progresses through puberty, producing active seizure and requiring change in either dose or type of medication. During these periods of medical change, the student's mood and school performance may be altered. There is also a slightly increased risk of having a seizure during school. Although the observation of a grand mal seizure may be very frightening, seizure is also self-limited and in and of itself is not life-threatening. An understanding of the basic principles of first aid will enable the teacher to protect the student while obtaining the help of the school nurse (*American Red Cross Standard First Aid Workbook*, 1988). Most students with spina bifida who develop a seizure in the classroom should be taken home for evaluation. If possible, the decision for further medical evaluation should be discussed with the parents. The occurrence of a seizure in a child with a known history of seizure may be familiar to the parents and require little additional medical evaluation, whereas the unexpected seizure or first occurrence of seizure will require further medical evaluation. A common cause of unexpected seizure during adolescence is failure on the part of the student to take the antiseizure medication faithfully. Other causes include problems with the spinal fluid shunt, fever, or infection. The isolated seizure may require only alteration in the dose of medication and the student may promptly return to school. More serious problems may require hospital evaluation and treatment.

The psychological stigmata associated with seizure activity in public cannot be overemphasized. Classmates who observe a seizure may become fearful and further withdraw from the student with spina bifida. Equally, the pupil with spina bifida may withdraw from peers because of embarrassment. If the teacher understands that seizure is an uncontrolled release of electrical impulses by the brain and that it usually does not indicate serious disease, he or she will be able to reassure the class that the student with seizure is not dangerous or abnormal, while simultaneously supporting the embarrassed and troubled student. An attitude of openness and warmth will help alleviate the fears of the classroom and school community.

The adolescent with spina bifida and hydrocephalus may develop failure or obstruction of the spinal fluid drainage system (cerebrospinal fluid shunt). There may be no symptoms to indicate this complication. However, subtle changes such as decreasing attention span and activity, decrease in visual acuity, mild headache, decreased appetite, change in personality, and declining school performance may indicate shunt problems. Persistence of these changes should be reported to the parents and school nurse. Deterioration of shunt function may also be heralded by severe headache, neck pain, vomiting, and somnolence. This combination of more serious symptoms requires prompt evaluation by the clinical team.

The operation to revise (restore function to) a shunt requires hospitalization. Most adolescents with hydrocephalus have had previous shunt revisions and are frightened and apprehensive about the possible need for an additional operation. The parents are equally anxious because of keen awareness of the fact that sudden failure of a shunt may, albeit rarely, take the life of the student with spina bifida. Therefore, sensitivity to this fear of the student and parents should be remembered when discussing the possibility of shunt failure. Whether urgent or elective, a shunt revision may be associated with slow recovery of previous levels of school performance. Although rare, performance may never return to pre-shunt failure levels. Therefore, teachers should take an observant and patient approach as the student first returns to school after hospitalization for a shunt revision. Although the complications associated with shunts may be frightening, the advent of the cerebrospinal fluid shunt was the single most important development leading to survival and normal intellectual development for people with spina bifida. It should be reassuring to educators that the frequency of shunt problems declines dramatically with increasing age.

Today tethered spinal cord will have been considered and treated during the first decade of life. Nevertheless, recurrent tethering is considered as a possible neurologic complication throughout adolescence and adulthood. The most frequent indications of retethering of the spinal cord are change in strength and orthopedic deformity of the legs. Alterations of function of the bladder may also suggest recurrent tethering. The treatment is the same as in earlier life and requires an operation on the spine. The changes of scoliosis have usually stabilized by adolescence and do not require further treatment.

Progressive obesity may be a problem for as many as 50% of young adults with spina bifida (Shurtleff, 1986). Obesity carries many risks to good health, interfering with ambulation and participation in social and educational activities. Furthermore, obesity tarnishes self-image and contributes to peer rejection. Studies indicate that, in order for the obese adolescent with spina bifida to achieve weight reduction, caloric intake of 800 calories or less per day may be required. Although we emphatically recommend vigorous nutritional counseling for teenagers, dietary instructions are tempered by the knowledge that for some, almost inhumane limitations of diet are required for weight loss. The cause of this metabolic efficiency is unclear. The concept that adolescents with spina bifida gain weight because they are not able to burn adequate calories by

using only their upper extremities is invalid. The support and cooperation on the part of the school for restriction of caloric intake can only
help with weight maintenance and reduction.

Sexuality is an important part of adolescent education. Studies have
confirmed that individuals with spina bifida have the interest and the capacity for sexual activity. There have been numerous reports of fertile
males and females with myelomeningocele. Pregnancy of women with
myelomeningocele has occurred and continues to occur (Cass, Bloom, &
Luxenberg, 1986). Since sexuality is an important part of our society and
is increasingly and openly discussed, all students with spina bifida should
be equally included in all sex education activities throughout the stages
of development.

It would be easy to conclude that all illness for students with spina
bifida is serious. However, children and adolescents with spina bifida are
no different than others. In fact, they are susceptible to the same common
diseases such as earaches, sore throats, common cold, and the flu. The
common diseases of children are far more common than crisis and can
be identified by the student's pediatrician or spina bifida clinic staff. Most
children with spina bifida have good attendance records and do not have
lengthy hospitalizations. Although there are exceptions, comprehensive
medical care has led to a general state of good health for students with
spina bifida. Some of the teacher's apprehension may be allayed by knowing that there is support and mutual interest in all aspects of care of the
adolescent with spina bifida within the team outlined in Figure 1.1. Just as
the parents realize that they are not alone in caring for these children, so
the education team becomes secure in this realization. Working together,
the team will be able to provide maximal educational opportunity for
each child with spina bifida. A future of reward and meaning depends
upon the success of our combined cooperative efforts.

GLOSSARY

Amblyopia   Form of blindness secondary to loss of visual perception of the
brain. It is not caused by diseases of the eye.

Amniocentesis   Needle aspiration of amniotic fluid (a clean, colorless fluid surrounding the fetus) from the uterus, usually performed toward the end of the
pregnancy. The fluid is analyzed for proteins (alpha-fetoprotein) which may
indicate the presence of spina bifida.

Amniotic fluid   Clean, colorless fluid within the membrane (amniotic sac) surrounding the fetus.

Cerebrospinal fluid (CSF)   Clear, colorless fluid within the ventricles and surrounding the brain.

Cesarean section   Delivery of a fetus through a uterine and abdominal
incision.

Arnold-Chiari malformation   Extension of the most posterior part of the brain
into the cervical canal.

Clean intermittent catheterization (CIC) Process of inserting a clean catheter (nonsterile hollow tube) to remove urine from the bladder.

Club foot Congenital deformity in which the foot turns and rotates inward (inversion).

Colon Large intestine. Continuation of intestine between the ileum and rectum.

Crede maneuver Bimanual compression of the bladder resulting in expulsion of urine.

Decubitus ulcer Interruption of the surface of the skin and subcutaneous tissues surrounded by redness and inflammation.

Dialysis Process of removing blood substances, ordinarily excreted by the kidney, with a system of membranes either artificial or natural (peritoneum).

Electroencephalogram (EEG) Graphic record of the electrical activity of the brain. Scalp surface electrodes are used to retrieve brain electric potentials which are then amplified and recorded by a special instrument (electroencephalograph).

External sphincter Bundles of muscle surrounding the urethra and rectum which contract or close to produce continence.

Hip dislocation Displacement of the head of the femur from the hip socket in the pelvis.

Hydrocephalus Abnormal accumulation of cerebrospinal fluid (CSF) in the ventricles (caves) of the brain. Excessive production, interference with flow, and absorption of CSF all may be causes.

Incontinence Inability to voluntarily control evacuation of the bladder (urine) or bowel (feces).

Meningocele Cystic protrusion of spinal meninges (membranes) through an opening in the spine. The cyst primarily contains cerebrospinal fluid. This is a form of spina bifida.

Myelomeningocele Severe form of spina bifida in which the meninges of spinal canal, nerves, and spinal cord protrude out of the spinal canal.

Neural tube Tube of primitive nerve tissue (neuroectoderm) that develops (differentiates) into the nervous system (brain, spinal cord, nerves).

Neuroectoderm Outermost of the three primary layers of tissue of the embryo. Forms the nervous system.

Neurogenic bladder Urinary bladder with abnormal function caused by pathologic changes of the nerves or brain.

Ophthalmologist Surgeon skilled in treatment of diseases of the eye.

Orthopedics Field of surgery dealing with disorders and deformities of bones, muscles, joints, ligaments, and muscles.

Renal dialysis See Dialysis.

Scoliosis Lateral (side to side) curvature of the spine. Named according to location (i.e., thoracic) and direction of convexity of the curve (right or left).

Shunt Small, silastic tube used to divert excessive spinal fluid from the ventricles of the brain to an alternate site of absorption such as the lining of the abdomen (peritoneum) or atrium of the heart.

Spina bifida occulta Failure of the posterior part of a vertebra (lamina) to form properly. This is the mildest form of spina bifida (Figure 1.2).

Spinal fusion Fusion of two or more vertebrae in order to prevent motion. Metallic rods and bone are frequently used as struts to create the fusion.

Strabismus Abnormality in which the eyes do not follow or focus in parallel. Caused by weakness of one or more of the muscles which move the eyes. The person appears to have crossed eyes.

Ultrasound image Image obtained by recording echoes of sound waves from anatomic structures of varying densities. The image obtained has an X-ray–like appearance. Structures of low density appear black; high density structures, white.

Ureter Long tube that passes urine from the kidney to the bladder.

Urethra Canal through which urine from the bladder flows to the outside of the body.

Urologist Surgeon skilled in the diagnosis and treatment of disorders of the urinary (kidney and bladder) and genital organs.

Ventricle One of four caves or pouches within the brain in which cerebral spinal fluid is produced by structures (choroid plexus).

Vertebra One of the 33 bones composing the spinal column (vertebral column).

REFERENCES

American Red Cross Standard First Aid Workbook. (1988). Norfolk, VA: National Chapter of the American Red Cross.

Bailey, R.B. (1991). *Urologic management of spina bifida.* In H.L. Rekate (Ed.), *Comprehensive management of spina bifida* (pp. 185–214). Boca Raton: CRC Press.

Biglan, A.W. (1990). Ophthalmologic complications of meningomyelocele: A longitudinal study. *Transaction of the American Ophthamological Society, 87,* 389–462.

Boone, D., Pansons, D., Lochman, S.M., & Sherwood, T. (1985). Spina bifida occulta: Lesion or anomaly? *Clinical Radiology, 36,* 159–161.

Cass, A.S., Bloom, B.A., & Luxenberg, M. (1986). Sexual function in adults with myelomeningocele. *Journal of Urology, 136,* 425–426.

Ehrlich, O., & Brem, A.S. (1982). A prospective comparison of urinary tract infections in patients treated with either clean intermittent catheterization or urinary diversion. *Pediatrics, 70,* 665–669.

Fraser, F. (1974). Genetic counseling in some common paediatric diseases. *American Journal of Human Genetics, 26,* 636–661.

Gilbert, J.N., Jones, K.L., Rorke, L.B., Chernoff, G.F., & James, H.E. (1986). Central nervous system anomalies associated with meningomyelocele, hydrocephalus and the Arnold-Chiari malformation: Reappraisal of the theories regarding the pathogenesis of posterior neural tube defects. *Neurosurgery, 18,* 559–564.

Gool, J.B., & Good, J.D. (1986). *A short history of spina bifida.* Netherlands: Society for Research into Hydrocephalus and Spina Bifida.

Greenberg, F., James, L.M., & Oakley, G.P. (1983). Estimates of birth prevalence rates of spina bifida in the United States from computer-generated maps. *American Journal of Obstetrics and Gynecology, 145,* 570–573.

Kass, E.J., & Koff, S.A. (1983). Bladder augmentation in the pediatric neuropathic bladder. *Journal of Urology, 129,* 552–555.

Khoury, M.J., Erickson, J.D., & James, L.M. (1982). Etiologic heterogeneity of neural tube defects: Clues from epidemiology. *American Journal of Epidemiology, 115,* 538–548.

Lapides, J., Prokno, A.C., Silber, S.J., & Lowe, B. (1972). Clean intermittent self-catheterization in the treatment of urinary tract disease. *Journal of Urology, 107*, 458–461.

Mayfield, J.K. (1991). Comprehensive orthopedic management in myelomeningocele. In H.L. Rekate, (Ed.), *Comprehensive management of spina bifida* (pp. 113–163). Boca Raton: CRC Press.

McLone, D.G., & Naidich, T.P. (1989). Myelomeningocele: Outcome and late complication. In R. McLaurin (Ed.), *Pediatric neurosurgery* (2nd ed., pp. 53–70). Philadelphia: W.B. Saunders.

McLone, D.G., Suna, J., Collins, J.A., Poznanski, S., & Knepper, P.A. (1983). Neurulation: Biochemical and morphological studies on primary and secondary neural tube defects. In R. Humphreys (Ed.), *Concepts in pediatric neurosurgery* (Vol. 4, pp. 15–19). Basel: S. Karger.

Menelaus, M.B. (1976). The hip in myelomeningocele. *Journal of Bone and Joint Surgery, 58-B*, (4), 448–452.

Milunsky, A. (1979). Alpha-fetoprotein and the prenatal detection of neural tube defects. *American Journal of Public Health, 69*, 552–553.

Quigley, M.R., Reigel, D.H., & Kortyna, R. (1989). Cerebrospinal fluid shunt infections. Report of 41 cases and a critical review of the literature. *Pediatric Neuroscience, 15*(3), 111–120.

Reigel, D.H. (1983). Tethered spinal cord. In R.P. Humphreys (Ed.), *Concepts in pediatric neurosurgery* (Vol. 4, pp. 142–164). Basel: S. Karger.

Reigel, D.H. (Ed.). (1989). Spina bifida. *Pediatric neurosurgery* (2nd ed., pp. 35–52). Philadelphia: W.B. Saunders.

Reigel, D.H. (1991). Relationship of tethered spinal cord to scoliosis in patients with spina bifida [Abstract]. *American Association of Neurological Surgeons Annual Meeting*, Dallas, TX.

Reigel, D.H., Stanitski, C., & Simpson, G. (in press). *The relationship of tethered spinal cord to scoliosis.*

Scheuer, M.L., & Pedley, T.A. (1990). The evaluation and treatment of seizures. *New England Journal of Medicine, 323*(21), 1468–1474.

Shurtleff, D.B. (1986). Dietary management. In D.B. Shurtleff (Ed.), *Myelodysplasias and extrophies: Significance, prevention and treatment* (p. 287). Orlando: Grune & Stratton.

Shurtleff, D.B., & Dunne, K. (1986). Adults and adolescents with meningomyelocele, In D.B. Shurtleff (Ed.), *Myelodysplasias and extrophies: Significance, prevention and treatment* (p. 435). Orlando: Grune & Stratton.

Shurtleff, D.B., Goiney, R., Gordon, L.H., & Livermore, N. (1976). Myelodysplasia: The natural history of kyphosis and scoliosis. A preliminary report. *Developmental Medicine and Child Neurology, 18*, (Suppl. 37), 126–133.

Shurtleff, D., Lemire, R., & Warkany, J. (1986). Embryology, etiology and epidemiology. In D.B. Shurtleff (Ed.), *Myelodysplasia and extrophies: Significance, prevention and treatment* (pp. 65–87). Orlando: Grune & Stratton.

Statistical Abstract of the United States. (1988). Washington, DC: Goverment Printing Office.

Stauffer, D.T. (1984). Catheterization—A health procedure schools must be prepared to provide. *Journal of School Health, 54*, 37–38.

Thompson, M.W., & Rudd, N.L. (1976). The genetics of spinal dysraphism. In T.P. Morley (Ed.), *Current controversies in neurosurgery.* Philadelphia: W.B. Saunders, pp. 126–146.

Warkany, J. (1977). Morphogenesis of spina bifida. In R. McLaurin (Ed.), *Myelomeningocele* (pp. 31–35). New York: Grune & Stratton.

Frequently Asked Questions

GENERAL

Q: Is there anything I might do that could harm the student with spina bifida?

A: No. The health problems associated with spina bifida are not caused by activities.

Q: Do these children have chronic pain?

A: No. Actually the inability to perceive pain may lead to problems such as pressure sores.

Q: Does spina bifida get worse with age?

A: No. The changes observed at birth are static. However, changes with development and associated health problems may suggest the possibility of deterioration.

Q: Is the back sensitive to pain?

A: No. If anything, it is insensitive.

HYDROCEPHALUS

Q: What are the symptoms of shunt problems?

A: Irritability, headache, neck pain, loss of appetite, vomiting, change in vision, and decreasing level of activity and school performance.

Q: Are there special precautions for children treated with shunts?

A: No. There are no special precautions or limits for activities.

Q: Does cognition of the student change following a shunt revision?

A: The child will demonstrate slow but steady cognitive improvement, which may initially require less demanding requests until the student catches up. An occasional child may not achieve his previous level of work. These children should be carefully reevaluated by all members of the education team. When the child returns, he may be sensitive about his incision area and missing hair. This may be overcome by understanding and permitting the pupil to wear a cap or scarf.

Q: Does hydrocephalus affect learning?

A: Yes. See Chapter 4—Conducting Psychological Assessments.

SEIZURE

Q: What is a seizure?

A: A seizure is a sudden uncontrolled electrical discharge from the brain which causes momentary loss of consciousness and a variety of uncontrolled muscle jerking, such as spasms of the head and neck and extension of the extremities. Seizures may also cause incontinence and temporary alteration in breathing patterns.

Q: How long does a seizure last?

A: Most seizures last less than 2 minutes and many forms are only seconds in duration.

Q: Do seizures stop spontaneously?

A: Yes. Usually within two minutes or less. Occasionally the duration may be prolonged. In this case, the child should be transferred to the nearest emergency room.

Q: What is the cause of seizure?

A: Seizures may have many causes such as injury or trauma, infection, hemorrhage, and metabolic disease. Seizure may be precipitated or appear with fever, fatigue, emotional distress, hyperventilation, and the use of drugs. For many, the cause may be unknown.

Q: How is seizure controlled?

A: With medication. The most common anticonvulsants are phenobarbital, Depakene, Tegretol, and Dilantin (Scheuer & Pedley, 1990).

Q: Are there side effects to seizure medication which would be evident in the classroom?

A: Yes. The side effects most commonly occur when the dose is excessive or changed. These include hyperactivity with phenobarbital and somnolence with Depakene and Tegretol. Questions about medication and seizure control should be referred to the school nurse or the spina bifida clinical team.

Q: How is the right dose of anticonvulsants determined?

A: By measuring the amount of drug in the blood. Standard levels which will control seizure have been defined.

Q: Can a seizure disorder affect learning?

A: Yes. Uncontrolled occurrence of seizure interferes with learning and acquisition of information. Equally, excessive amounts of anticonvulsant medication interfere with learning.

Q: What should be done for the student who has a seizure within the classroom?

A: If a petit mal occurs, there is no treatment other than to inform the parents and the school nurse. If the seizure is grand mal in type, the first responsibility of the teacher is to the student. The primary goal is to avoid injury by preventing a fall or hitting or striking objects.

This can be accomplished by moving furniture and placing pillows under the student. Do not attempt to restrain the child. Second, attempt to maintain the airway by placing a padded or soft structure between the teeth. Do not attempt to place anything in the mouth if the jaw is rigid. Do not put your fingers in the mouth. Once the seizure is complete, place the pupil on his or her side and clear the airway, summon the school nurse, and prepare to transfer the student to the student health center. Following transfer of the student, reassure classmates (*American Red Cross Standard First Aid Workbook*, 1988).

CLEAN INTERMITTENT CATHETERIZATION

Q: Where can I read about CIC?
A: Donald T. Stauffer's "Catheterization—A Health Procedure Schools Must Be Prepared To Provide." It is published in *Journal of School Health*, (1984), *54*, pp. 37–38.
Q: Must school personnel provide assistance for the student who requires help with catheterization?
A: Yes. Public Law 94-142, now updated as the Individuals with Disabilities Education Act (IDEA).
Q: Does CIC cause infection or injury?
A: No. CIC *prevents* infection.

ORTHOPEDICS

Q: How can I tell if a student's braces don't fit properly?
A: By observing the pupil for indentations or marks on the skin beneath the brace, or complaints of brace discomfort.
Q: Must a child wear the braces all the time?
A: No. However, they should be used enough so that the orthosis becomes comfortable and part of the child's life. See the chapter on physical management in the education setting (Chapter 2).
Q: How do I put braces and other orthotic devices on the student?
A: See the chapter on physical management in the education setting (Chapter 2).
Q: Can I cause a fracture of the leg?
A: Fractures occur for a variety of reasons including improper transfers and falls. Braces help prevent fractures. When a child's muscle strength is adequate for walking with minimal or no bracing, it can be assumed that the bones are less fragile. If the child is confined to a wheelchair, caution is needed when a child transfers into and out of the wheelchair or performs activities out of the chair. Out-of-chair activities are recommended to maintain arm strength and functional independence.

Access to the School

Suzanne Benintend Baker
and Mary A. Rogosky-Grassi

Seventy-five percent of students with spina bifida require some form of adaptive equipment to achieve an acceptable level of mobility, although some can function without the use of wheelchairs, braces, or crutches. Because control of the bowel and bladder is located at the end of the spinal column, almost all students with spina bifida lack control of the bladder, the bowel, or both, and require an adaptive toileting program. When a school is preparing to enroll a student with spina bifida, a program of physical management that provides for these needs is usually one of the first requirements. This chapter provides information about the variety of services that a school can incorporate into its program of physical management.

Besides a change in attitude on the part of society to recognize the abilities and rights of the handicapped, new services and methods of delivery must be developed to maximize the independence of students with spina bifida.

Services related to the management of the physical needs of children with spina bifida begin at birth and are continuous through early intervention and preschool programs. Occupational and physical therapists, child development specialists, and preschool teachers focus on gross and fine motor skills, language acquisition, and socialization (Williamson, 1987). When the child reaches the age of school entry, the school becomes a primary site for the delivery of services that maximize independence.

Ideally, the school will be in communication with the child's parents as well as the specialists who have helped the child to achieve functional independence and who continue to work with the child. In addition to coordinating services with parents and other professionals, school personnel will need to possess specific information in their own right. The following sections of this chapter provide information on accessibility, adaptive equipment, mobility in the school setting, creating a functional environment, and involvement of the student in the routines of the school.

The discussion of "accessibility" reviews the current legal guidelines for structural modifications, in addition to the less obvious, but equally important, guidelines for reducing social barriers.

The section on "adaptive equipment" presents descriptions and illustrations of various types of bracing and walking aids. The parts of a wheelchair are also reviewed along with wheelchair accessories.

Following this, mobility in the school setting as it relates to both the ambulatory student and the student who uses a wheelchair for mobility is discussed. This section provides information on gait patterns, proper methods of assisting the students, and a review of techniques employed in stair and curb management.

"Creating a Functional Environment" introduces practical suggestions for eliminating classroom obstacles, such as reaching and storing books and crutches, finding a suitable desk, and transporting supplies. Finally, the student's educational world in the classroom and beyond is assessed. Involvement in class routines, bathroom needs, library use and assemblies, the cafeteria, and general school layout are discussed. Additional special areas of concern reviewed are field trips, physical education, transportation, and fire and safety procedures.

DEVELOPING A POSITIVE ATTITUDE TOWARD ADAPTIVE EQUIPMENT

The perception of a student with adaptive equipment is the first area to be considered in access to the school environment. When a person who requires adaptive equipment appears among a group of nondisabled students, the teacher's attitude toward the equipment makes a critical difference in the quality of the access that will be provided. The equipment can be viewed as a mark of difference and as something that sets the person who needs it apart from the group. In this view the person who comes with the equipment is seen as having special problems that the group will have to accommodate, probably at some inconvenience. Alternatively, the equipment can be viewed more productively, in its positive aspect, as a set of tools that make it possible for this person to come and be with the group, in school, where all young people belong. The choice between these two views is open to each teacher and student as they regard the student with spina bifida and the equipment that comes with that student (Clopton, 1981).

This chapter advocates the second view and the attitude of acceptance that accompanies it. It cannot be denied that accepting a student with spina bifida will require physical adjustments. With the information in this chapter, educators will be able to make these necessary adjustments with a minimum of inconvenience so that all concerned can quickly move their focus of attention away from the new procedures and equipment and toward the student who is in school because of them. When this change of focus has been achieved, the equipment ceases to be a mark of difference that causes the student with spina bifida to be, and to feel, excluded. The equipment itself becomes welcome because it enables the student to be included in school activities. Once this occurs, the truly important work of education can begin.

LEGAL REQUIREMENTS OF ACCESSIBILITY

Since the passage of The Rehabilitation Act of 1973, federal law has required that access be given to persons with disabilities in federally funded buildings and programs. Section 504 of The Rehabilitation Act of 1973, as reported in a pamphlet produced by the U.S. Department of Education, Office for Civil Rights, states that:

> No qualified handicapped person shall be denied the benefits of, be excluded from participation in, or be otherwise subjected to discrimination under any program or activity because a recipient's facilities are inaccessible or unusable. The Section 504 regulation requires all recipients of Federal financial assistance from the Department of Education to operate their federally assisted programs or activities so that when viewed in their entirety they are readily accessible to handicapped persons. (p. 2)

Furthermore,

> In meeting the objective of program accessibility, a recipient must take precautions not to isolate or concentrate handicapped persons in settings away from nonhandicapped participants, since the regulation prohibits unnecessary segregation of handicapped people. As an example, it would be a violation to make only one facility or part of a facility accessible if this resulted in segregating handicapped persons. (p. 3)

For example, if a student with a disability elects typing, he or she cannot legally be denied participation in this element of the program on the grounds that the typing room is in a part of the school building not accessible by wheelchair. More recently, the Americans with Disabilities Act, passed in 1990, mandates access for all persons with disabilities to buildings, programs, and services used by the public. Specific information about accessibility is available from the U.S. Department of Education, Office for Civil Rights. (See the appendix at the end of this chapter for the complete mailing address.)

ACCESS TO MEET DEVELOPMENTAL NEEDS

Even partial exclusion from part of a school program can have lasting effects on a student's social and emotional development. In one case, a student was included on a field trip, but had to stay behind when the other students went down the hill to play. He repressed his disappointment for 3 weeks, and finally released it with great force in family counseling, telling his father how horrible and lonely he felt. The father later succeeded in reducing these intense feeling when he took the boy back to the spot and down the hill. Unfortunately, all such incidents are not resolved so successfully. Students may not always display their feelings of rejection and isolation when adults exclude them. Their passive behavior does not necessarily mean they have not been hurt.

Perhaps the least obvious effects of being left out of school activities are the long-term economic and social consequences (Blum, 1983; Hanson & Graves, 1987). Far too many students with spina bifida graduate from high school only to feel estranged from the adult world of work and higher education. This feeling of estrangement may be avoided during the school years through a consciously applied program of guaranteed access. Providing accessibility to the entirety of the school program lets the student know that he or she has the same opportunity and right of access to the world as everyone. Although it may cost tax dollars to provide accessible education programs that lead to independence and vocational productivity, teaching students with spina bifida that they are excluded may relegate them to the role of tax users instead of tax payers for the rest of their lives.

TYPES OF ADAPTIVE EQUIPMENT

Students with spina bifida may have varying degrees of physical impairment and paralysis depending upon the location of the lesion along the spinal column (Carroll, 1987; Dias, 1978) (see Figure 2.1). In addition, sensation such as perception of touch and pain also may be diminished or absent. Students with less extensive paralysis may require bracing only for the ankles and feet. Students with higher lesions (more toward the head, i.e., thoracic) will generally have a greater degree of impairment. They may need more leg bracing, and possibly trunk bracing, in order to walk with crutches (Bahnson, 1982; Kupta, Geddes, & Carroll, 1978). It should be noted that even when extensive bracing is required, students with spina bifida are capable of participating in some form of most school activities, including field trips and those activities commonly done on the floor or playground. The following is a review of the types of equipment and their applications.

Braces

Types of Braces   Braces are used to support weak or paralyzed muscles and assist in mobility. They are named for the major body joints they control. Students with sacral level lesions causing minimal muscle weakness often do not require bracing (Dias, 1978; Gaff, Robinson, Parker,

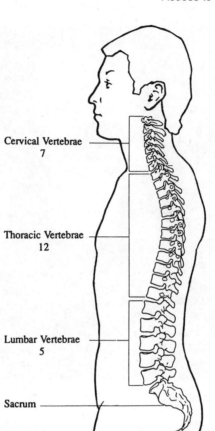

Figure 2.1. Anatomic areas of the human spine. Spina bifida is most commonly located in the lumbar area.

1984; Lough, 1984). A "low" lumbar lesion, one occurring at the level of the fourth and fifth lumbar vertebrae, results in paralysis of the feet and ankles. These students generally use a molded plastic ankle/foot orthosos (AFO) for stability (see Figure 2.2). Students whose lesion occurs in the area of the first three lumbar vertebrae exhibit the greatest variability in bracing. Some may require the support of bracing extending to the hips and attached to a pelvic band, while others may have adequate hip control so that bracing extends only above the knee. This latter type, shown in Figure 2.3, is called a knee/ankle/foot orthosis (KAFO). Children whose lesion occurs in the thoracic area have complete paralysis of the legs. They require full bracing to provide trunk and leg support. This type of bracing, shown in Figure 2.4, is referred to as hip/knee/ankle/foot orthosis

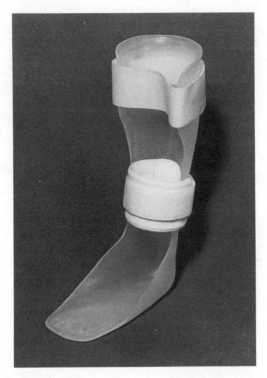

Figure 2.2. Ankle/foot orthosis (AFO).

(HKAFO), and is attached to a spinal orthosis. This spinal orthosis may be of two types. One is referred to as a thoraco-lumbo-sacral orthosis (TLSO) and is fabricated of molded plastic, either as a one-piece, with front or back closure model (Figure 2.5) or as a two-piece "clam-shell" version (Figure 2.6). Frequently these "body jackets" are used to control progression of spinal curves, such as scoliosis or kyphosis (Dias, 1978). If spinal curvature is not a major concern, the spinal orthosis may consist of two metal bands, one at mid-chest and one in the pelvic area connected to the leg braces with a metal upright on each side. The abdominal, or front, portion of this type of orthosis is made of cloth with Velcro straps. When a molded body jacket is used, a metal frame that is attached to the leg braces fits over the jacket and incorporates it into the total brace, as shown in Figure 2.7. There is also a category of bracing that has been described as dynamic and includes the reciprocating gait orthosis (RGO) and floor reaction orthoses. These are similar to the HKAFO and AFO described above. If braces other than the types described are used, questions should be referred to the parents or therapist for more specific guidelines.

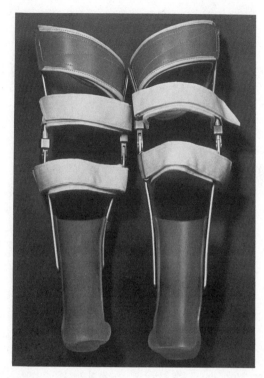

Figure 2.3.   Knee/ankle/foot orthosis (KAFO).

Using Braces   Braces are used to provide the support and control lacking in the lower extremities of the student with spina bifida. Daily use is important in order to maintain maximal mobility and function. Molded plastic braces for the feet and ankles (AFO) can be worn inside regular shoes. The upper leg braces (KAFO) are also worn under clothing. Each student is encouraged to be as independent as possible in putting on and taking off his braces (Clopton, 1981). If assistance is needed, the teacher should refer to the guidelines that follow. Further specific questions may be answered by the child's parents or physical therapist. To apply leg braces, the steps outlined below are followed:

1. The skin is first examined for reddened areas. If any are noticed, the braces should not be used until the parents, physical therapist, or nurse is consulted.
2. All straps are opened, locks disengaged, and shoes unfastened as much as possible. (See Figure 2.8 and 2.9.)
3. The student assumes a position within the braces, such that the hips and knees are flexed. The feet are placed into the molded plastic form of the foot with the heels inside. The shoes are then put on and tied.

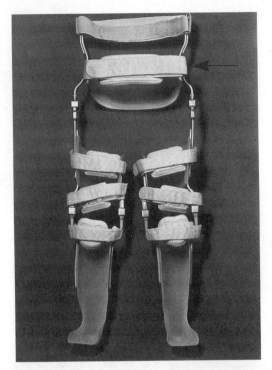

Figure 2.4. Hip/knee/ankle/foot orthosis (HKAFO)—Arrow shows pelvic band.

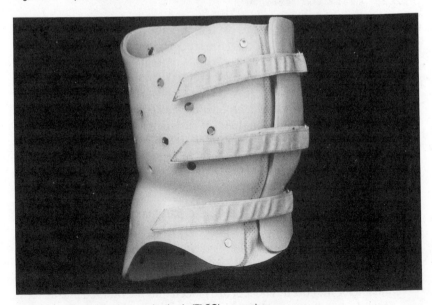

Figure 2.5. Thoraco-lumbo-sacral orthosis (TLSO)—one-piece.

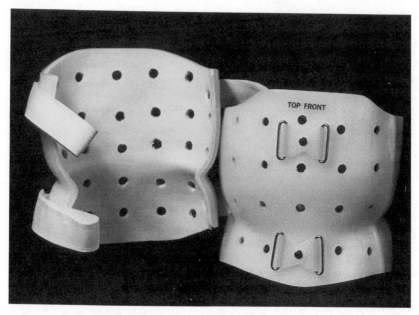

Figure 2.6.   Thoraco-lumbo-sacral orthosis (TLSO)—clam-shell.

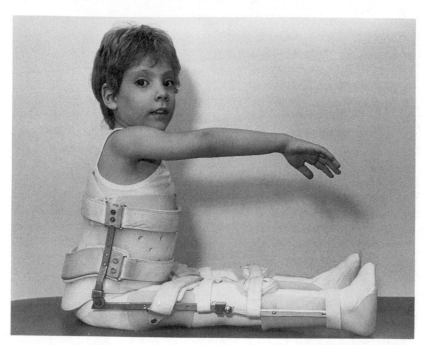

Figure 2.7.   Spinal frame.

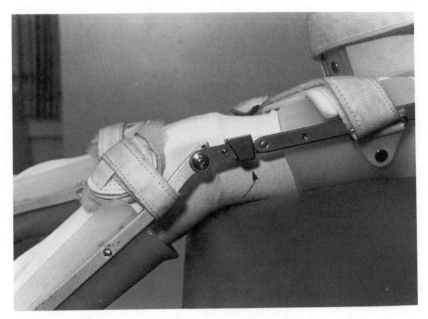

Figure 2.8. Knee lock, unlocked. See arrow.

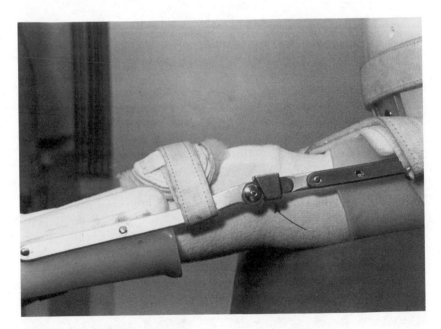

Figure 2.9. Knee lock, locked. See arrow.

4. The legs are then straightened and the remaining straps are fastened, beginning at the feet and progressing to the pelvic band. Knee pads, if present, are buckled with the knees slightly flexed to reduce pressure when the student is seated. The pelvic band is fastened with the child in a seated position, again to reduce pressure when sitting.

5. To remove leg braces, the above steps are reversed.

To apply a body jacket, the steps outlined below are followed:

1. The skin is first examined for reddened areas. If any are noticed, the body jacket should not be applied until the parents, physical therapist, or nurse is consulted.

2. A two-piece, or clam-shell, thoraco-lumbo-sacral orthosis (TLSO) is then applied in the following manner:
   a. The student lies face down; the back portion of the brace is positioned on the student so that the waist indentations correspond to the student's waist. Carefully roll the student onto his back and adjust the undershirt so that no wrinkles will occur between the student's skin and the brace (Figure 2.10a).
   b. The front portion of the brace is then positioned over the student's chest and abdomen. The waist indentations must be aligned again and the undershirt smoothed (Figure 2.10b).
   c. Once both sections are in place, the straps are tightened. If there are three straps on each side, fasten the middle ones first, then the top, and finally the bottom. If there are only two straps, tighten the top one first and then the bottom. To make sure that the front section will overlap equally on the back section, the straps on each side should be tightened simultaneously (Figure 2.10c).

3. A one-piece style of body jacket is applied as follows:
   a. The student lies on his or her back with the hips and knees flexed. The waist indentations on either side are positioned between the top of the hip and the lower edge of the ribcage. The body jacket is then spread and placed around the student. After the positioning is checked, the undershirt is smoothed.
   b. The student is then rolled onto his or her stomach and the brace position is again aligned with the waist indentations.
   c. The straps are tightened beginning with the middle strap, then the top, and finally the bottom strap.

Skin Care   The student is expected to examine his or her skin for areas of pressure. These may occur if minor brace adjustments are needed or if the student has grown. Early identification of skin pressure helps to prevent skin breakdown. If open areas of skin develop, it will be

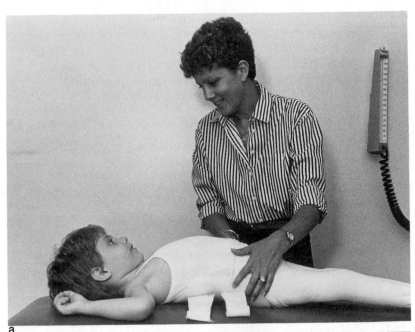

a

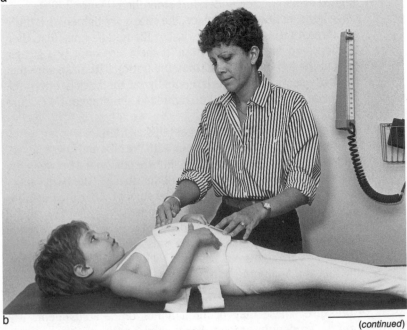

b

(continued)

Figure 2.10. Application of two-piece TLSO. a) Placement of back piece. b) Placement of front. c) Fastening straps.

Figure 2.10. *(continued)*

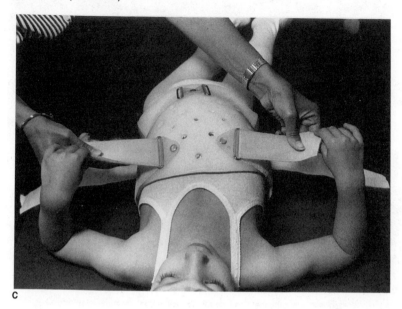

c

necessary for brace wear to be discontinued until healing occurs (Clopton, 1981; Shurtleff, 1986a) (see Figure 2.11).

Crutches and Walkers

An early goal for students with spina bifida is mobility in the environment (Dias, 1978; Shurtleff, 1986b; Yngve, Douglas, & Roberts, 1984). Once appropriate braces are obtained, walking aids are introduced. Initially, walkers may be used to provide increased stability. There are generally two types. The rollator resembles a conventional walker with small wheels replacing the front legs (Figure 2.12a). The wheels enable the student to maneuver the walker without the need to lift it. The second type of walker is the reverse, or posture walker. This style also incorporates small wheels. It encircles the student from behind and in some cases may facilitate a more erect posture (Figure 2.12b).

After the student has mastered the use of a walker, he or she will progress to crutches. Triceps-cuff crutches are constructed of wood with leather cuffs. When properly sized, the cuff encircles the upper arm, providing additional support in ambulation (Figure 2.13a). Forearm crutches are made of aluminum with a molded plastic semicircular cuff. The cuff of this style encircles the lower arm below the elbow. Both types allow the student to stand in a balanced position with at least one hand free for activity (Figure 2.13b) (Hoberman, 1965).

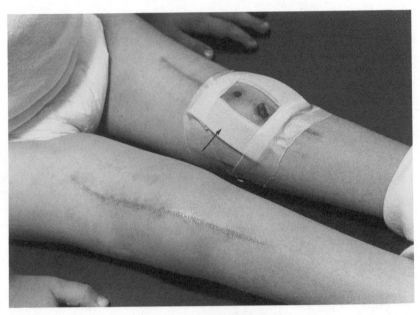

Figure 2.11. Pressure sore at left knee. Foam padding protects from pressure. (See arrow.)

Recommendations for Crutch Use in the Classroom

1. Explain the proper use and function of crutches to other students to satisfy their curiosity. Students should be discouraged from playing with crutches.

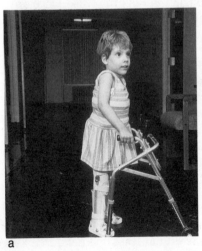
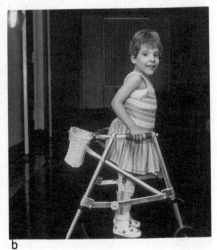

Figure 2.12. a) Rollator walker. b) Posture walker.

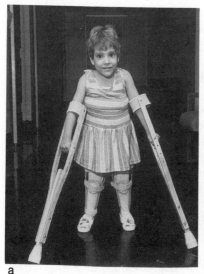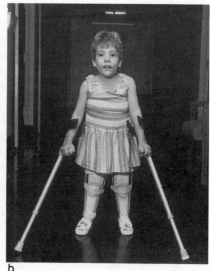

a   b

Figure 2.13. a) Triceps-cuff crutches. b) Forearm crutches.

2. Store crutches near the person who uses them; suitable places include on the wheelchair or under the desk.
3. Keep crutches out of the aisles and pathways of others to prevent tripping.
4. Encourage caution on wet or slippery floors, particularly near outside doors, bathrooms, and water fountains.
5. Floor mats and loose rugs can be a hazard for tripping and falling and should be removed.

The teacher should be aware that ambulation with braces and crutches requires the expenditure of a great deal of energy (Agre et al., 1987; Shurtleff, 1986b; Williams et al., 1983). It has also been noted that the maintenance of long distance ambulation is affected by actual muscle strength. As a result, students requiring bracing over the hips and knees are less likely to remain ambulatory into adolescence (Dudgeon, Jaffe, & Shurtleff, 1991; McDonald, Jaffe, Mosca, & Shurtleff, 1991). These students may prefer to discontinue bracing and rely solely on the use of a wheelchair as a more effective means of mobility. This change in mode of locomotion often occurs in early adolescence (Asher & Olson, 1983; Carroll, 1987; DeSouza & Carroll, 1976; Gaff et al., 1984).

Wheelchairs

A wheelchair is often used by the student with spina bifida as an additional means of independent mobility. For some students, the wheelchair may be used as the only means of mobility. Other students may use a wheelchair for only part of the school day, usually to travel long distances (Findley et al., 1987; Klein, 1983; Williamson, 1987). The wheelchair enables the student to have independent mobility and, therefore, contributes to the development of responsibility and maturity. "A wheelchair can provide ways for the child to be as independent as possible, to do things for himself, and to be involved in a variety of activities" (Klein, 1983, p. 20). Students using wheelchairs are able to participate in most classroom and school activities (Schultz-Hurlburt & Tervo, 1982).

There are several different models and sizes of wheelchairs and it is important that the student be fitted for a chair by a qualified professional such as a physical therapist, occupational therapist, or equipment sales representative (Klein, 1983). School personnel should have a good understanding and working knowledge of the parts and use of a wheelchair to assist the student in achieving full participation in school activities.

Parts of a Wheelchair

Brakes   The brakes are the major safety feature of a wheelchair. Brakes are located on both rear wheels of the chair, at or below seat level. They should always be locked when the chair is not in motion and when the student transfers into or out of the wheelchair. Most students with spina bifida will be able to operate the brakes without assistance, but reminders may be needed (Figure 2.14a).

Armrests   Armrests on the wheelchair are another safety feature for the student with spina bifida. By resting one arm or the other, the student is able to improve balance. The armrests also permit the student to lift up and change position in the chair. Frequent changes in position help to prevent the development of pressure sores or skin breakdown caused by sitting in one position for long periods of time (Okamoto, Lamers, & Shurtleff, 1983). The armrests can be removed or swung away for side transfers. In most cases, the student will be familiar with armrest function.

Footrests   Footrests provide support, positioning, and protection for the student's feet. For safety, the student's feet should always be placed on the footrests. Usually they can be swung away from the chair and are removable, but some types only lift up and out of the way. When the student is transferring in and out of the chair, the footrests must be out of the way. Most students with spina bifida will be able to move the footrests independently or with a little assistance (Figure 2.14b).

Push Handles   Push handles or handgrips are located on the back of most wheelchairs and are used to push the chair. The majority of students propel their chairs independently and will need this assistance only when going up steep hills or over long distances. Some students will need help when propelling up or down ramps if the angle is too steep (Figure 2.14c—curved arrow).

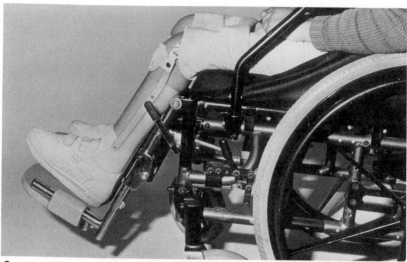

a

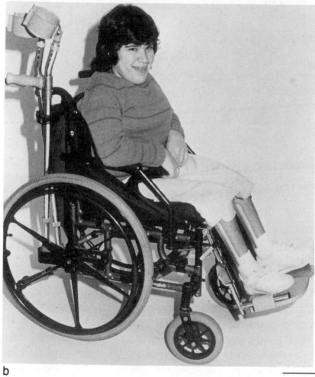

b

(continued)

Figure 2.14. a) Wheelchair parts: brakes, footrest, armrest. b) Wheelchair with child properly positioned. c) Wheelchair accessories: crutch holder, push handles carrying pouch, tipping lever. (See arrows.)

Figure 2.14.   *(continued)*

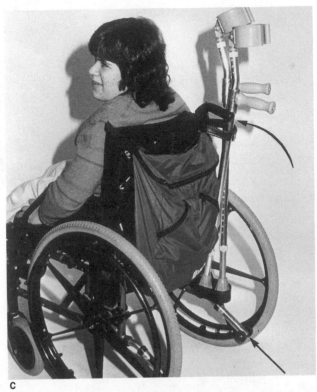

c

Tipping Lever   A tipping lever is located at the base of the rear of the wheelchair below the push handles. By pressing down on the tipping lever with the foot, the pusher can tip the wheelchair backward to cross curbs or other obstacles (Figure 2.14c—straight arrow).

Seat Belt   A seat belt is an essential safety feature for the student. The seat belt should be fastened at all times when the student is using the wheelchair.

Wheelchair Accessories

Crutch Holder   A crutch holder (Figure 2.14c), usually consisting of a Velcro strap and support base, is essential for storage. This device enables the student to keep crutches available for ambulation as needed.

Carrying Pouches   Carrying pouches can be placed on the wheelchair to store books and other school supplies. There are commercially available pouches made for wheelchairs, but many students use backpacks strung across the wheelchair push handles. Pouches placed at the back of the chair are often difficult for students with high bracing as they cannot reach their supplies independently. These students may need alternative places for supply storage or some assistance in retrieving and storing books and supplies.

Wheelchair Cushions All students with spina bifida using wheelchairs should use some type of cushion on the wheelchair seat. Because of impaired skin sensation, they are at high risk for development of pressure sores (Okamoto et al., 1983; Shurtleff, 1986a, Chapter 14). A wheelchair cushion is important to protect the buttocks from the effects of sitting for long periods of time (Stewart, Eng, Palmieri, & Cochran, 1980).

The type of cushion the student uses is determined by his or her activity level. The ambulatory student, who uses a wheelchair only for long distances (e.g., cafeteria for lunch) may use a simple foam cushion. The student using a wheelchair for mobility full-time should use a gel cushion or air-filled cushion to provide sitting support and skin protection (see the appendix at the end of this chapter). All students using wheelchairs must be careful to shift position every 7–10 minutes for pressure relief. The presence of a cushion does not eliminate the need for frequent position changes.

MOBILITY IN THE SCHOOL SETTING

Students walking with braces and crutches display a variety of gait patterns. These include the following—*reciprocal:* the crutch and leg movement alternate in a pattern similar to walking; *swing-through:* the student swings his/her body between and beyond the crutches which are then moved forward and the "swing-through" is repeated; *swing-to:* the body is lifted forward to a point between, or a bit behind, the crutches, the crutches are then advanced, and the "swing-to" is repeated (Hoberman, 1965; Williamson, 1987). If there is a question about the student's gait or about safety, it is best to talk to the parents or a physical therapist.

Ambulatory Student

Entering Doorways The student with braces and crutches can usually manage to open and close doors independently, although a young student or one with weak arms may need assistance. When approaching a door, the student positions himself or herself close to the door, maintains support by balancing with one crutch, and turns the doorknob or handle with the opposite hand. The student then pushes or pulls the door open, propping it open with one crutch while passing through the doorway.

Stairs The method of stair management with braces and crutches will vary depending upon the student's muscle strength and size, the type of braces and crutches, the height of the step, and the position of the rail. The following process is for the student using braces unlocked at the hip.

Ascending   The student stands with feet close to the next higher step, holding the rail with one hand while keeping the remaining crutch on the same step as his feet. The crutch not being used is transferred to the other hand and held with the shaft parallel to the handgrip. It may also be given to an aide or another student. To mount the step, the student lifts himself up using the crutch and rail for support (Figure 2.15a). Balance is maintained by keeping the trunk straight. This maneuver is repeated for each step. If assistance is needed, the aide should stand directly behind the student on the next lower step and hold the top of the braces (Bromley, 1976) (Figure 2.15b).

Descending   The student transfers the crutches to one hand, stands as close as possible to the edge of the step, holding the rail with one hand while placing the opposite crutch on the step below. The pupil then lowers himself or herself down each step, maintaining an erect posture. If assistance is needed, the aide should stand one step below the student and position both hands at the student's waist. The person giving assistance must have good footing and anticipate the movements of the student (Bromley, 1976) (Figures 2.16a–b).

Crossing Curbs

Ascending   When ascending a curb, the student uses his crutches to lift himself onto the curb. To assist, stand behind the student, grasp the top of the braces, and lift the student onto the curb.

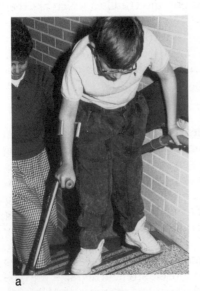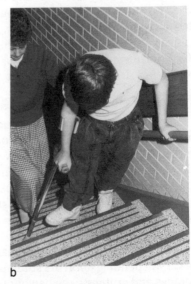

a   b

Figure 2.15.   Ascending steps. a) Student holds rail and one crutch. b) Student lifts himself using the crutch and rail.

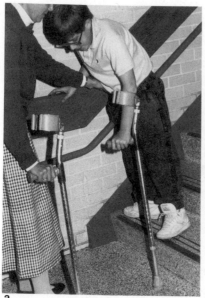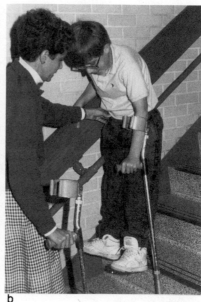

Figure 2.16. Descending steps. a) Student holds rail and places crutch on step below. b) Student lowers himself using crutch and rail for balance.

Descending   When descending a curb, the student stands at the edge and lowers both crutches to street level and then swings both legs down, keeping the trunk erect. If assistance is needed, stand at the student's side and assist with recovery of balance.

Floor Mobility

Getting Down to the Floor   With the braces locked or unlocked at the hips, the student slowly "walks" the crutches forward away from the feet. As the upper trunk nears the floor, he or she reaches out with both hands, lowering to the floor. Assistance is given by holding the student at the hips. He or she then unlocks the hip joints if needed, turns over, and assumes a sitting position (Bromley, 1976) (Figures 2.17a-e).

Getting Up from the Floor   As the student lies face down, the braces are unlocked at the hips and the crutches are placed at the sides in line with the body and with the tips away from the body. After doing a push-up, the student walks his hands toward the feet assuming a jack-knife position. While balancing on one hand, the student grasps the handpiece of the opposite crutch. After shifting weight to this crutch, the student can then grasp the handpiece of the remaining crutch. He or she then "walks" the crutches toward the feet as the trunk is straightened. The braces are then locked at the hips. Assistance is provided by holding the student at the hips (Bromley, 1976).

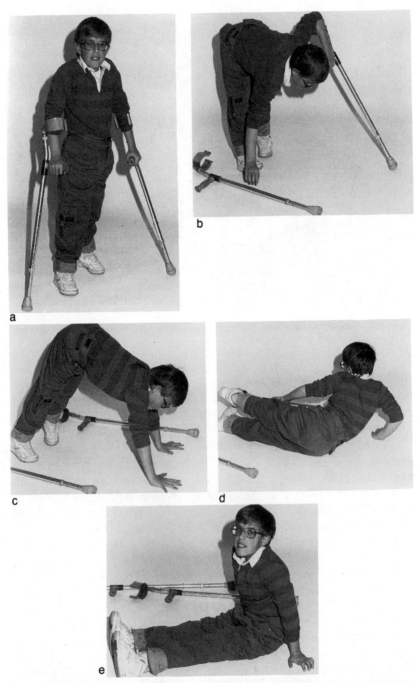

Figure 2.17.   a) Student in full upright position. b) Student walking crutches forward. c) Student in jack-knife position, lowering self to floor. d) Student rotating to sit. e) Student sitting. This process is reversed when moving from floor to stand.

Wheelchair-Mobile Student

Entering Doorways The student in a wheelchair approaches a door in a parallel fashion (Figure 2.18a). He or she then uses one hand to open and hold the door, while using the other hand to move the wheelchair through the doorway (Figure 2.18b). A young student, or a student with weak arms, may need assistance to wheel through doorways.

Stairs

Ascending Two people are needed to lift a wheelchair up stairs. Steps are ascended one at a time by backing the wheelchair up the steps. One person leads from above, controlling and pulling the chair at the handgrips, while the other stands below holding the frame and assisting with a lifting motion. The person at the handgrips directs the movement (Figure 2.19).

Descending The process is similar to that described above. However, the person standing below gently guides the wheelchair down while the person holding the handgrips controls its descent.

Crossing Curbs

Ascending To ascend curbs, begin with the wheelchair facing the curb. Grasp the handgrips and tilt the wheelchair backward. Once the front casters are on the curb, lift the back of the wheelchair and roll it forward onto the sidewalk (Figure 2.20).

Descending To descend curbs, begin by facing the wheelchair away from the curb. Tilt the wheelchair back, and lower it to the street while holding the handgrips. Guide the wheelchair backward until the front casters clear the curb and can be lowered to the street.

Transfer from Sitting to a Standing Position The student with braces and crutches may use various methods to come to a standing position from a wheelchair. For safety the wheelchair must be stabilized, the brakes of the wheelchair must be locked, the footrests must be out of the way, and the student's crutches must be accessible. With the knees of the braces locked, the student leans forward, pushing on the crutches or armrests to lift up and out of the chair. Crutch support is then used to straighten the trunk and lock the hip joints of the braces. Some students may prefer to turn and face the chair, pushing to an upright stance from the armrests, reaching for the crutches, and then straightening to lock the hip joints. To assist, stand at the side and slightly behind the student and help by lifting and stabilizing the student at the hips while the braces are locked. In the bathroom the procedure to stand from the commode is the same, using grab bars and other permanently secured fixtures for support when available, and as necessary (Figures 2.21a–e).

Transfer from Standing to Sitting As with moving to the standing position from a wheelchair, the chair must be stabilized with the brakes locked and the footrests out of the way. The student backs up to the chair until contact is made. Support is provided by the crutches or other stable

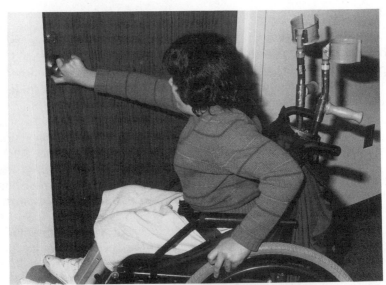

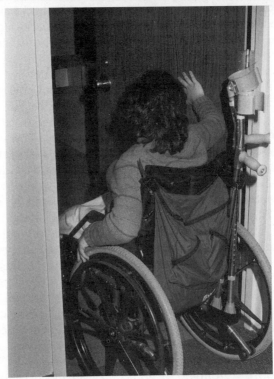

Figure 2.18.   a) Entering a doorway with a wheelchair. b) Holding door open.

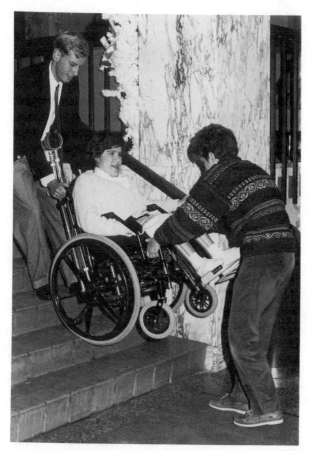

Figure 2.19. Ascending, descending stairs with a wheelchair.

furniture, as the student unlocks the hip joints of the braces, leans forward, and lowers or lifts into the chair. Some students walk forward to the chair, hang the crutches on the handgrips, unlock the hips, and use the armrests for support to lift and turn into the sitting position. To assist, stand at the side and slightly behind and guide the student into the chair. In the bathroom the procedure to sit on the commode is the same, utilizing grab bars and other permanently secured fixtures for support where available, and as necessary.

Creating a Functional Environment

Just as all students learn to take care of their possessions, the student with spina bifida can and should assume responsibility for organizing

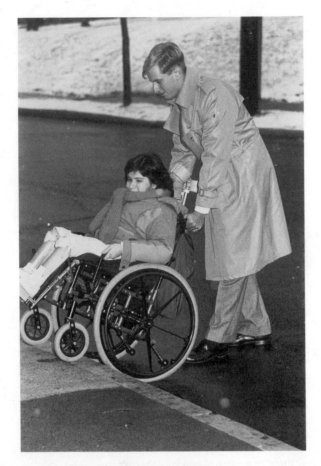

Figure 2.20.   Ascending, descending curb with a wheelchair.

and transporting materials. Experience with this task is especially important for students with spina bifida who will always need to adapt in order
to function within society.

   Organizing the Desk Area   It is important for the student with
spina bifida to have a workable desk area to aid in the development of
organizational skills. These students often have difficulty organizing their
work and belongings and need to learn methods to organize themselves
and their surroundings (Hurley, Dorman, Laatsch, Bell, & D'Avignon
(1990); Mattson, 1982; Tew & Lawrence, 1975). The student should take an
active role in designing these modifications.

   A one-piece desk with a lift top may be used without modifications
(Figure 2.22). However, a desk with storage underneath the chair may cre-

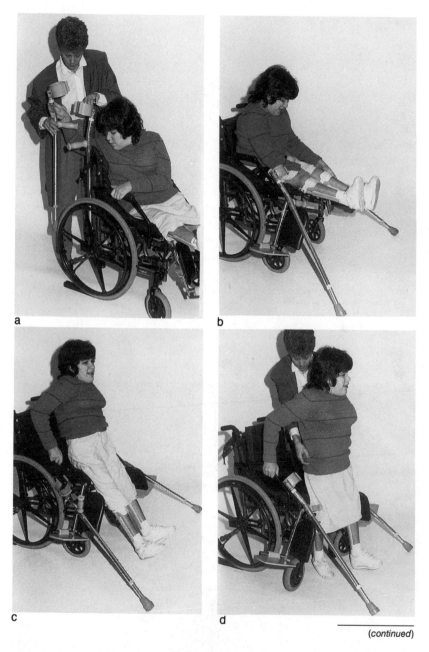

(continued)

Figure 2.21.   Sit-to-stand sequence. a) Student removes crutches from crutch holder. b) Student locks knee joints of braces. c) Student slides forward out of wheelchair. d) When standing, assistance is given to lock hip joints of braces, if needed. e) Student in stance with crutches. This process is reversed when moving from stand to sit.

Figure 2.21. (*continued*)

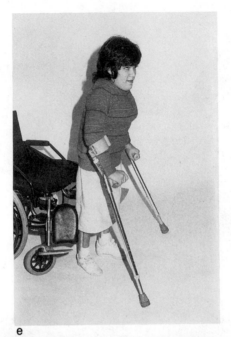

e

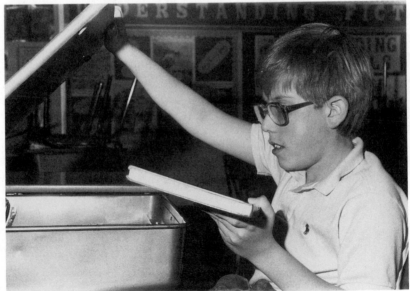

Figure 2.22.   Desk with lift-top.

ate difficulties in managing books for the student with bracing, impaired trunk musculature, and poor balance. If this is the case, school supplies can be kept on the desk top in a bin. Alternatively, another desk, chair, or study carrel may be placed beside the student. The storage area should be high enough to make supplies easily accessible.

If the student remains in the wheelchair during class, a table the size of a desk will provide the best working area. The table should be no higher than chest level with the wheelchair positioned as close as possible and the wheels kept locked. A table with a cut-out area may work better for some students by allowing them easier access to their work. At times, it may be advisable for the student to stand during a part of the school day. Tables with adjustable height allow for growth and enable the student to work from a standing position. These tables are commercially available or can be constructed by a carpenter (see the appendix at the end of this chapter).

Additional specific desk adaptations may be required to allow the student to achieve optimum work abilities. Pencils often tend to roll off a desk onto the floor where they cannot be readily retrieved by the student. Tying a string around the pencil will enable the student to retrieve it independently and an edge on the desk surface may prevent its loss (Figure 2.23). Frequently, items on the desk top will slide about, making it difficult for the student to work. Nonskid matting known as Dycem is commer-

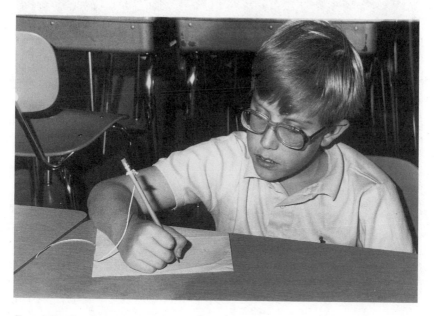

Figure 2.23.   Pencil attached to desk with string.

cially available and may alleviate many of these problems (see the appendix at the end of this chapter). Dycem may be used on the desk top to keep books in place or under a desktop bin or cafeteria tray to keep them from sliding (Figure 2.24). It may also be placed on the seat of a wheelchair or desk chair to prevent the student from sliding forward in the seat.

Storing Crutches Crutches are often an object of curiosity to other students who may be tempted to play with them, but they should always be kept within reach of the student who depends upon them. Students with good trunk balance and mobility are able to store their crutches flat on the floor under their desk. Crutches should be kept out of aisles and classroom walkways to prevent tripping. Crutches can also be strapped to the desk or table with a Velcro strap (Figure 2.25). Another alternative is to use a clamp, such as those commercially available to hold mops and brooms, to attach the crutches to the desk. Some students who are ambulatory may also use a wheelchair for part of the school day. Wheelchair crutch holders keep crutches readily accessible to the student.

Transporting Books and Papers The student who walks with crutches, uses a walker, or propels a wheelchair needs both hands for

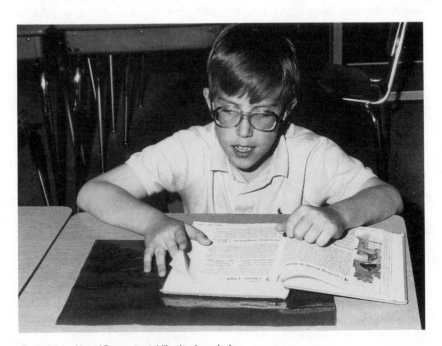

Figure 2.24.   Use of Dycem to stabilize book on desk.

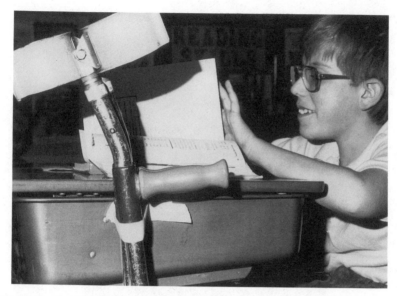

Figure 2.25. Crutches attached to desk with Velcro strap.

mobility and is unable to carry books, papers, and school supplies. A method should be developed for the student with spina bifida to transport these items to and from school independently. A variety of devices are available to meet this need. Book bags can be attached to walkers for holding school work. These bags should be large enough to hold books and small enough so that the student can reach the bottom of the bag. Commercially made bags are available to attach to crutches, but their small size limits their functional use. Often the student using crutches or a walker is able to use a backpack which distributes weight evenly and minimizes loss of balance (Figure 2.26). Backpacks can also be attached to the back of the wheelchair. Many students will also have two sets of books, one kept in school and one at home, to reduce the need to carry books back and forth.

INVOLVEMENT OF THE STUDENT IN SCHOOL ENVIRONMENT

With this understanding of types of equipment, mobility, development of a work space, and related issues, it is appropriate to discuss the physical management of the student with spina bifida in a variety of school environments. These include the classroom, bathroom, cafeteria, gymnasium, library, hall and locker areas, assemblies, and field trips. Because these are all aspects of the social environment of the school, social needs

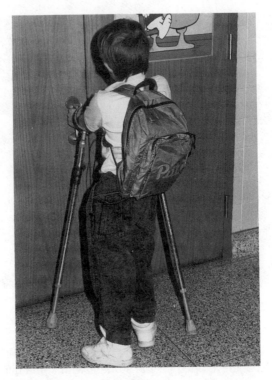

Figure 2.26.   Use of backpack to transport supplies.

will be given consideration in the discussion of the management of the environments. Social and interpersonal development is a key goal of education, and integration of the student as fully as possible into the normal daily school experience significantly contributes to self and group identity (Blum, 1983). These social dimensions are discussed in greater detail in Chapter 9.

Students should begin to assume responsibility for managing crutches and school supplies as early as kindergarten. They should be encouraged to use their backpacks when moving to different classrooms, the bathroom, the cafeteria, and to and from school. These methods enable students with spina bifida to be responsible for their own belongings and function more independently in the school environment.

In the Classroom

The student with spina bifida should be seated in an area of the class that is accessible, but not separated from the rest of the students. Aisles should be clear enough to permit wheelchair or crutch access. Students should have a clear view of the teacher and the blackboard. Students with spina bifida have as much or more need to change positions throughout the day as their nondisabled peers (Klein, 1983). Moving about increases bone growth, prevents pressure areas on the skin, and increases circulation (Clopton, 1981; Myers, Cerone, & Olson, 1981; Williamson, 1987; Yngve et al., 1984). These students should take their turn at the blackboard, pass out papers, and move between areas of the school with their class. The classroom should be organized to permit independent access to pencil sharpeners, the blackboard, the aisles, doorways, and the wastebaskets. These special considerations enable the student to be an equal participant instead of a spectator. With responsibility and competence in these areas comes a valuable sense of belonging.

In the Bathroom

As discussed in Chapter 1, most students with spina bifida have a neurogenic bowel and bladder and require an adaptive toileting program. Most use the clean intermittent catheterization program described in Chapter 1. All will need special provisions to accommodate their hygiene needs. Bathrooms should be wheelchair accessible with a separate stall and door to insure privacy. Grab bars, a raised toilet seat, or ring adaptor to make the seat smaller will ease toilet activities and contribute to independence. The school may want to supply a closed container for disposable diapers. Personnel who assist should be provided with disposable gloves.

To avoid painful embarrassment for the student, a convenient storage area near the bathroom is desirable. Otherwise diapers and catheters should be carried in a bookbag. It could be very embarrassing for a student to be observed walking down the hall carrying a disposable diaper or accompanied by an aide carrying these supplies. Assistance with personal hygiene provided by aides should be within the confines of a private toilet facility in distinction to a public restroom. An empty locker may provide supply storage. Supplies should not be kept in the bathroom unless they can be secured. Every effort should be made to preserve privacy and avoid a sense of shame about the student's toileting program. Whenever possible, toileting activities should occur in the bathroom rather than the nursing station to more closely match the normal situation. If the assistance of an aide is required, it is extremely important that the aide be of the same sex as the student.

It is often possible to change a disposable diaper while the student is standing in a previously identified private area. This saves time in the bathroom, and makes it possible to avoid having the student fully undress or lie on a cot in a passive position. A grab rail or supporting surface is essential for this procedure. If the student wears the diaper under the braces and wears underpants over the braces, the changing procedure is simplified by the following routine:

1. Pull down the slacks or pull up the skirt.
2. Pull down the underpants.
3. Release the tabs of the diaper.

The student may then remove the diaper from front to back. Unlocking the hips and bending over may help. The procedure is then reversed:

1. Put on the fresh diaper front to back and fasten the tabs.
2. Lock the hips.
3. Pull up the underpants and slacks or pull down the skirt.

Communication in a spirit of cooperation between aides, school nurses, teachers, and parents will lead to understanding for all people concerned. The elimination of waste is a biological fact and reduction of emotion and stress around this activity will be enhanced by open and positive communication.

Outside of the Classroom

The Library and Assembly Activities   Students with spina bifida should be as involved in classroom activities as any other student. They should join others on the floor during story time and be outside during recess (Klein, 1983). Forming "wheelchair wagon trains" by placing all students in wheelchairs together during assemblies or other large scale activities should be avoided since this leads to isolation and segregation.

The Cafeteria   Lunchtime may be an appropriate time for the student crutch walker to use a wheelchair if the cafeteria is a long distance away and if time is a factor. Seating students at the end of a table in a separate chair or in a wheelchair allows them to eat with their peers. Lunchtime is an important part of the school day and the student with spina bifida also has a need for this form of socialization.

General School Layout   When scheduling classes, give special consideration to the location of classrooms and lockers. It is suggested that as many classes as possible be located on one floor. The student's locker should be assigned centrally in relationship to classes and located on the end of a row to allow better access. The hooks and shelves in the locker may need to be lowered. Long distances between classes may require releasing the student a few minutes early in order to permit arrival at the next class on time.

Field Trips   Just as for class activities, the student with spina bifida should be included in all field trips. These students need diverse learning experiences as much or more than other students. Field trips may require advance planning to review architectural barriers that may be present. Although parents are good resources for solving problems, the school should not rely on parents to accompany their child on field trips. This reliance would only reinforce differences and the student's tendency to remain dependent on his or her parents. Students lose equal status and independent identity among peers when accompanied by a parent on class field trips.

Physical Education   Because of mandated physical education requirements, students with spina bifida must be included in the school's physical education program (Buckanavage, 1980; Clopton, 1981). There are countless methods of adapting and modifying existing curricula to include the student with spina bifida and make physical education a meaningful portion of the school program. Every effort should be made to give each student an opportunity for active participation in the regular program, ambulating when possible, or using a wheelchair when necessary. Depending on the extent of paralysis, students with spina bifida may participate in general locomotor skills, ball activities, group games, team sports, calisthenics, conditioning, aerobic exercise, dance and rhythm activities, swimming, recreational sports such as bowling and archery, and even tumbling and gymnastics (Buckanavage, 1980; Cratty & Breen, 1972).

Adaptations and modifications do not require special equipment, extensive training, or extraordinary time and energy. They do require an attitude of openness, resourcefulness, and acceptance of the challenge and responsibility. Remember that simply keeping score or watching the other students in gym class does not fulfill mandated requirements. Most importantly, participation in physical education does help the student with spina bifida learn the value and joy of exercise and group sports, develop a sense of peer identity and acceptance, and aid in the development of leisure activities for adult life (Brown & Gordon, 1987; Morrissy, 1978; Schleien & Ray, 1988).

Fire Drills   As with all school activities, students with spina bifida need to be included in regular fire drills. It is obvious that their handicaps will require *advanced* planning in case of an emergency. Exit in a wheelchair is generally faster and safer, and therefore the student's wheelchair should always be readily accessible. One individiual, preferably an adult, in each of the student's classes should be responsible for assisting in rapid exit. The escape plan should be established according to Labor and Industry Fire and Panic Regulations for public schools.

Bus Rides   The bus ride to and from school can be an important social time in the student's day. As with all students, bus safety is a priority. The ambulatory student with spina bifida may only need to "buckle-up." The student using a wheelchair has several other considerations. The wheelchair should be stabilized in the bus or van and the student should wear his wheelchair seatbelt. Utilization of the bus or van wheelchair lift should always be supervised by an adult (Azrael & Klein, 1989).

SUMMARY

With recent efforts to expose the disabled and physically normal populations to one another, differences are becoming increasingly minimized. In time and with this effort, it should be possible for us to see the 'person' in the wheelchair rather than the wheelchair with the person in it. Disabled people are beginning to say, "Our bodies may make us disabled, but it is society which makes us handicapped." It is the willingness of the physically normal to change their perceptions and the disabled to fight for changes which gives us hope for an enlightened future. (Myers, Cerone, & Olson, 1981, p. 62)

In summary, it is hoped that the practical information found in this chapter will aid in the inclusion of the student with spina bifida in all areas of school life. Braces, crutches, and wheelchairs need not be a barrier, but should be a bridge to a more rewarding school experience because they permit the full participation of another human spirit.

GLOSSARY

Adaptive equipment   Modified equipment that enables the student to perform daily tasks.
Cervical   Seven vertebrae in the neck.
Gait   Pattern of walking.
Kyphosis   Spinal curvature with the convexity to the back.
Lordosis   Spinal curvature with the convexity to the front.
Lumbar   Five vertebrae in the low back area.
Occupational therapist   Health care professional with training in the evaluation and treatment of upper limb function, fine-motor skills, perceptual-motor skills, self-care skills, and the use of adaptive equipment.
Orthosis   External means of support for weakened or paralyzed body parts; a brace.
Physical therapist   Health care professional with training in the development of motor function, ambulation, and use of mobility aids and adaptive equipment.
Sacral   Five vertebrae that attach to the pelvis at the end of the spine.
Scoliosis   Spinal curvature with the convexity to the side; may also involve some rotation of the vertebrae.
Thoracic   Twelve vertebrae extending from the neck to the waist.

REFERENCES

Agre, J., Findley, T., McNally, M.C., Habeck, R., Leon, A., Stradel, L., Birebak, R., & Schmalz, R. (1987). Physical activity capacity in children with myelomeningocele. *Archives of Physical Medicine and Rehabilitation, 68*, 372–377.

Asher, M., & Olson, J. (1983). Factors affecting the ambulatory status of patients with spina bifida cystica. *Journal of Bone and Joint Surgery, 65-A* (3), 350–356.

Azrael, A., & Klein, S. (Eds.). (1989). School bus safety: Tie-downs and restraints. *Exceptional Parent, 19*(6), 60–63.

Bahnson, D. (1982). Myelomeningocele and its problems. *Pediatric Annals, 11*(6), 528–540.

Blum, R. (1983). The adolescent with spina bifida. *Clinical Pediatrics, 22*(5), 331–335.

Bromley, I. (1976). *Tetraplegia and paraplegia: A guide for helping the child with spina bifida.* Springfield, IL: Charles C Thomas.

Brown, M., & Gordon, W. (1987). Impact of impairment on activity pattern of children. *Archives of Physical Medicine and Rehabilitation, 68*, 828–832.

Buckanavage, R. (Ed.). (1980). *Adapting physical education: A guide for individualizing physical education programs.* Harrisburg: Pennsylvania Department of Education, Bureau of Curriculum Service, Division of Health, Science and Technology.

Carroll, N. (1987). Assessment and management of the lower extremity in myelodysplasia. *Orthopedic Clinics of North America, 18*(4), 709–724.

Clopton, N. (1981). *Caring for your child with spina bifida.* Oak Brook, IL: Eterna Press.

Cratty, B., & Breen, J. (1972). *Educational games for physically handicapped children.* Denver: Love Publishing.

DeSouza, L., & Carroll, M. (1976). Ambulation of the braced myelomeningocele patient. *Journal of Bone and Joint Surgery, 58-A* (8), 1112–1118.

Dias, L. (1978). Orthopedic management of the myelomeningocele child. In J.M. Wilson (Ed.), *Orthopedic aspects of developmental disabilities* (pp. 84–101). Chapel Hill University of North Carolina at Chapel Hill, School of Medicine, Department of Medical Allied Health Professions, Division of Physical Therapy.

Dudgeon, B., Jaffe, K., & Shurtleff, D. (1991). Variations in midlumbar myelomeningocele: implications for ambulation. *Pediatric Physical Therapy, 3*(2), 57–62.

Findley, T., Agre, J., Habeck, R., Schmalz, R., Birkebak, R., & McNally, M.C. (1987). Ambulation in the adolescent with myelomeningocele. I: Early childhood predictors. *Archives of Physical Medicine and Rehabilitation, 68*, 518–522.

Gaff, J.E., Robinson, J.M., & Parker, P. (1984). The walking ability of 14 to 17 year old teenagers with spina bifida—A physiotherapy study. *Physiotherapy, 70*(12), 473–474.

Hanson, R., & Graves, M. (1987). Current concepts: Care and habilitation of the child with myelomeningocele–a multidisciplinary approach. *Journal of Mississippi State Medical Association, 28*(6), 145–150.

Hoberman, M. (1965). Crutch and cane exercises and use. In S. Licht (Ed.), *Therapeutic exercise* (pp. 275–405). Baltimore: Waverly Press.

Hurley, A., Dorman, C., Laatsch, L., Bell, S., & D'Avignon, J. (1990). Cognitive functioning in patients with spina bifida, hydrocephalus and the "cocktail party" syndrome. *Developmental Neuropsychology, 6*(2), 151–172.

Klein, S.D. (Ed.). (1983). Wheelchairs: Aids for participation and discovery. *Exceptional Parent, 13*(1), 17–28.

Kupta, J., Geddes, N., & Carroll N., (1978). Comprehensive management of the child with spina bifida. *Orthopedic Clinics of North America, 9*(1), 97–113.

Lough, L.K. (1984). Bracing. In J.A. Blackman (Ed.), *Medical aspects of developmental disabilities in children, birth to three* (pp. 15–30). Rockville, MD: Aspen Systems.

Mattson, B. (1982, July/August). Learning problems of children with spina bifida. *Clinical Proceedings Children's Hospital National Medical Center, 38*, 225–230.

McDonald, C., Jaffe, K., Mosca, V., & Shurtleff, D. (1991). Ambulatory outcome of children with myelomeningocele: Effect of lower extremity muscle strength. *Developmental Medicine and Child Neurology, 33*, 482–490.

Morrissy, R. (1978). Spina bifida: A new rehabilitation problem. *Orthopedic Clinics of North America, 9*(2), 379–389.

Myers, G., Cerone, S., & Olson, A. (Eds.). (1981). *A guide for helping the child with spina bifida*. Springfield, IL: Charles C Thomas.

Okamoto, G., Lamers, J., & Shurtleff, D. (1983). Skin breakdown in patients with myelomeningocele. *Archives of Physical Medicine and Rehabilitation, 64*, 20–23.

Schleien, S., & Ray, M.T. (1988). *Community recreation and persons with disabilities: Strategies for integration*. Baltimore: Paul H. Brookes Publishing Co.

Schultz-Hurlburt, B., & Tervo, R. (1982). Wheelchair users at a children's rehabilitation center: Attributes and management. *Developmental Medicine and Child Neurology, 24*, 54–60.

Shurtleff, D. (1986a). Decubitus formation and skin breakdown. In D. Shurtleff (Ed.), *Myelodysplasias and exstrophies: Significance, prevention and treatment* (pp. 299–311). New York: Grune & Stratton.

Shurtleff, D. (1986b). Mobility. In D. Shurtleff (Ed.), *Myelodysplasias and exstrophies: Significance, prevention and treatment* (pp. 313–356). New York: Grune & Stratton.

Stewart, S., Eng, M., Palmieri, B., & Cochran, G. (1980). Wheelchair cushion effect on skin temperature, heat flux, and relative humidity. *Archives of Physical Medicine and Rehabilitation, 61*, 229–233.

Tew, B., & Lawrence, K. (1975). The effects of hydrocephalus on intelligence, visual perception, and school attainment. *Developmental Medicine and Child Neurology, 17*(Suppl. 35), 129–134.

U.S. Department of Education, Office for Civil Rights. (1986). *Section 504 of the Rehabilitation Act of 1973: Handicapped persons' rights under federal law*. Washington, DC: U.S. Government Printing Office.

Williams, L., Anderson, A., Campbell, J., Thomas, L., Felwell, E., & Walker, J. (1983). Energy cost of walking and of wheelchair propulsion by children with myelodysplasia: Comparison with normal children. *Developmental Medicine and Child Neurology, 25*, 617–624.

Williamson, G. (Ed.). (1987). *Children with spina bifida: Early intervention and preschool programming*. Baltimore: Paul H. Brookes Publishing Co.

Wright, B.A. (1983). *Physical disability: A psychological approach*. New York: Harper & Row.

Yngve, D., Douglas, R., & Roberts, J. (1984). The reciprocating gait orthosis in myelomeningocele. *Journal of Pediatric Orthopedics, 4*, 304–310.

Equipment and Accessibility Resources

ACCESSIBILITY LITERATURE

U.S. Department of Education
Office of Civil Rights
Washington, D.C. 20202
(215) 596-6112

ADAPTIVE EQUIPMENT

Achievement Products, Inc.
P.O. Box 547
Mineola, New York 11501
(516) 747-8899

Danmar Products, Inc.
221 Jackson Industrial Drive
Ann Arbor, Michigan 48103

Flaghouse, Inc.
150 No. MacQuesten Parkway
Mt. Vernon, New York 10550
(914) 699-1900

Fred Sammons
Box 32
Brookfield, Illinois 60513
(800) 323-5547

J.A. Preston Corporation
60 Page Road
Clifton, New Jersey 07012
(800) 821-9319

North Coast Medical, Inc.
450 Salmar Avenue
Campbell, California 95008
(800) 821-9319

**Rifton Equipment for the
  Handicapped**
Route 213
Rifton, New York 12471
(914) 658-3141

Southpaw Enterprises, Inc.
800 West Third Street
Dayton, Ohio 45407
(513) 223-7510

Sportime in the Mainstream
2905-E Amvoiler Road
Atlanta, Georgia 30360
(800) 241-9884

AMBULATION AIDS

Guardian Products
780 Easy Street
Box 549
Simi Valley, California 93065
(800) 524-1703

Kaye Products, Inc.
535 Dimmocks Mill Road
Hillsboro, North Carolina 27278
(919) 732-6444

WHEELCHAIRS

Everest & Jennings, Inc.
3233 E. Mission Oaks Boulevard
Camarillo, California 93010
(805) 987-6911

WHEELCHAIRS (*continued*)

Invacare Corporation
899 Cleveland Street
P.O. Box 4028
Elyria, Ohio 44036
1-800-INVACARE

Sunrise Rehabilitation
2842 Business Park Avenue
Fresno, California 93727
(209) 292-2171

WHEELCHAIR CUSHIONS

Embracing Concepts
76 Woodside Drive
Pennfield, New York 14526
(716) 381-9229

Jay Medical, Ltd.
P.O. Box 18656
Boulder, Colorado 80308
(800) 648-8282

ROHO, Inc.
100 Florida Avenue
Belleville, Illinois 62221
(800) 851-3449

Accommodations for Students via School Nursing

Ruth E. Leo

School nurses must prepare themselves to work with children who are physically and mentally challenged. Students with special needs require the expansion of the traditional school health program to afford them maximum benefit from their educational experiences. To enable the student with spina bifida to do this, the school nurse must design a plan for care in collaboration with the student, parents, school personnel, and community resources. The school nurse can be an adult friend to and advocate for the student. This chapter traces some of the changes in school nursing to accommodate students with special needs; explores some of the professional mandates for nurses; uses the ANA Standards of School Nursing Practice as a framework for nursing intervention; identifies an approach to the use of the nursing process advocated by the School Nurse Achievement Program; and gives illustrations of the work of school nurses with students with spina bifida.

SETTING THE STAGE

The prekindergarten round-up was going to be a busy day for the school nurse. She enjoyed the eagerness of the new pupils and enjoyed her interactions with the parents who were generally excited about this milestone

---

While teaching courses in school nursing at Slippery Rock University, the writer has worked with many nurses who have cared for children with special needs. The nurses have shown that the school nurse can effectively help these children. In particular, the writer acknowledges the following nurses whose work with students with spina bifida inspired some of the examples in this chapter: Marcie Dexter, Patsy Frankle, Christine Gelacek, Alda Kerschner, Michelene Neubert, Deborah Slater, and Debbie Waddell.

in their children's development. As she walked down the corridor, she noticed one beautiful blonde girl seated with her parents. The child's winning smile attracted the nurse's attention right away; the second thing she noticed was that the child was wearing short leg braces and had her cuffed crutches under the bench. The nurse felt a moment of panic. No one had told her to expect a student with braces and crutches today. Could this be a child with spina bifida? She knew that children with spina bifida were being mainstreamed, but she had not realized she might have a student with the condition in her school this coming school year. She had so many questions for the child's parents; would they be able to answer them? Many unanswered questions were racing through her mind, and she realized that there were many things which she did not know about helping a child in school when the child had spina bifida.

Many school nurses are finding themselves in this situation today. According to the CDC Birth Defects Monitoring Program, each year a growing number of children with spina bifida will be in school, and "the number of surviving children born with spina bifida since 1980 will be approximately 13,000 by the end of 1990" (Economic burden, 1989). This chapter will address ways in which the school nurse may work more effectively with the student with spina bifida.

CHANGES IN SCHOOL NURSING

When school nursing services began in the United States at the turn of the century, there was a great emphasis upon public health practice and the maintenance of wellness to enable children to attend school and to benefit from their education. This required much contact between the school nurse and the child's home. But changes have occurred that did not foster the early precepts, as Wold (1981) summarized. "Over the past 50 years, the role of the school nurse has diminished in scope and value. It has emphasized episodic care and record-keeping at the expense of preventive care, health education, and community involvement" (p. 3).

The impact of the passage of PL 94-142, the Education for All Handicapped Children Act of 1975, on the placement of students with special needs in regular classroom settings, as well as PL 101-476, its reauthorization in 1990 under the new name of the Individuals with Disabilities Education Act (IDEA), with additional transition planning, has necessitated changes in school nursing. This may have served as a stimulus to returning school nursing to its original roots with an increased awareness of the role of the nurse in collaborating with the parents, school personnel, and the community.

School Nursing and IDEA

School health services for students with special needs are included under the "related services" portion of the Individuals with Disabilities Education Act (IDEA) that are specified in Chapter 13. Since original passage of this legislation in 1975 as PL 94-142, the law "requires public schools to identify and assure provision of special education and related services to children with educational, developmental, emotional, or physical disabilities that adversely affect educational performance" (Burkett, 1989, p. 251). There has been controversy regarding which related services are required in the schools and who is eligible for them, especially if a student requires *only* "related services." In their book, Hobbs, Perrin, and Ireys (1985) state, "Children with chronic illnesses, especially those with spina bifida, often find themselves at the center of the controversy" (p. 114). In a summary of a 5-year Collaborative Study of Children with Special Needs (*Serving handicapped children*, 1988), the authors state, "Although PL 94-142 neither mandates nor regulates health services for the handicapped, it assumes that children with educational handicaps deserve those health services that may enable them to benefit from their public education" (p. 12). Many health needs of children with handicaps may overwhelm the school nurse who is not prepared to address those needs.

> Maintaining and expanding the capacity of the public education system to serve handicapped children will depend on parents' continued vigilance and on the hard work of education and health professionals who design and implement programs addressing the day-to-day needs of individual children. (*Serving handicapped children*, 1988, p. 18)

In 1980, to address the role of the school nurse with students with special needs, the American Nurses' Association Divisions on Nursing Practice, the American School Health Association, and the National Association of School Nurses joined together to identify the special health care needs of children with special needs and the nurse's role in meeting those needs while at school. The recommended solutions to meeting the special needs of students who required care during school hours were prepared by a task force and published as a document entitled "School Nurses Working with Handicapped Children" (1980).

The task force presented the following recommended solutions:

1. School health services to handicapped students should be provided by school nurses. The ratio of nurse to student should be based on the nature and severity of the handicapping conditions of the children to be served. Trained health aides, supervised by the school nurse, should be employed to assist the nurse in providing adequate health services to students requiring special care.

2. The initial evaluation of handicapped students should include in each instance a comprehensive health and developmental history as well as a health assessment, including a physical examination to determine health status. The school nurse should assume responsibility for obtaining this information and coordinating health management. Individual nursing care plans should be developed for each handicapped student to identify needs and project a course of nursing intervention during the school day. In the construction of the individual educational

plan, the school nurse should provide the health information and make specific recommendations related to managing health problems.

3. Individual nursing care plans for handicapped children requiring special health services or procedures at school should be recorded. These plans should reflect a holistic view of a child's health while in school and should identify priorities of care and continued evaluation. Each record should indicate the type of service provided.

4. The school nurse, in collaboration with other school and community personnel, should determine the safety program necessary for each handicapped student and should facilitate implementation of this plan.

5. Because the school system is a group of interrelated parts working together to achieve a common goal, it is strongly recommended that children, parents, teachers, school nurses, and other members of the school health system continue to work together as a team in providing assistance to students with handicaps. Each member of this team contributes a particular expertise or perspective without which the goal of providing appropriate public education to all cannot be realized.

6. A nationwide program of continuing education for school nurses to expand and update rehabilitation knowledge and skills should be instituted within the near future, with support and direction from the American Nurses' Association Divisions on Nursing Practice, the American School Health Association, and the National Association of School Nurses. Consideration must be given to the accessibility and sponsorship of this program. (pp. 4–5)

Progress Toward the Recommended Solutions

Although the above statement was made in 1980, all school nurses have not attained the type of programming to meet the health needs of children with disabilities at the level defined by the task force. This may, in part, be due to the ratio of students to school nurse, the role definition of the school nurse, and the preparation of the school nurse for working with children with disabling conditions.

School Nurse:Student Ratio

The ratio varies markedly throughout the United States; as part of an educational needs assessment conducted as an aid to the development of a continuing education program at the School Nurse Achievement Program (SNAP) at the University of Colorado School of Nursing, school nurses from 44 states participated in a survey in 1980. "The average overall school nurse-to-student ratio reported by these school nurses was 1:2137" (Smith & Goodwin, 1982, p. 536). Depending upon the numbers of schools one nurse must cover for health services, the numbers of students, and numbers of students with special needs in each school, it may be extremely difficult to give care or do the necessary planning for care required by the student with spina bifida. It may be necessary to change from previously established ratios to give safe, effective, and thorough care in the schools. Nurses should become advocates for change of ratios in their own schools and in their districts; working with school nurse organizations in one's own area may aid in changing the ratio. Since the advent of mainstreaming of students with special needs, nurses have been advocating change in the ratios. In an addendum to the American Nurses' Association Standards of School Nursing Practice (*Standards of School Nursing Practice,* 1983, p. 18), the authors state:

> The establishment of school nurse staffing patterns in school settings varies across the United States, dependent upon identified needs of students and available resources. In general, these staffing decisions are made based on one or a combination of the following criteria:
> 1. Numbers of students in an area of responsibility
> 2. Population density
> 3. Numbers of handicapped students
> 4. Health services and education to be provided to all students or a portion of students
> 5. Federal, state, and local funding
> 6. Federal, state, and local regulations
> 7. Identified health care delivery personnel (public health department, consultant services) (p. 18)

> The overall complexity of establishing school nurse staffing patterns is very individualized to state agencies and local education departments and therefore, most appropriately, their responsibility. The authors of the Standards of School Nursing Practice reached consensus regarding the general guidelines for school nurse staffing patterns. The following ratios are presented as general guidelines:

> 1:750 in general school populations
> 1:225 in mainstreamed populations
> 1:125 in severely/profoundly handicapped populations (p. 19)

Variables in Defining the School Nurse Role

Another reason that the recommended solutions have not been realized in more school districts relates to the variables in definition of the school nurse's role from district to district. A 5-year study was conducted to examine the interface between health and education services for children with special needs in five school districts in the United States by a research team from Children's Hospital, Boston (*Serving handicapped children,* 1988). While the role of the school nurse was not one of the specific areas studied, much data was generated about the role. The types of nurses who staffed the schools were varied. They included community health nurses assigned to the schools, nurses hired by the districts, and school nurse practitioners. Some practitioners were hired to work specifically with children with special needs. By reviewing the reports of the five schools studied, it was evident that there was much variability as to what actual care was given by the nurses to the students with special needs. There was much diversity in the nurse's role in involvement in the staffing teams and in input to the health component of the individualized education program (IEP). The areas where nurses' roles could be expanded to assist students with disabilities included: giving explanations to teachers and other school personnel about the child's condition and what signs and symptoms were important to report, giving information about community resources, giving explanations about medication effects and potential side effects, working more closely with parents, communicating with clinics and other health care providers, and giving more health education to the students with special needs (*Collaborative study of children,* 1984). In one area studied, "It was believed by school and health department personnel that nurses could play a larger part in case advocacy, case management, related service provision, supervision of medication and health education" (*Collaborative study of children,* 1984, p. 32). School nurses must ascertain that working with students with special needs is part of their job description.

Preparing To Work with Students with Special Needs

Another reason that the recommendations have not been implemented may relate to school nurses not having adequate preparation for the tasks at hand. "Between 1981 and 1985, 4000 nurses from 26 states completed SNAP" (Smith, 1987, p. 30). Smith reported that nurses who completed SNAP (The School Nurse Achievement Program, a continuing education program offered by the University of Colorado School of Nursing) identified:

> that they increased and improved nursing activities in the following areas: 1) Use and modification of screening procedures to detect handicaps, 2) performance of specific procedures and use of adaptive/assistive devices required by some children, 3) writing the health component of the IEP, 4) modifying the environment to meet safety requirements for the handicapped, 5) instruction/counseling of handicapped children and their families, teachers, and classmates regarding health needs and treatment, 6) participation in school staffings as a member of the multidisciplinary team, and 7) evaluation of the effectiveness of nursing interventions implemented with handicapped children. (p. 32)

School nurses need to take courses such as SNAP to prepare to meet the needs of children with special needs. Goodwin, Igoe, and Smith (1984) state:

> The school nurses' need for continuing education and their success in locating what they consider suitable offerings are, however, two separate issues. . . . Most of these nurses maintain that they have no alternative or that nursing schools simply do not offer courses germane to the needs of school-age youth. (p. 338)

Assertiveness and enthusiasm go far in creating opportunities for learning. University schools of nursing may offer workshops for school nurses or may be willing to do so if contacted by school nurses. For example, for the last five summers, the author has taught an interactive summer workshop for registered nurses in a camping setting with children and teens with spina bifida through a cooperative arrangement between the Spina Bifida Association of Western Pennsylvania and Slippery Rock University. School nurses could become much more familiar with the unique needs of these children in such a setting. Intermediate units often offer courses for school nurses. Getting release time to attend conferences and workshops may present challenges to the school nurse. However, if the needs of the students are to be met, nurses must be prepared.

Preparing To Work with the Student with Spina Bifida

To prepare to work with the student with spina bifida, the school nurse should confront his or her own attitudes about persons with disabilities, explore resources to learn about the condition, identify some of the unique needs of the students, and clarify the skills the nurse will need to plan for the students' health needs in the school.

Attitudes of the School Nurse

It is important to get in touch with one's own feelings about children with spina bifida. The nurse may look at the child with pity for what he or she does not have or cannot do because he or she cannot run and play as "normal" children can. The child can be viewed from the perspective of weaknesses or deficits but should especially be viewed from the frame of reference of the strengths. The child has had the disability since birth so is not being rehabilitated but is being habilitated to live with the condition. Bramadat and Melvin (1987) identify habilitation as "including all the activities and interactions that enable an individual with a disability or dysfunction to develop new abilities and to achieve his or her maximum potential" (p. 76). The school nurse has an active role in the habilitation process and can be an adult friend who believes in the student's ability to achieve and accomplish. An attitude of looking for abilities and strengths gives encouragement and caring. It is necessary to see beyond the disability to tap the strengths. It will take a concerted effort on the part of the nurse to identify what specific challenges confront him or her in the care of the student with spina bifida. The nurse should not depend upon preconceived ideas about the children, but should get to know them as individuals. For example, the school nurse may be fearful that the student will fall. While it is very important to be watchful for the child's safety, the nurse should not assume that the child will be injured, but should talk with the child and parents about how the child manages falls and tries to prevent them. The student has lived with his or her alteration in mobility prior to school, and has learned ways to fall and ways to get back up. One should ask the child how he or she handles falls and what kind of assistance he or she needs. One school nurse used a creative strategy for assisting students with special needs by creating a buddy system in which willing preadolescents who had parental consent, teacher endorsement, and training were paired with a student with special needs. This enabled the nurse to know that a specific person would know how to get assistance if necessary (Guynn, 1983).

There is a tendency on the part of adults to "mother" children with disabilities. It has been the writer's observation that in initial interactions, in an attempt to be kind or perhaps to deal with their own feelings of inadequacy, nurses used terms of endearment more appropriate to younger children, or tended to hover over the children, rather than giving them room to try things on their own. The nurse must strive to identify the fine line between supervision and "smothering."

Nurses who worked with children in a university course at a spina bifida summer camp summed up some of the attitude changes which occurred in establishing relationships with children with spina bifida. One commented: "I started out doing too much for her until I caught on to the fact that she could do so much more for herself. She seemed content to have others do for her; it was important to give her independence." Another stated: "After getting to know the girls, I no longer saw them as girls with disabilities but as girls who play, laugh, argue, and talk about boys." And another summed up her changed attitude in this way: "I came to see her as a young girl who has dreams like all young girls, she needs the doors opened to her to accomplish them" (R.E. Leo, personal communication, June 1989). Two resources regarding attitudes that the school nurse may find useful include the puppeteer group, "Kids on the Block, Inc.," which has a specific program on students with spina bifida (1-800-368-KIDS) and the videotape, "The Same Inside" (March of Dimes, 1983). Both would be appropriate for adults and students alike as a springboard for discussion of attitudes towards persons with disabilities. Robert Perske (1988) has written *Circle of Friends,* a book of short stories illustrating how people with disabilities and their friends enrich the lives of one another. This, too, is an appropriate reference for students, nurses, and teachers about attitudes.

Resources for School Nurses

Resources to learn about spina bifida are many, including references noted in this book. School nurses should maintain a personal library of references on current treatment and management of conditions likely to be encountered in the school-age population. Block (1989) identified five categories of essential references for school nurses; however, the list did not include specific information on children with disabling conditions.

The regional Spina Bifida Association may offer assistance to families and school personnel. The Spina Bifida Association of Western Pennsylvania serves as a valuable resource (1-800-548-7110). Often conferences detailing the most recent information on treatment, management and education, and nursing approaches are sponsored by the Spina Bifida Association. A national listing of associations is available from the National Information Center for Children and Youth with Disabilities, which may be of assistance to the school nurse. Their number is 1-800-999-5599. They list the national Spina Bifida Hotline as 1-800-621-3141.

Nurses in a geographic area could develop support and information networks to ease the transition for students with spina bifida. For example, one school nurse in a district may have developed plans and techniques for managing the in-school catheterization for students and could serve as an excellent resource to other nurses in the area who have not worked with children with spina bifida previously. These networks may be organized through local school nurse organizations.

Nurses who have not worked in acute care pediatrics in recent years are often surprised by the new treatment modalities and the quality of life available for children with spina bifida (Reigel, 1989). The clinic staff at the facility where the student with spina bifida receives care is an excellent source of information, and also may provide guidance in realistic goal setting for the student. It is important to communicate with the clinic staff in order to have coordination of care. For the student who has required hospitalization, Burkett (1989) states, "A school visit by the pediatric rehabilitation nurse and other team members, often coupled with a home visit, can help to reassure education and school personnel that this child can be safely and optimally managed within the education setting" (p. 252).

UNIQUE NEEDS OF STUDENTS WITH SPINA BIFIDA

Some of the unique needs of the students with spina bifida are addressed in this section. It would be impossible to predict the potential needs for each student with spina bifida with whom the nurse may work, just as it is impossible to predict the needs of any students. Each student must be assessed individually. By using the North American Nursing Diagnosis Association listing of diagnoses (Gordon, 1991–1992), the author identifies that students with spina bifida are at high risk for needing nursing intervention in many areas. Only a selected sample of possible diagnostic problem statements will be listed here, as they are those that the school nurse may encounter with students with spina bifida.

Because of their impaired neurologic state, students with spina bifida, with or without hydrocephalus, may have alterations in mobility necessi-

tating the use of braces, crutches, other assistive devices, and wheelchairs. They may be at high risk for impaired skin integrity and for injury
necessitating assessment, frequent repositioning, and the use of protective techniques. This is especially so in transferring in and out of the
wheelchair, and in any areas where injury could occur such as in swimming pools or cooking classes, or if positioned too close to sources of
heat or cold. If students have shunts for hydrocephalus, they must be observed for signs of shunt failure such as headaches, seizures, somnolence, declining school performance, repetitive vomiting, or change in
vision or coordination. If they have seizures or are on medication for seizures, precautions must be taken to prevent injury should seizures occur.
The nurse should obtain information about the medications used for seizures. Students with spina bifida are also at high risk for hypothermia and
hyperthermia for which the nurse must be alert. Some students have difficulty swallowing and must be monitored at meals. Alterations in urinary
elimination necessitating clean intermittent catheterization in the school
may require actual care, teaching, or supervision; side effects of medications given for assistance with continence are important to know. Many
are at high risk for infection because of the neurogenic bladder. Alterations in bowel elimination need to be monitored by the nurse in cooperation with the parents. Depending upon the child's disability, he or she
may have self-care deficits which need to be addressed for optimal functioning in the school. Other types of areas to which the nurse should
be alert include an awareness of knowledge deficits which the student
may have. These knowledge deficits may be about his or her condition,
treatment, medications, restrictions, and such concerns as early pu-
bertal changes, including menstruation at an age younger than other
classmates.

For any student with a chronic illness, the nurse should realize that
he or she may be at high risk for an alteration in growth and development,
for noncompliance with treatment regimens, for home care problems that
may affect school performance, for diversional activity deficits; potential
for social isolation; and potential for self-esteem disturbances, powerlessness, and spiritual distress (Perrin & Gerrity, 1984). Nutritional alterations may affect school performance and may need the attention of
the school nurse. These could be more or less than body requirements
and need to be monitored and addressed in the plan of care. Family and
individual coping styles may affect the student in school. Meeropol
(1991) reported on a small study of adolescents with chronic illness
and identified their concerns at being different from their peers, and
"more vulnerable to disturbance of their psychosociosexual development" (p. 248). It is obvious from this listing that the nurse must be alert
to a wide range of high risk areas needing nursing attention.

SKILLS THE SCHOOL NURSE NEEDS

The school nurse will need many skills to work effectively with the student with spina bifida. The acceptance of premises to guide nursing activities is a good first step. Both the American Nurses' Association document, "School Nurses Working with Handicapped Children" (1980, p. 5) and the SNAP Program on Physical Disabilities (Grunfeld, 1984, p. vi.) suggest premises that are appropriate for school nurses working with children with spina bifida. They include:

a. The handicapped child is first and foremost an individual with a particular complement of strengths and needs.
b. In addition to needs arising from his handicap, each handicapped student has normal maturational, situational, and physical crises that must be addressed in the provision of care.
c. Cognitive, physical, and psychosocial aspects must all be attended to in the provision of holistic care for the handicapped student.
d. The ultimate goals of intervention are promotion of health and the attainment of the highest possible level of individual development and independence.

Throughout the school nurse's anticipation of working with students with spina bifida as well as in the actual interactions and care, there should be a genuine respect and caring for the individual.

The school nurse should be willing to view his or her role to encompass the challenges which may come. Improving and refining one's communication skills is imperative to facilitate effective communication among and between school personnel, health care personnel, families, and students to act as a liaison person. The school nurse should create an atmosphere within the health room to encourage the maintenance of wellness rather than viewing the health room as a center for sickness. In such an environment, the student can view the health room as a "safe haven" and can come there for assistance with the self-care he or she needs to stay well. The school nurse should be equipped to teach self-catheterization and aspects of safety. Knowledge of teaching techniques and principles is important. Assessment of the child's motivation to learn, mental age, fine motor control, and self-help skills is essential.

In teaching self-catheterization, emphasis on one step at a time, cleanliness of equipment and hands, correct positioning, emphasis on consistently carrying out the procedure, and signs of a urinary tract infection should all be included (*Clean intermittent catheterization,* 1986; Stauffer, 1984). The nurse should obtain instruction in the techniques used in clean intermittent catheterization. Larson (1988, pp. 207–212) has a helpful chapter on the techniques. Useful pamphlets and brochures on clean intermittent catheterization and effective bowel management have often been prepared at clinics for children with spina bifida. A telephone call to the clinic requesting educational materials and information may be helpful. Monitoring the student's ability to transfer and ambulate safely as well as inspecting the fit of orthoses is an area for collaboration with other health professionals. Helpful information regarding mobility and orthoses is available for the school nurse in Larson (1988, pp. 241–252 and 267–280). Knowledge of nursing process is necessary to manage care effectively in the school setting.

USING THE NURSING PROCESS

The Standards of School Nursing Practice (1983, pp. 3–15) is used as an organizing framework for a discussion of the role of the school nurse with children with spina bifida, especially Standards I–VIII. The reader is referred to the original source for the in-depth discussion of each of the standards. SNAP suggests a format for the analysis of health needs and the nursing process for use with children with disabilities. Sections of SNAP are used to illustrate the use of nursing process.

THE STANDARDS OF SCHOOL NURSING PRACTICE

   I. The school nurse applies appropriate theory as basis for decision making in nursing practice.
  II. The school nurse establishes and maintains a comprehensive school health program.
 III. The nursing process includes individualized health plans which are developed by the school nurse.
       A. Collection of Data
           The school nurse collects information about the health and development status of the student in a systematic and continuous manner.
       B. Nursing Diagnosis
           The nurse uses data collected about the health and educational status of the student to determine a nursing diagnosis.
       C. Planning
           The nurse develops a nursing care plan with specific goals and interventions delineating school nursing actions unique to student needs.
       D. Intervention
           The nurse intervenes as guided by the nursing care plan to implement nursing actions that promote, maintain, or restore health, prevent illness, and effect rehabilitation.
       E. Evaluation
           The nurse assesses student responses to nursing actions in order to revise the data base, nursing diagnoses, and nursing care plan and to determine progress made toward goal attainment.
  IV. Interdisciplinary Collaboration
       The school nurse collaborates with other professionals in assessing,

planning, implementing, and evaluating programs and other school health activities.

V. Health Education

The nurse assists students, families, and groups to achieve optimal levels of wellness through health education.

VI. Professional Development

The school nurse participates in peer review and other means of evaluation to assure quality of nursing care provided for students. The nurse assumes responsibility for continuing education and professional development and contributes to the professional growth of others.

VII. Community Health Systems

The school nurse participates with other key members of the community responsible for assessing, planning, implementing, and evaluating school health services and community services that include the broad continuum of promotion of primary, secondary, and tertiary prevention.

VIII. Research

The school nurse contributes to nursing and school health through innovations in theory and practice and participation in research.

The nursing process, composed of assessment, diagnosis, planning, intervention, and evaluation, should be used as the organizing element for nursing practice. The school nurse may wish to do additional study on the nursing process and its use in school nursing today.

APPLYING THEORY AS BASIS FOR DECISION MAKING

The school nurse uses a broad base of knowledge from the social, behavioral, and natural sciences as well as the humanities to work with students. The nurse's knowledge base should be updated frequently so that information used as the basis for nursing practice is current and based upon research studies.

The school nurse should be able to define the pathophysiology of spina bifida and hydrocephalus and the potential manifestations in the student. The rationale for various initial and long-term treatments and therapies should be related to the pathophysiology. Familiarity with the ethical dilemmas confronting health care providers will assist the school nurse to understand some of the differences in treatment in various centers. Revell and Liptak (1991) state that, "Integrating knowledge of developmental theories with knowledge of childhood chronic health care conditions into the framework of nursing theory can also lead to better anticipatory guidance and the prevention of secondary complications" (p. 266). Knowledge of growth and development and its potential alterations; family dynamics and coping styles; response patterns; societal responses to people with disabilities, and information of strategies for teaching, helping, and caring are but a sampling of the knowledge base which may be used in decision making.

PROGRAM MANAGEMENT

The school nurse is responsible for developing and managing the health care program for all students in his or her assigned school(s). This includes coordinating the program for the assessment and plan of care for students with special health needs. In an article redefining school nursing practice to include the developmentally disabled (Rustia, Hartley, Hansen, Schulte, & Speilman, 1984), the authors state:

> The kinds of health problems students bring to school or that develop while they are in school cannot be predicted. School personnel cannot be expected to have more than a basic knowledge of health. It is the specific nursing function to be the expert on matters of health in school settings and the use of that knowledge in ways which transpose what they already know about client care in health care settings to nonhealth care settings. (p. 61)

Preparedness for many possible events is important because of the unpredictability of situations which may arise.

The school health program should include: Cooperative planning with other school personnel to meet legal requirements and the desires of parents; developing policies and procedures for emergency care, administration of medication, or other therapies; maintaining records with accuracy and confidentiality; arranging for in-service training regarding student health needs and the supervision of any health care functions to be performed by anyone other than the nurse; establishing channels of communication with other school personnel, parents, and the community; and working within an established budget (*Self-assessment for school nursing*, 1986).

Collection of Data

As complete a data base as possible should be systematically collected and updated as necessary. Data should be collected by reviewing existing records, conducting parent interviews, consulting with other school personnel, and contacting health care personnel in the community who care for the child. It is advisable to interview the parent either in the home or the school prior to school entry to be able to prepare well in advance of the start of school. Bramadat and Melvin (1987), in discussing the value of the home visit for data collection, state:

> Although these visits can be completed in the nurse's office, assessments on pre-schoolers and young school age children may be richer and more accurate when done in the child's home. Home visits also lay the foundation for rapport that facilitates team interventions. (p. 78)

Numerous assessment tools may be used such as are contained in current nursing textbooks dealing with nursing history-taking and physical assessment. One assessment tool which the writer has found helpful assesses the client's human functional patterns (Gordon, 1987). It was developed to assess adults in one format (pp. 438–440) and infants and children in another (pp. 443–445). The 11 functional patterns common to all clients, which are useful in formulating nursing diagnoses, are addressed. For the school nurse familiar with the work of the North American Nursing Diagnosis Association, this may be an assessment tool appropriate for use. If the nurse has not had a strong background in nursing process, he or she may find the assessment tools developed by the SNAP program of use. Included in the assessment should be both objective and subjective data which can be analyzed. See Appendix—Worksheet 1. Assessment Phase (Data Collection).

Nursing Diagnosis

The data are analyzed and synthesized using a thorough data base including searching the literature to arrive at a conclusion of what is occurring with the student at this time. The North American Nursing Diagnosis Association defines *nursing diagnosis* in this way:

> A nursing diagnosis is a clinical judgment about individual, family, or community responses to actual or potential health problems/life processes. Nursing diagnosis provides the basis for selection of nursing interventions to achieve outcomes for which the nurse is accountable. (Carlson, Craft, McGuire, Popkess-Vawter, 1991, p. 6)

Gordon (1987) suggests the use of the PES format for the diagnostic statement that includes the (P) Problem statement (drawn from the NANDA listing), the (E) Etiology or Related Factors leading to the problem, and (S) Signs and Symptoms or Defining Characteristics of the diagnosis. Weber (1991) states, "Identifying the signs and symptoms as part of the diagnostic statement may help in defining desired outcomes and in evaluating progress toward achievement of the outcomes" (p. 425).

The SNAP Module on Physical Disabilities (Grunfeld, 1984) identifies diagnosis as "a summarizing statement which forms the basis for the health care plan. The diagnosis is based on three elements:
1. Subjective data
2. Objective data
3. List of Human Responses, Health Trait Influences, Practices and Responses" (p. 21).

As part of the analysis of data, the nurse examines each of the three elements and combines them to formulate the diagnosis. The letters of each portion (S.O.L.D.) help the nurse to remember the parts to be analyzed for the diagnosis. See Appendix—Worksheet 2. Assessment Phase (Nursing Diagnosis [S.O.L.D.]).

To state the nursing diagnosis after data has been thoroughly analyzed, include the statement of the health problem, factors to which the problem may be related, and how it is evidenced or manifested. For example, a student's problem might be summarized as a nursing diagnosis of: Actual high risk for injury related to inattentiveness to her lack of sensation in her lower extremities manifested by frequent bumping of legs, previous history of injury to her legs, and failure to wear her seatbelt when in the wheelchair. This clearly states the problem, the factors to which it is related, and how it is manifested in the student. Another example is that the student may be at a high risk for infection related to not understanding the importance of regular, every-3-hour catheterizations. This gives the nurse direction and guidance for the rest of the nursing process because the problem statement is addressed in the planning phase; the factors to which the problem is related can be approached in the interventions; the specific human responses manifested in the student should change if the plan is effective, and thus be examined in the evaluation (Price, 1980).

The process of making a nursing diagnosis is a complex one. It is beyond the scope of this chapter to teach the school nurse all of the elements of the diagnostic process. However, review of the references in this section should help considerably.

Planning Specific Goals and Interventions

Much goal setting must occur in this phase of the nursing process. The school nurse should be able to write clear, succinct, measurable goals and objectives. Priorities must be set; constraining factors identified; resources located; and general guidelines for care established.

In what the SNAP Curriculum identifies as the "management-planning phase," the questions, "What?", "Which?", "Who?", "When?", "Where?" and "How?" are suggested as an organizing aid. See Appendix—Worksheet 3. Management-Planning Phase.

As an example, in planning to assist a student at high risk for injury related to the need to use assistive devices and impaired neurological functioning, a list of *what* factors need to be addressed may include: environmental factors dealing with access to the building and to rooms within the building; steep slopes; potentially dangerous places such as the lunch room, chemistry lab, swimming pool, home economics lab; emergency evacuation plans; safe passage between classes; and the correct use of a seatbelt in a wheelchair (Grunfeld, 1984).

An element in addressing "Who?" in the planning may mean that the nurse will need to structure instructional sessions for other school personnel. It may mean securing, instructing, and supervising an aide. To answer the question of "Which?" of these problems belong in the IEP, many elements related to safety may need to be addressed. This is described further under the heading "Interdisciplinary Collaboration."

Another element in planning is to identify some possible strategies for intervention. Wesolowski (1988) details a contracting system for use with students to complete self-care. The use of contracting could be a valuable approach in care. Another strategy that may be useful is described by Dimmock (1987) in which 11 children between 5 and 7 years of age attended a camping program prior to entering the regular school system. Many feelings of the children were addressed as well as self-care skills of bladder and bowel management. Details of bowel problems encountered by children with myelomeningocele are explored and various treatment measures identified in another source (Coffman, 1986). White (1990) identified the need for school nurses to cooperate with health care agencies to promote independence with the management of continence from an early age.

The nurse may need to become equipped to carry out interventions such as clean intermittent catheterization or to identify the best ways to teach a student to do the procedure. Locating resources such as a videotape and reference text developed at the University of Colorado School of Nursing, SNAP, and available through Learner Managed Designs, 2201 K West 25th Street, Lawrence, Kansas 66047, may be helpful. Entitled, "Clean Intermittent Catheterization," it demonstrates the procedure and teaching the procedure to the student in the school setting.

Intervention To Implement Nursing Actions

In intervention, how the school nurse will provide the necessary health services required during school must be determined. The nurse will need to specify what he or she will do in the form of direct service, what will be necessary to coordinate, how referrals will be done, and what time frames will be set. The specific types of instruction which personnel need will be determined. For example, if students are on medication during school hours, it may be advisable to prepare a notecard for the teacher detailing the name of the drug, the reason it is being given, the expected effect, side effects to observe for, and reasons to call the nurse. The teacher may need information about necessary precautions to take in the classroom; giving that information may alleviate fears. In a study reported by O'Hagan, Sandys, and Swanson (1984):

> 79% of parents felt either very strongly or quite strongly that teachers should be given more medical information about their child's condition. Some expressed the view that if the teachers were better informed they would know what warning signs to look for if the child's condition deterio-

rated. They felt more knowledge would be helpful in reducing any initial anxiety a teacher might have about the physically disabled child. (p. 36)

In a discussion on the support families need during chronic illness, Woods, Yates, and Primomo (1989) state that "professionals can provide the types of support that families have said they need: information, opportunities to share concerns and support services" (p. 48). The needs of the teachers can be likened to the needs of the families described by the authors. The school nurse can be the support to the teachers who need information and assistance. For interventions to be effective, accurate assessments are necessary.

If environmental modifications are required to implement the plans, the school nurse should be available for consultation for aspects such as preparation of bathrooms to accommodate children using assistive devices, or modifications of the classrooms to accommodate wheelchairs. See Appendix—Worksheet 4. Management-Implementation Phase.

Evaluation

The student, family, teacher, other school personnel, and the nurse should be involved in the evaluation process. Evaluation is dynamic and continuous within the nursing process; many factors affect one another. In this phase the nurse examines whether or not the expected outcomes were realized and how they were measured. The way the health problem was managed or resolved must be examined. Following evaluation, the plan may need to be revised or additional information may need to be obtained. New approaches may need to be used once all factors are considered. See Appendix—Worksheet 5. Evaluation Phase.

INTERDISCIPLINARY COLLABORATION

There should be extensive cooperation between and among the school nurse and school personnel, other health care personnel in the school, and health care personnel in the community. The school nurse works interdependently with others to accomplish goals.

> Maintaining open lines of communication among home, school and medical treatment staff is essential. Designation of a liaison person who is knowledgeable about both medical and school issues is ideal. Medical personnel may lack knowledge of what schools can and must provide. (Perry & Flanagan, 1986, pp. 335)

The school nurse should have much information and expertise to offer in regard to the health needs of the student during school. There should be channels for communication and feedback established among and between the school nurse and other school personnel.

Communication should also occur in interdisciplinary team meetings and in IEP conferences. There should be school policies developed for inclusion of the nurse in these conferences. If the nurse is not being included, it may be that others are not aware that the addressing of the health component could significantly affect the child's school performance. The nurse should assertively make known his or her interest in having input into conferences and actively participate. Those areas addressed by the nurse should have an influence upon the child's school performance. Specific objectives should be formulated in behavioral terms. As part of the outcome criteria for the achievement of the ANA standard on interdisciplinary collaboration within the Standards for School Nursing Practice (1983), the authors state:

> Review of nursing care plans and Individualized Educational Plans reflect collaboration and team functioning. This is demonstrated by a shared formulation of a problem statement and goals, an integrated plan with a common focus, and shared responsibility for implementation and evaluation. (p. 12)

General areas on which the nurse should have data prior to interdisciplinary meetings for the student with spina bifida include: environmental changes needed such as access to bathrooms, school desks, and exits; plans for coordination of services such as transportation, physical therapy, and nursing services; specific safety measures; use of assistive devices; self-care measures including clean intermittent catheterization; medications; health education needs of the student while in school; instructional needs of school personnel including health care aides; and the need for adapting health screening techniques. It is also important to identify ways to incorporate needed special assistance in the regular activities of the classroom and school. See Appendix—Worksheet 6. Forecast of Health Needs for the IEP.

HEALTH EDUCATION

Health education is an accepted role of the school nurse (Wold, 1981). To assist the student with spina bifida, it may be necessary to give one-on-one instruction regarding specific health care needs in school or to work with parents or other school personnel to implement teaching. The nurse may serve as a resource person to teachers and other school personnel regarding information on spina bifida, hydrocephalus, medications, treatment modalities, and safety measures, as well as observations to make in the classroom. Materials on attitudes regarding the children with disabilities may be useful to the teacher in presentations to the students. Specific teaching by the nurse, on invitation by a student's classroom teacher, to talk about the braces and other assistive devices may be appropriate for optimal school adjustment. It behooves the nurse to be watchful for teaching opportunities in formal and informal settings. One other dimension of health teaching may be supervision and monitoring of student's self-care techniques to prevent problems from developing.

PROFESSIONAL DEVELOPMENT

Professional development must be a continuous goal for the school nurse to be of assistance to the student with spina bifida. Evaluation of one's performance in meeting the health needs of students should be an integral part of the overall evaluation process. Seeking out continuing education opportunities is essential to assisting the student with special needs.

COMMUNITY HEALTH SYSTEMS

The school nurse is in an advantageous position to identify community resources and services that are either adequate or inadequate to meet the needs of the student with spina bifida. The nurse may need to become an advocate for the student in some areas to get necessary assistance. For example, if the student would benefit from an after-school recreation program because he or she is isolated from peers except at school, the nurse may be able to identify a way the student could attend a program in another community. This means that the nurse must know community resources and funding sources very well. The school nurse works actively on behalf of the student with spina bifida to promote health, to identify problems early, and to be actively involved in activities and services that foster the student's habilitation.

RESEARCH ACTIVITIES

School nurses can make significant contributions to the improvement of school health services to students with spina bifida through basing practice on theories tested in practice and sharing successes and failures with peers. Opportunities for peer review should be created as well as networking with other school nurses for the purpose of improving practice. School nurses should have opportunities to conduct research in their own settings to improve the quality of care for students with special needs.

USING THE NURSING PROCESS WITH STUDENTS

Four examples of school nurse/student interactions follow. These represent a deliberative use of the nursing process to accomplish the goal of assisting the student so he or she can benefit from the educational experience.

Example—Student and School Nurse Interaction #1

An 11-year-old boy, who was able to ambulate with only his ankle-foot-orthoses (AFO), was to use the rest room in the nurse's office for his self-catheterization as it afforded more privacy. The student seemed very confident that he could carry out the procedure well as he had been doing his own self-care for several years. As part of an ongoing assessment process, the nurse became aware of two changes. The student was evidently wet between catheterizations because of the saturated pads he left on the floor and the odor of urine on his clothes. The nurse also noted that there were hard fecal masses in the incontinent pads.

Based on these changes, the nurse asked the student to come for a conference. She discovered that he enjoyed school very much and especially enjoyed playing ball with his friends at recess. It was obvious that to be involved with his peers in these physical activities was important to him. He indicated that he was hurrying through his catheterizations and sometimes not doing them at all. He was unaware that the wetness might indicate an infection. His bowel control had been well established previously with enemas given every other night with some assistance from his mother. Because of his mother's new work schedule, he was not getting the same supervision and his pattern had been interrupted for several days. He did not seem aware of the urine odor and indicated that none of his friends had said anything.

Following an analysis of the data that she had obtained, the nurse formulated the following nursing diagnoses. These are stated using the PES format described in the chapter under "Nursing Diagnosis." Included are the Problem, Etiology, and Signs and Symptoms or Defining Characteristics.

Problem: alteration in urinary elimination
Etiology: related to a knowledge deficit about the importance of adhering to the every-3-hour cathing schedule
Signs and symptoms: manifested by: 1) spending a very brief time in the bathroom, 2) admitting to not cathing at times, 3) wetness between catheterization, and 4) urine odor to his clothes.

Problem: alteration in bowel elimination: incontinence, constipation
Etiology: related to noncompliance with previous successful program and to altered supervision
Signs and symptoms: manifested by: 1) incontinence of hard stool, and 2) Statement: "I do not have time to do them (enemas) sometimes lately"

Problem: knowledge deficit about the need for thoroughly carrying out his bowel and bladder program

Etiology: related to having altered priorities for play with peers and other activities at home

Signs and symptoms: manifested by: 1) incontinence, and 2) statements about other priorities.

The objectives the nurse formulated with the student included:

1. Reestablishing his every-3-hour self-catheterization schedule
2. Being dry between catheterizations
3. Demonstrating thoroughly emptying his bladder by measuring the amount voided at each self-catheterization for 3 days
4. Stating three signs of urinary tract infection to observe for
5. Identifying another helper present in his home to assist with his bowel program
6. Reestablishing his every-other-night enema program
7. Being continent during school following the reestablishing of the program
8. Stating three reasons he should carry out his bowel and bladder program on a regular basis

Through a concerted effort, over time, the nurse and the student were able to effect change. Basing her interventions on a respect for the student and an appreciation of his need to establish other priorities and to be involved with his peers, she created opportunities for him to be involved in the decision making. He agreed to try a schedule for cathing which would start at awakening and continue every 3 hours. This meant that he would cath twice during school hours. The nurse made arrangements with the classroom teacher to permit the student to leave for the nurse's office earlier with the stipulation that he could accomplish his assignments later in the day. This enabled him to perform his catheterizations and still have time for recess with his friends. The nurse and student reviewed the cathing procedure including handwashing and care of equipment. He agreed that he would like to have some help with his enema at home, so with the student's permission, the nurse contacted the family and the boy's dad agreed to assist him when the mother was away. Within 2 weeks there was resolution of the problems. Because of the nurse's early efforts, the student's educational and social patterns were not adversely affected. His self-esteem was protected by the nurse's sensitivity to his need to be involved in decisions affecting his health.

Example—Student and School Nurse Interaction #2

When a new school nurse was assigned to a school, she reviewed the previous nurse's plan of care for the self-catheterization program for a third grader named Alice. Alice had been doing her own catheterization since the start of school in September. She told the nurse she had no problems; however, in reviewing the procedure with her, the nurse identified that Alice did not clean her perineal area prior to the procedure; was not bringing clean catheters to school until after crystallization had occurred; did not wash her catheter after the procedure; and had no special cleaning process which was followed at home for the catheters.

The nurse formulated the following nursing diagnosis: Knowledge deficit about intermittent self-catheterization procedure related to inadequate reinforcement and lack of a consistent plan manifested by not cleansing the perineum prior to catheterization, failure to care for the catheters at school and at home, and report of *E. coli* cultured with last urinary tract infection.

The nurse formulated the following objectives with the student:

1. Consistently following through in the self-catheterization procedure when supervised by the nurse
2. Demonstrating care of her catheter at school
3. Identifying an adult to assist her in catheter care at home

The nurse developed a teaching plan for the student which included an index card with a simplified guide for the procedure of cathing and another for the cleaning procedures. The student participated in a demonstration/return demonstration on two different occasions. Because of the relationship which the nurse was able to establish with the student and her grandmother, the care of the catheters at home improved as well. In this situation by careful assessment and follow through with the nursing process, problems with urinary tract infections may have been minimized for this student.

Example—Student and School Nurse Interaction #3

Because students with spina bifida have neurological deficits, problems with mobility may affect participation in activities in school. Following an assessment of a student's alterations, the school nurse identified that because the student had a contracture of her left knee, her orthopedist at the clinic had asked her to keep her braces locked and her legs in an extended position as much as possible when she was seated. She was in an adaptive gym class but did not participate actively in the class. The student expressed to the nurse that she often felt left out in her gym class because she had to stay in her wheelchair. She was able to walk with her braces and assistive devices; she could walk well but because of the contractures, she needed to be supervised. She received physical therapy twice each month in school.

The nurse formulated the following nursing diagnoses: Impaired physical mobility related to the need to keep her braces locked and the need for supervision as manifested by not being as actively involved as previously and expressions of being left out in gym class, where she had been active previously. A second related problem was an alteration in skin integrity related to a combination of her locked braces, the angle of the contracture, and the seated position in class as manifested by excoriated areas on her upper thigh.

In an attempt to solve the two above problems, the nurse consulted with the classroom teacher, the physical therapist, and the adaptive gym teacher. Several interventions were used including the use of a low footstool in the classroom when at her desk to avoid pressure on the thighs while still maintaining the locked position of the braces. The adaptive gym program was changed to include more time on mats for the student to do range-of-motion exercises and time to do walking as had been supervised by the physical therapist. The physical therapist and nurse worked out an arrangement whereby the student could practice walking up stairs with the nurse at least twice a week. This example demonstrates the need for coordination and a liaison person in the school as an advocate for the student with spina bifida. The nurse has the expertise to be both the liaison and the advocate.

Example—Student and School Nurse Interaction #4

A student returned to school in September and began to have an increased number of tonic-clonic seizures. Just prior to a seizure, the student became pale, and had drowsiness and mental confusion. At times she was irritable and hard to please. She had difficulty describing recent events and complained of headaches frequently. In class the student did not concentrate well even on simple tasks. Clearly, the student was at high risk for injury related to her increasing numbers of seizures which were no longer controlled by medication as manifested by her loss of consciousness for 2–3 minutes and the fact that she fell to the floor when she had a seizure.

The school nurse developed a plan whereby mats were placed near the student's desk; the student and her best friend were moved to the back of the classroom where the aide could more easily assist the child if she had a seizure.

The school nurse also felt that the student needed to be evaluated by her primary care physician and the clinic where she was seen for spina bifida. The referral occurred after a meeting of the parents and school caregivers.

Because of the school nurse's alertness, the student was protected from injury during a seizure and was referred for care. She needed a revision of her shunt for hydrocephalus. Once her shunt was functioning, her behavior changed. This is an example of how the nurse must make decisions about what can be managed in the school and what must be referred quickly.

SUMMARY

The role of the school nurse has changed in recent years to include caring for the student who has special health care needs. Since 1980 professional nursing organizations have advocated changes as are illustrated in this chapter using materials from the American Nurses' Association and the School Nurse Achievement Program. These changes stress using the nursing process holistically in the school setting, and collaborating with students, parents, school personnel, and the community. The goal is to maximize the benefit of the educational experience for the student by providing optimal health care in the school. Students with spina bifida present a broad range of potential and actual health needs while in the school. School nurses should be equipped to be caregivers, teachers of self-care, supervisors of the health plan, liaisons, advocates, and leaders for change for these students.

GLOSSARY

Advocate   One who knows the facts and speaks or acts on behalf of the client/ family or one who makes certain that the client/family has the facts and supports them in the decisions which they make.

American Nurses' Association   Professional organization representing nurses in the United States.

Registered Nurse   A legal term indicating that the person is licensed to practice in a specific state as evidenced by completion of an approved educational program and the successful completion of a national examination validating knowledge to be a safe caregiver.

School Nurse   Registered nurse, usually prepared at the baccalaureate level, who has had advanced education and experience to meet the health care needs of students to facilitate their attendance in school. School nurses direct the health care program in the school. They act as resource people and collaborate with parents, school administrators, and personnel and act as a liaison with health care providers in the community.

School Nurse Practitioner   The school nurse practitioner is a registered nurse with an advanced educational degree who has completed further education and training to enable him or her to do more in the area of physical assessment and decision making. The SNP must obtain a second license from the state verifying that he or she is a certified nurse practitioner who is qualified to carry out the expanded nursing role.

REFERENCES

Block, C.E. (1989). The school nurse's need for reference materials. *School Nurse, 5,* 9–13.

Bramadat, I.J., & Melvin, C.L. (1987). Habilitation: Application of a concept. *Clinical Nurse Specialist, 1*(2), 76–79.

Burkett, K.W. (1989). Trends in pediatric rehabilitation. *Nursing Clinics of North America, 24,* 239–255.

Carlson, J., Craft, C., McGuire, A., & Popkess-Vawter, S. (1991). *Nursing diagnosis: A care study approach.* Philadelphia: W.B. Saunders.

Clean intermittent catheterization: An educational unit designed for school nurses, parents, teachers and health aides. (1986). Denver: School Nurse Achievement Program, University of Colorado School of Nursing.

Coffman, S. (1986). Description of a nursing diagnosis: alteration in bowel elimination related to neurogenic bowel in children with myelomeningocele. *Issues in Comprehensive Pediatric Nursing, 9*(3), 179–191.

Collaborative study of children with special needs. (1984). Boston: Children's Hospital, I–V.

Dimmock, W. (1987). An approach to bladder and bowel management in children with spina bifida. *American Urological Association Applied Journal, 8*(1), 9–12.

Economic burden of spina bifida—United States, 1980–1990. (April 21, 1989). *Morbidity Mortality Weekly Report, 38*(15), 264–267.

Goodwin, L., Igoe, J., & Smith, A. (1984). Evaluation of school nurse achievement program: A follow-up survey of school nurses. *Journal of School Health, 54*(9), 335–338.

Gordon, M. (1987). *Nursing diagnosis* (2nd ed.). New York: McGraw Hill.

Gordon, M. (1991–1992). *Manual of nursing diagnosis.* St. Louis: C.V. Mosby.

Grunfeld, C. (1984). *Physical disabilities.* Denver: School Nurse Achievement Program at the University of Colorado School of Nursing.

Guynn, J. (1983). The buddy system: An integrated health plan. *Journal of School Health, 53*(10), 624–625.

Hobbs, N., Perrin, J., & Ireys, H. (1985). *Chronically ill children and their families.* San Francisco: Jossey-Bass.

Larson, G. (Ed.). (1988). *Managing the school age child with a chronic health condition.* Wayzata, MN: DCI Publishing (A division of Diabetes Center).

Meeropol, E. (1991). One of the gang: Sexual development of adolescents with physical disabilities. *Journal of Pediatric Nursing, 6*(4), 243–250.

Nursing process worksheet and forecast of health needs for IEP. (1985). Denver: School Nurse Achievement Program at the University of Colorado School of Nursing.

O'Hagan, F., Sandys, E., & Swanson, W. (1984). Educational provision, parental expectation and physical disability. *Child: Care, Health, Development, 10*(1), 31–38.

Perrin, E., & Gerrity, P. (1984). Development of children with a chronic illness. *Pediatric Clinics of North America, 31,* 19–31.

Perry J., & Flanagan, W. (1986). Pediatric psychology: Implications to the school needs of children with health disorders. *Techniques: A Journal for Remedial Education and Counseling, 2*(4), 333–340.

Perske, R. (1988). *Circle of friends.* Nashville: Abingdon Press.

Price, M. (1980). Nursing diagnosis: Making a concept come alive. *American Journal of Nursing, 80*(4), 668–671.

Reigel, D. (1989). *Pediatric neurosurgery: Surgery of the developing nervous system* (2nd ed.). Philadelphia: W.B. Saunders.

Revell, G., & Liptak, G. (1991). Understanding the child with special health care needs: A developmental perspective. *Journal of Pediatric Nursing, 6*(4), 258–268.

Rustia, J., Hartley, R., Hansen, G., Schulte, D., & Speilman, L. (1984). Redefinition of school nursing practice: Integrating the developmentally disabled. *Journal of School Health, 54*(2), 58–62.

School nurses working with handicapped children. (1980). Kansas City, MO: American Nurses' Association.

Self-assessment for school nursing–school health services. (1986). Harrisburg: Pennsylvania Department of Education, Division of Student Services.

Serving handicapped children: A special report. (1988). Princeton: Robert Wood Johnson Foundation.

Smith, A. (1987). School nurse achievement program: 1980–1985. *School Nurse, 3,* 28–32.

Smith, A., & Goodwin, L. (1982). Program development in twelve states. School nurse achievement program. *The Journal of School Health, 52*(12), 535–538.

Standards of school nursing practice. (1983). Kansas City: American Nurses' Association.

Stauffer, D. (1984). Catheterization—a health procedure schools must be prepared to provide. *Journal of School Health, 54*(1), 37–38.

Weber, G. (1991). Making nursing diagnosis work for you. *Nursing and Health Care, 12*(8), 424–430.

Wesolowski, C. (1988). Self contracts for chronically ill children. *MCN, The American Journal of Maternal Child Nursing, 13*(1), 20–23.

White, M. (1990). Independence for the handicapped child. *Nursing Times, 86*(7), 69–72.

Wold, S. (1981). *School nursing: A framework for practice.* St. Louis: C.V. Mosby.

Woods, N., Yates, B., & Primomo, J. (1989). Supporting families during chronic illness. *Image: Journal of Nursing Scholarship, 21*(1), 46–53.

Nursing Process Worksheet and Health Care Plan

WORKSHEET 1. ASSESSMENT PHASE (DATA COLLECTION)

I. Subjective Data
  A. List of human responses, health trait influences, practices, and resources
    1. Human responses to health problem
      a. type, consistency, effectiveness
      b. previous experience with health problems and coping ability
      c. factors influencing response (e.g., energy level, self-concept sense of integrity, problem-solving ability)
    2. Health trait influences
      a. health knowledge, beliefs, attitudes, interest, values
      b. preferred type of health consumer/provider relationship (active/passive, mutual participation)
    3. Health practices
      a. disease prevention, health promotion, and health protection practices
      b. curative practices
      c. restorative (rehabilitative) practices
    4. Health resources
      a. source of health care
      b. nature of/and effectiveness of support system
      c. availability of health education
  B. Presenting complaint and expectations for the visit
  C. Present illness
    1. onset
    2. duration
    3. positive and negative symptoms
    4. aggravating and alleviating factors
    5. medication/treatments used

From Grunfeld, C. (1984). *Physical disabilities,* pp. 60–80. Denver: School Nurse Achievement Program at the University of Colorado School of Nursing; reprinted by permission.

   D. Previous health
1. antenatal
2. natal
3. neonatal
4. infancy/toddlerhood
5. preschool
   E. Development
1. milestones
2. urinary continence
3. bowel control
4. teeth eruption
5. comparison with siblings, parents
6. unusual growth (gain, loss)
7. present developmental status (physical cognitive, language, motor, social)
8. school
9. learning style
   F. Nutrition
1. infancy and preschool
2. present
   G. Illnesses/disabilities/handicaps
1. infections
2. contagious diseases
3. other
   H. Immunizations
1. age
2. number
3. type
4. boosters
5. reactions
   I. Operations
1. type
2. age
3. complications
4. reasons
   J. Accidents and injuries
1. nature
2. predisposing factors
3. sequelae
   K. Family history
1. father—mother
2. siblings

        3. miscarriages/abortions
        4. illnesses among family members
  L. Personality history
        1. nature
        2. effectiveness
  M. Social history
        1. income
        2. housing
        3. caregivers
        4. peers (including dating and sexual activity)
        5. delinquency
  N. Habits
        1. eating
        2. sleeping
        3. exercise
        4. elimination
        5. dental care
        6. stress management
        7. disturbances
  O. Systems review
        1. ears, nose, throat
        2. cardiorespiratory
        3. gastrointestinal
        4. genitourinary
        5. neuromuscular
II. Objective Data
  Height _____ (_____%)   Weight _____ (_____%)
  B/P _____ T _____ P _____ R _____
  Visual acuity _____ Hearing acuity _____
  A. Physical exam:
        1. general appearance
        2. skin
        3. lymph
        4. HEENT
        5. cardiorespiratory
        6. abdomen
        7. genitalia
        8. anus
        9. spine and extremities
       10. neurological:
            a. overall cerebral (judgment, orientation, memory, affect, calculation ability)

    b. specific cerebral (sensory interpretation, motor integration, language)

    c. cranial nerves

    d. cerebellar function
- eyes
- tongue
- upper extremities
- lower extremities

    e. motor function
- ability
- tone
- strength
- size

    f. sensory function

    g. reflexes

  11. musculoskeletal

B. Lab tests

C. Developmental examination (results of any developmental testing, psychological evaluations performed)

D. Health maintenance examination (results of health knowledge tests; locus of control tests; physical endurance testing; nutritional diary information, biofeedback evaluation; results from first aid, life events, and self-concept questionnaires)

WORKSHEET 2. ASSESSMENT PHASE (NURSING DIAGNOSIS [S.O.L.D.])

Subjective findings, positive-health history

Objective findings, positive-physical examination, lab tests, developmental examination, health maintenance examination

List of human responses, health trait influences, practices, and resources-health history

Diagnosis—a statement of the health problem plus etiology plus human response

WORKSHEET 3. MANAGEMENT-PLANNING PHASE

1. *What* are the priority health problems and maladaptive human responses that need to be addressed; the treatment goals associated with these problems; the expected outcomes of these goals (physiological change, behavior change, affective/emotional change, skill acquisition, or knowledge acquisition), and the activities that will be undertaken to achieve these outcomes?

2. *Which* of these problems (if any) belong in the individualized education program (IEP)?
3. *Who* will be involved in the health care plan proposed by the school nurse?
4. *When* will the health care plan take place (timetable) and which activities have priority?
5. *Where* will the health care plan proposed by the school nurse be implemented?
6. How will I modify this plan if it doesn't work? (What are my alternative plans?)

WORKSHEET 4. MANAGEMENT-IMPLEMENTATION PHASE

1. How will *the nurse* provide the preventive, curative, restorative health services that are planned to alleviate the health problems defined in the nursing diagnosis?
   - Specify direct services.
   - Include information related to coordination efforts.
   - Note how referrals will be handled.
   - Specify time-frame during which activities should occur.
2. What *self-care* measures will be handled by student/family; how will the nurse provide the necessary education and supervision?
3. Which of the student's health needs will be *delegated to school personnel;* what type of education and supervision will the nurse need to provide to these people?
4. What *environmental modifications* are needed to execute the care plan; how will these modifications be made? (School health clinic; entrance ways, halls; toilet facilities; classroom; cafeteria; gymnasium/locker room; outside areas such as playground, sports field; bus.)
5. What kind of *counseling* is needed to modify attitudes of the student or others in the school setting?

WORKSHEET 5. EVALUATION PHASE

1. What were the expected outcomes?
2. How were these outcomes measured?
3. Did the expected outcomes happen?
4. What was the impact of these outcomes on the health problem?
   a. Problem(s) resolved.
   b. Immediate problem(s) resolved but not intermediate or long-term problems.

    c. Anticipated or potential problem(s) not resolved.
    d. Problem(s) not resolved.
    e. Behavioral manifestations indicate new problems.
5. Did the student and his/her family concur in the evaluation of the plan?
6. What factors contributed to the progress of the plan?
7. What factors adversely affected the progress of the plan?
8. What modifications in approach are now needed?
    a. Further building of the consumer/provider relationship
    b. Additional assessment and revision of the diagnosis
    c. Revision of the plan
    d. Introduction of new techniques/actions/procedures for implementing the plan

WORKSHEET 6. FORECAST OF HEALTH NEEDS FOR IEP

Name _____

Nursing diagnosis(es): _____

_____

_____

Do health problems require:	Yes	No	N/A	Yes— not at school
1. Special training and supervision of school personnel				
2. Counseling for student or classmates				
3. Change in school environment (e.g., removal of barriers in lunch room, play area)				
4. Change inside classroom (e.g., lighting, special desks)				
5. Added safety measures (e.g., on bus, in classroom, in gym)				
6. Measures to relieve pain and discomfort (e.g., suctioning, skin care)				
7. Special diet				
8. Assistance with activities of daily living (e.g., toileting, feeding, dressing)				
9. Medications				

(continued)

WORKSHEET 6. FORECAST OF HEALTH NEEDS FOR IEP *(continued)*

Do health problems require:	Yes	No	N/A	Yes— not at school
10. Regular contact between physician and school personnel				
11. Adaptation of school health program (services and education)				
12. Maintenance of special equipment, records				

This checklist sorts out those problems appropriate for inclusion in the IEP. Only those health problems with direct influence on learning should be part of the IEP.

Tailoring the Academic Program

Conducting Psychological Assessments

Anne DesNoyers Hurley

With the passage of PL 94-142 in 1975, public schools were mandated to provide appropriate educational programs for all children with spina bifida. Special educators, physical and occupational therapists, school nurses and physicians, psychologists, health care providers, and parents of children with spina bifida have worked with regular classroom teachers to share new discoveries about the specialized needs of these children. For example, mathematics deficits occur with great frequency in children with spina bifida despite normal intelligence and success in language-related areas (Shaffer, Friedrich, Shurtleff, & Wolf, 1985; Tew, 1989). However, it is also not uncommon for children with spina bifida to be passed along in school for years while falling behind in academic skills. Parents and educators may have unrealistic expectations that the child fails to meet. These experiences lead to declining self-esteem and limited opportunity for future growth and independence.

Recent research on the cognitive and learning status of children with spina bifida has begun to shed light on the nature of their learning problems and to offer solutions for appropriate remedial and educational services. These studies show that the cognitive abilities of children with spina bifida are the result of a number of factors including the presence of hydrocephalus, the history of shunting and complications from shunting, educational history, and medical leaves from school (Anderson, 1975; Badell-Ribera, Shulman, & Paddock, 1966; Raimondi & Soare, 1974; Shaffer et al., 1985; Shurtleff, Folz, & Loeser, 1973; Soare & Raimondi, 1977; Tew & Laurence, 1979, 1983; Thompson et al., 1991). While many children with spina bifida function well in school, a great number have learning problems in at least one area (Shaffer et al., 1985; Tew & Laurence, 1975,

1984). Many have learning disabilities but are seen to be normal and without special educational needs because of their ability to freely generate sentences with good articulation.

In order to ensure academic success, a thorough multidisciplinary evaluation of the child with spina bifida should be conducted as part of the educational plan. This multidisciplinary review team should include a psychologist, speech-language clinician, occupational therapist, physical therapist, teacher, and medical personnel. A comprehensive psychological assessment, beyond standard IQ testing and achievement tests, is necessary: the presentation of learning disorders in the child with spina bifida can be subtle and can go undiagnosed if based on routine assessments alone, leaving the child with inappropriate educational programming. Thus, the psychological assessment's importance to this process is that it combines an overall developmental evaluation with cognitive and emotional assessment. If problems are identified, appropriate remediation and treatment strategies can be recommended.

THE PSYCHOLOGICAL ASSESSMENT PROCESS

The assessment of the child with spina bifida should be viewed as a multifaceted process that includes the collection of extensive data obtained by observation, interviews, informal assessment, and administration of norm-referenced tests that have been standardized with a defined group and scaled in such a way that the individual's score reflects a rank within the normative group (Sattler, 1988). For students who are already enrolled in school, curriculum-based assessment should be included in the evaluation process to determine the instructional needs by using the curriculum as a diagnostic tool.

Establishing Rapport

The evaluation process begins with establishing rapport between the evaluator and student. The evaluator should approach the student as a child who happens to have a disability, not as a disabled child. Due to their many special needs, students with spina bifida are best assessed over several sessions: this lessens fatigue and also provides multiple samples of behavior. In addition, the testing room should be arranged prior to the session so that the student will be comfortable and any needs for adaptive equipment can be met. For example, not all offices can accommodate wheelchairs. In addition, when seated, the student in a wheelchair is often not able to sit comfortably at the testing table and table height must be adjusted. Thus, the psychologist must make arrangements ahead of time for the child with spina bifida by asking the teacher and parents what special needs for equipment or comfort are required and then making the proper arrangements.

Initial Assessment

The first psychological assessment should occur prior to the student's entering school. This evaluation should include extensive observation of the student, combined with assessment of developmental status. The psychologist should also review all of the child's medical records to understand any physical impairments or difficulties the student may have encountered. It is also important to speak with the student's preschool teachers and, if possible, to observe the child in class. Observing the child in his or her home is also a key part of the developmental assessment. Through discussion with the child's family, the psychologist can learn the extent of medical involvement (e.g., previous surgical procedures and complications) that may have affected the child's development and limited opportunities for typical family and community experiences. The child with spina bifida may also have had limited opportunity to socialize with neighborhood children and participate in household life due to his or her medical and physical disabilities. Such limitations will alter the interpretation of developmental assessments.

Whether the placement of the child with spina bifida is in a regular education (mainstream) kindergarten or in a special education program, a multidisciplinary team meeting should be scheduled to include: all of the teachers who will work with the child, the child's parents, the building principal, the guidance counselor, the school nurse, the school psychologist, and all other school personnel who have a legitimate educational interest in the student. At this meeting, all available developmental data should be exchanged. This opportunity should also be used to provide general background information about spina bifida and to alert personnel for possible problems that are unique to and may interfere with the education of the student with spina bifida.

Subsequent Assessments

Once the child has entered school, subsequent assessments will be required. Children with spina bifida may have a changing medical status and it can affect educational achievement and abilities. Disrupted educational histories occur due to medical problems such as surgery or pressure sores, for example. The effects of such leaves from school cannot be minimized. In addition to actual time missed from school, children may lose energy and concentration for long periods of time after surgery.

Children may also have variable psychological status due to the problems associated with hydrocephalus. Subtle continuing loss in abilities may occur because of hydrocephalus; after a shunt revision, the child may have a gain in cognitive abilities (DeMol, 1977; Hammock, 1976; Hammock, Baron, & McCullough, 1983; Jacobs, 1976; Milhorat, 1972; Raimondi & Soare, 1974; Tew & Laurence, 1975; Torkelson, Leibrock,

Gustavson, & Sundell, 1985). Some children may have more marked, permanent losses if they develop a seizure disorder or contract a brain infection during shunting (McLone, Czyzewski, Raimondi, & Sommers, 1982; Shurtleff et al., 1973). Approximately 40% of children with spina bifida have seizures. (For further discussion of hydrocephalus and seizures, see Reigel, chap. 1, this volume.) Also, active seizures and antiseizure medications may alter levels of activity, concentration, and performance. Some students may have marked, permanent losses if they develop an uncontrolled seizure disorder or if ventriculitis (inflammation of the lining of the ventricles of the brain) occurs following a shunting operation (McLone et al., 1982; Shurtleff et al., 1973). Recognition of change in the child's performance by parents or teachers should be followed by an updated psychological evaluation.

Developmental Assessment

When evaluating young children, it is important to include a developmental assessment of general functioning to assist in generating an appropriate educational placement. Published developmental assessments were standardized on nonhandicapped populations and must be interpreted cautiously when used with children who have major physical and medical disabilities (Sousa, Gordon, & Shurtleff, 1976). Nonetheless, such assessments provide valuable information regarding the functioning of the child with spina bifida in relationship to his or her peers.

The developmental assessment should be conducted by a psychologist familiar with the child's particular age group. Personal observation combined with administration of a standardized questionnaire, such as the Vineland Adaptive Behavior Scales (Sparrow, Balla, & Cicchetti, 1984), will provide the most balanced picture of the child's functioning. Scales such as the Vineland Adaptive Behavior Scales provide many independently rated areas of development, separating communication skills from motor skills, for example, enabling the psychologist to dispense with certain areas affected by the child's particular disabilities.

Overall developmental competence must be considered in classroom placement. The child with spina bifida must have a reasonable fit with his or her peers to promote successful socialization experiences. The psychologist can also make valuable recommendations to assist the child in making friendships, dealing with nonhandicapped peer competition, and in acquiring age-appropriate skills in many activities of daily living.

DISABILITIES AFFECTING THE PSYCHOLOGICAL ASSESSMENT PROCESS

Students with spina bifida may have a number of disabilities that directly affect their cognitive functioning or their performance on standardized test measures. These disabilities may require the psychologist to alter the selection of tests for assessment, the administration of psychological tests, and the interpretation of test data. The following major categories of disabilities are helpful to consider in planning to evaluate the student with spina bifida.

Motoric Disabilities

In addition to problems with lower limbs, many students with spina bifida often have loss of motor control in the upper extremities, affecting the use of their arms and hands. These motoric problems are due to hydrocephalus, abnormal brain development, and/or spinal cord problems. Many children with spina bifida have poor eye-hand coordination and perform poorly on tasks that require persistent motor control, execution of fine motor tasks, or speed in production (Anderson & Plewis, 1977; Dennis et al., 1981; Hurley, Laatsch, & Dorman, 1983; Mazure, Aylward, Colliers, Stacey, & Menelaus, 1988; Pearson, Carr, & Halliwell, 1988; Turner, 1985). Due to the effects on the motor centers of the brain, hydrocephalus causes children to be left handed or ambidextrous more often than the general population (Dennis et al., 1981; Lonton, 1976). Poor penmanship is common in students with spina bifida and hydrocephalus. Many students respond to structure and cueing to improve their writing and referral to an occupational therapist may aid in developing a program (Pearson, Carr, & Halliwell, 1988; Shaffer et al., 1986).

Many cognitive assessment tasks involve the use of the hands, including bimanual manipulation. When administering such tests, it is ordinarily assumed that hand function is not impaired and that any slowness or abnormality is the result of cognitive problems. For the student with spina bifida, this cannot be assumed as impaired fine motor speed and dexterity can result from problems limited to motoric skills or the spinal cord alone. (See Culatta, chap. 7, this volume for further discussion.) The psychologist should account for these difficulties when interpreting the results of timed tests or tests that require drawing, reproduction of figures, or visual–constructive abilities. The student should also be allowed to complete tasks after formal time limits have elapsed. Furthermore, there are also a variety of tests that assess cognitive functions without requiring the use of the hands such as the Visual Form Discrimination Test and the Judgment of Line Orientation Test (Benton, des-Hamsher, Varney, & Spreen, 1983). These tests often use a four-choice format, in which the student indicates which of four choices is the correct solution to a specific problem. It is useful to consider adding such tests to current assessment batteries. (Table 4.1 provides a list of tests.)

Difficulties with motor planning skills, in contrast, tend to be related to visual-perceptual and organizational deficits. When evaluating the child with spina bifida, the psychologist should carefully attend to the

Table 4.1.   Tests useful in evaluating the child with spina bifida

Title	Publisher
Overall Cognitive Functioning	
Goodenough-Harris Drawing Test	The Psychological Corporation
Kaufman Assessment Battery for Children	American Guidance Service
McCarthy Scales of Children's Abilities	The Psychological Corporation
Stanford-Binet Intelligence Scale, 4th Edition	Riverside Publishing Company
Vineland Adaptive Behavior Scales	American Guidance Service
Wechsler Adult Intelligence Scale—Revised	The Psychological Corporation
Wechsler Intelligence Scale for Children— Revised	The Psychological Corporation
Wechsler Preschool and Primary Scale of Intelligence	The Psychological Corporation
Wisconsin Card Sorting Test	Psychological Assessment Resources
Language Skills	
Peabody Picture Vocabulary Test—Revised	Riverside Publishing Company
Illinois Test of Psycholinguistic Ability	Slosson Educational Publications
Visual-Perception Skills	
Hooper Visual Organization Test	Psychological Assessment Resources
Judgment of Line Orientation Test	Psychological Assessment Resources
Raven's Progressive Matrices	The Psychological Corporation
Test of Nonverbal Intelligence	PRO-ED
Visual Form Discrimination Test	Psychological Assessment Resources
Visual-Motor Skills	
Beery Test of Visual-Motor Integration	Modern Curriculum Press
Bender Visual Motor Gestalt Test	American Orthopsychiatric Association
Goodenough-Harris Drawing Test	The Psychological Corporation
Emotional Functioning	
Self-Esteem Inventory	Consulting Psychologists Press
Emotional Problems Scales	Psychological Assessment Resources
Rorschach inkblot technique	The Psychological Corporation
Tasks of Emotional Development	TED Associates
Thematic Apperception Test	Harvard University Press

way in which the child organizes his responses to motoric tests. This qualitative assessment, rather than a reporting of scores alone, allows for a meaningful interpretation of abilities. For example, while deficits in speed may compromise execution of an assembly task, disorganization and confusion in placing parts or approaching the task signal organizational deficits rather than motoric problems.

Visual Disabilities

Students with spina bifida and hydrocephalus often have a number of visual defects (Dennis et al., 1981; McLone et al., 1982). Common deficits are abnormal eye gaze, poor visual acuity, and strabismus. Such problems, because they occur during early developmental periods, may be partially responsible for poor development of visual perceptual skills. It is also common for students who have strabismus left untreated to lose vision in one eye (amblyopia) as they grow older. Because the eyes appear normal, teachers and therapists may be unaware of the loss.

Prior to the evaluation sessions, the psychologist must be familiar with any medical information and should check ophthalmology reports. If any visual defect is present, testing materials should be chosen accordingly and placed within the appropriate range. Interpretation of the results of any testing that involves visual skills should also be adjusted.

Serious problems in visual perception are common among students with spina bifida and hydrocephalus (Dennis et al., 1981; Tew & Laurence, 1975). These students have difficulty understanding the position in space of objects in their environment and this may lead to problems maneuvering, driving a car, or in adjusting personal space in social situations. Organization of materials in class, study materials, or belongings at home may also be affected. Additionally, students may have difficulty organizing tasks that involve assessing the relationship of objects in space, such as organizing the cooking of a meal or oganizing catheter equipment properly. Deficits in visual perception may be related to a general nonverbal learning disability that even affects social skills (Semrud-Clikeman & Hynd, 1990). If deficits in visual perception are diagnosed, the psychologist should consult with the school personnel and family in order to ensure that the student has proper expectations developed for him or her. Additional consultation with an occupational therapist will assist in providing aids to the student and in designing compensatory strategies to achieve optimum independent living skills. (See Culatta, chap. 7, this volume, for further discussion.)

Speech and Language Disabilities

The language development of students with spina bifida may be delayed or abnormal (Culatta, 1980; Culatta & Culatta, 1978; Dennis, Hendrick, Hoffman, & Humphreys, 1987). Many children with spina bifida tend to be verbose, with good articulation, but poor understanding of abstract concepts. (See the section on "cocktail party syndrome" below.) If any language deficit is present, the student should be referred to a speech-language pathologist for a full evaluation. Occasionally, students with spina bifida also have more serious language problems, such as dysarthria, due to medical complications such as meningitis. In such an instance, consultation with the speech-language pathologist prior to the psychological evaluation is essential to obtain guidelines for assessment and to have effective communication with the student. (See Culatta, chap. 6, this volume, for further discussion.)

The presence of a language deficit often causes the child to be perceived by others as "slow." In addition, language deficits often are related to poor development of reading and spelling skills, further affecting academic achievement and compounding the appearance of lack of ability. The psychologist is in a critical position to document a wide range of cognitive skills and to emphasize strengths and potential in other areas. Language problems, per se, need not deleteriously affect long-term outcome for employment or independent living, and the strong areas of cognitive functioning can be used for education and rehabilitation programming.

Cocktail Party Syndrome

The "cocktail party syndrome" is a cognitive/behavioral disorder that can be found in students at any level of intelligence who have a history of hydrocephalus. This syndrome is not exclusive to spina bifida and is found in other conditions associated with hydrocephalus (Hagberg, 1962; Hagberg & Sjorgen, 1966; Hurley, Dorman, Laatsch, Bell, & D'Avignon, 1990; Ingram & Naughton, 1962; Tew, 1979; Tew & Laurence, 1979). It can affect an individual with a history of hydrocephalus, whether it was treated or not, or even if it remitted and is no longer a problem. The neurological etiology of the syndrome is not well understood, although it was originally thought to be a special type of frontal lobe syndrome (Hagberg & Sjorgen, 1966). The "cocktail party syndrome" is currently a changing concept and may be related to more subtle and diffuse dysfunction in individuals with brain injury (Hurley et al., 1990).

Children with "cocktail party syndrome" have well articulated speech and are quite verbose. Close examination of the content of speech reveals that such children have excessive and inappropriate use of jargon and clichés (e.g., *My sense of direction flew out the window*). Individual words may also be used inappropriately (Culatta, 1978; Schwartz, 1974). In addition to the striking verbosity, there is a tendency to be overly friendly. Although this is initially seen as quite a social advantage, it is often inappropriate and too personal. Thus, while the child is superficially quite skilled in verbal areas, actual verbal performance is lacking. Moreover, the child's overall actual performance in daily life is quite impaired when compared to verbal performance (Hurley et al., 1990). However, because our society often judges others' skills on the basis of verbal abilities, family and teachers may have high expectations that the child cannot meet. This causes frustration for those who work with the student and confusion and loss of self-esteem in the student.

Students with "cocktail party syndrome" often obtain relatively higher Verbal than Performance IQ scores, although equal Verbal and Performance IQ scores are also found (Badell-Ribera et al., 1966; Hurley et al., 1990; Tew, 1979). While many children with "cocktail party syndrome" are also mentally retarded, many have tested IQs in the average range with commensurate reading and spelling skills. If it is suspected that a child has "cocktail party syndrome," a full neuropsychological assessment should be conducted. Periodic follow-up will be needed because some children who show the syndrome when young become normal with age. If the child has "cocktail party syndrome," a conference should be held with all teachers and the parents to discuss the situation and to reconsider the goals for the child. Expectations should be adjusted and greater structure provided. Often, the child performs better if he or she has a behavior chart outlining all daily duties with a reinforcement-consequence component. Upon transition to the adult service network, a full neuropsychological evaluation should be performed again. Few individuals with "cocktail party syndrome" can fully manage themselves independently in adulthood, putting them at medical risk should they live alone. Thus, supervised living situations or acquisition of a case manager to assist the individual may be needed.

Attention, Concentration, and Memory Disabilities

Many children with spina bifida show difficulties in applying sustained attention to a task, in focusing on relevant information, and in memory (Abercrombie, 1968; Cull & Wyle, 1984; Horn, Lorch, Lorch, & Culatta, 1985; Shaffer et al., 1985). These difficulties can occur in any range of intelligence. Many children with spina bifida show some deficit in this area, even when they are free of other learning disabilities and have little physical impairment.

If a student appears to have an attentional problem, testing should be altered to obtain the best performance. Formal assessment may occur over a number of short sessions and this may improve performance. Taking short breaks in testing and varying the content and type of task may help. Throughout the assessment, the student may need frequent cues to stay on task as well as praise for completing the tasks.

Students with spina bifida may also have attention deficit hyperactivity disorder (ADHD). If the student is considered for such a diagnosis, the psychologist should make a referral to a neurologist or pediatrician who specializes in developmental problems. It is important that ADHD be recognized because it can be successfully treated with medication and specialized education and remediation strategies. Additionally, problems in conduct, interpersonal skills, and impulsivity often accompany ADHD and respond well to proper treatment. Problems with impulsivity and sustained attention have been noted in the cognitive assessment of children with spina bifida (Lollar, 1990).

There is no one psychological test that assesses ADHD, and patterns of performance on the Wechsler Intelligence Scales do not predict this disorder (Barkley, 1990). In order to determine if the child with spina bifida has ADHD, a full evaluation should be conducted. Measures of continuous performance are helpful, as well as the administration of questionnaires to teachers and parents (Barkley, 1990). Measures of hyperactivity are difficult to utilize for the child in a wheelchair. Thus, the psychologist must interpret data without the usual measures of motoric activity.

Emotional Problems

Some children with spina bifida may have emotional difficulties due to coping with their disability, family problems, or problems adjusting to surgical and medical procedures (Anderson, 1979; Connell & McConnel, 1981; Dorner, 1976; Friedrich & Shaffer, 1986; McAndrews, 1979; Tew & Laurence, 1985). Students with spina bifida may feel isolated and rejected by peers, despite the best efforts of schools to integrate students and provide fertile ground for friendships (Rinck, Berg, & Hafeman, 1989). Periodic hospitalizations can be particularly disruptive and frightening, and it can be anticipated that increased dependency and inability to concentrate may be evident following these absences from school. Further, hospitalizations isolate the child and disrupt family routine and structure which in turn contribute to regression and insecurity for the child. (See Rowley-Kelly, chap. 9, this volume, for further discussion.)

When a child has a major disability, the emotional problem is sometimes overlooked by mental health professionals, in addition to school personnel and family. The phenomenon, termed "diagnostic overshadowing," was developed through work with developmentally disabled individuals (Reiss, Levitan, & Szyszko, 1982). Briefly, this phenomenon occurs when a professional is so overwhelmed with the individual's disability that it "overshadows" the problem behaviors. The mental health professional then attributes any clinically significant symptoms and signs to the disability. For example, if an individual with a major cognitive impairment were withdrawn, somber, noncommunicative, and displayed little eye contact, rather than immediately considering a diagnosis of depression, a clinician would see those behaviors as a typical part of the cognitive impairment (Sovner & Hurley, 1983). For the child with spina bifida, the salience of the many manifestations of the disability has the same effect. Rather than seeing problems as a unique part of the child, clinicians and school personnel may see problems as a typical result of spina bifida. Thus, children with spina bifida may not receive the supportive mental health services they need to thrive and persevere. The psychologist must be alert to the many challenges faced by the child with spina bifida and select proper assessment tools to address adjustment issues.

Assessment of emotional status begins with an interview of the child and parents. Following this, discussions with the classroom teachers as well as classroom observations should occur. A formal psychological assessment using projective instruments and/or paper and pencil inventories should conclude the evaluation. The results should be shared with the parents, child, and all relevant teaching personnel to develop a plan to assist the child in stabilizing and progressing in school.

COGNITIVE AND LEARNING DISABILITY PROFILES

Students with spina bifida exhibit many types of cognitive and academic skill levels (Anderson, 1975; Halliwell, Carr, & Pearson, 1980). Intellectual ability levels may range from superior, to average, to mentally retarded. Academic skills may be advanced or deficient; some students with demonstrated average intellect can show significant learning deficits in one or more areas as a result of having spina bifida. The following subgroups may be identified through the psychological assessment process and are meant to serve as a general guide.

1. **Normal intelligence: Normal skills.** These students function in the normal range of intelligence with average reading, spelling, and arithmetic skills. They are well organized and have social skills similar to their peers. Such students are successful, can attend college, and can manage their own affairs as adults.

2. **Normal intelligence: Mathematics deficit.** These students function in the normal range of intelligence, but have poor arithmetic skills. They may perform adequately in elementary school, but as more complex mathematics skills are taught, these students begin to fall behind. Algebra may be the highest level of mathematics able to be learned. Special education programming in the area of mathematics computation and/or mathematics reasoning may be required. (See Culatta, chap. 6, this volume, for further discussion.)

3. **Normal intelligence: Visual-perceptual and organizational deficits.** These students function in the normal range of intelligence and acquire acceptable reading and spelling skills, but have poor reading comprehension, poor ability to write stories and paragraphs, poor mathematical abilities, and major deficits in their ability to organize their work. These children speak well, and are, therefore, consistently judged by others to be more capable than they are. Multiple basic education classsroom modifications and/or special education programming for students with learning disabilities may be necessary in order for these students to achieve their full potential. (Subsequent chapters discuss these concepts.)

4. **Low normal intelligence: Poor academic skills.** These students function in the low normal/borderline range of intelligence with

verbal skills that are more impaired than visual perceptual and organizational skills. Mathematics skills are typically poor but there may or may not be reading and spelling disabilities, and academic skills are usually consistent with Verbal IQ scores. Basic education classroom modification and/or special education programming for students with learning disabilities will be required. The psychologist must make specific recommendations for programming based on the child's strengths in nonverbal areas. Such a child may have good potential in many vocational areas, and these skills must be developed early to enhance skills and preserve self-esteem.

5. **Low normal intelligence: Poor academic skills, perceptual deficit, and organizational deficit.** These students function in the low normal/borderline range of intelligence with visual-perceptual and organizational skills that are more impaired than verbal skills. They are often judged to be more competent than they are based on their verbal abilities. These students tend to have deficits in mathematics with reading and spelling skills consistent with their Verbal IQ scores. Poor reading comprehension and writing skills are common. Such children are quite disorganized in their approach to their work and daily living skills. They require basic education classroom modifications and/or special education programming emphasizing structure and cues to help them organize tasks.

6. **Mental retardation.** These students function at all levels within the mentally retarded range of intelligence. Organizational skills are usually related to the level of visual perceptual abilities in each student. Reading recognition and comprehension are usually related to the level of verbal abilities. Many children show a lack of initiative and poor executive functioning relative to better verbal abilities, leading to the need for constant structure and supervision to attain educational and rehabilitation goals. Many students in this range may also show the "cocktail party syndrome." School programs should start training in vocational skills and independent living skills early in order to maximize the potential of these youngsters.

SUMMARY

The challenge for the psychologist is to obtain information about the student with spina bifida that will be of benefit to the student, parents, and all personnel involved in the student's education. The unique problems that interfere with a particular student's progress may be overcome, but first they must be *identified* and second, the parents and teachers must be *informed.*

If these requirements are met, solutions to learning delay are within reach. Sincere efforts and possible aspirations for students with spina bifida will lead to full educational attainment for all. The future of each child is dependent upon success in this venture.

GLOSSARY

Ambidextrous   The ability to perform manual skills well with both hands, some skills performed better with one or the other hand.

Amblyopia   An impairment of vision due to a number of conditions with obvious impairment to the eye itself.

Attention   The activity of selectively directing oneself toward a particular task.

Attention deficit hyperactivity disorder   A disorder in which the child has pervasive deficits in the ability to attend to tasks. It is associated with hyperactivity and academic achievement is usually poor. The disorder often responds to medication and/or remediation strategies.

Bimanual   Referring to the simultaneous use of both hands.

Cognition   A general term encompassing all forms of thought, memory, learning, perception, reasoning, and judgment.

Concentration   The fixing of attention with great intensity on a particular task.

Dysarthria   A motoric difficulty in producing speech due to defective coordination of the neuromuscular apparatus involved.

Frontal lobe syndrome   A term that refers to a wide range of dysfunctional personality characteristics that result from damage to the frontal lobes of the brain, e.g., apathy or irrelevant verbosity.

Intelligence   A general term with no agreed-upon definition, but referring to the abilities to meet and assess situations, develop action plans, adapt to the environment, and perform a wide variety of tasks.

IQ   Intelligence quotient, a number obtained after administration of a formal test thought to measure aspects of intelligence and based on normative data. Originally was the ratio of mental age to chronological age.

Learning disability   A difficulty in cognitive processing, resulting in problems with language, learning, and/or academic tasks but not primarily due to deficits in intelligence or sensory, motoric, emotional, or cultural disadvantages.

Mental retardation   A classification of severely impaired intellectual functioning that occurs during the childhood-developmental period and manifests itself in intellectual, social, and vocational deficits.

Neuropsychological assessment   The evaluation of cognitive, social, and daily functioning of a child conducted by a psychologist who specializes in neuropsychology, the study of brain-behavior relationships.

Organizational deficit   A skill deficit in which a person has impaired abilities to organize information or tasks, especially affecting learning, socialization, and daily living skills.

Performance IQ   The IQ score obtained by administering the performance portion of the Wechsler intelligence scales, involving a number of subtests that require visual-perceptual and visual-motor skills.

Strabismus   A deviation of the eye, sometimes referred to as "squint."

Verbal IQ   The IQ score obtained by administration of the verbal subtests of the Wechsler intelligence scales.

Visual constructive   The ability to manipulate objects manually or draw.

Visual perception   The ability to perceive visual stimuli correctly (e.g., in spatial relationships or directionality of objects).

REFERENCES

Abercrombie, J.L.J. (1968). Some notes on spatial disability: Movement, intelligence quotient and attentiveness. *Developmental Medicine and Child Neurology, 10,* 206–213.

Anderson, E. (1979). The psychological and social adjustment of adolescents with cerebral palsy or spina bifida and hydrocephalus. *International Journal of Rehabilitation Research, 2,* 245–247.

Anderson, E.M. (1975). Cognitive deficits in children with spina bifida and hydrocephalus: A review of the literature. *British Journal of Educational Psychology, 45,* 257–267.

Anderson, E.M., & Plewis, I. (1977). Impairment of a motor skill in children with spina bifida cystica and hydrocephalus: An exploratory study. *British Journal of Psychology, 68,* 61–70.

Badell-Ribera, A., Shulman, K., & Paddock, N. (1966). The relationship of nonprogressive hydrocephalus to intellectual functioning in children with spina bifida cystica. *Pediatrics, 37,* 787–793.

Barkley, R.A. (1990). *Attention-deficit hyperactivity disorder: A handbook for diagnosis and treatment.* New York: Guilford Press.

Benton, A.L., desHamsher, K., Varney, N.R., & Spreen, O. (1983). *Contributions to neuropsychological assessment: A clinical manual.* New York: Oxford University Press.

Connell, H.M., & McConnel, T.S. (1981). Psychiatric sequelae in children treated operatively for hydrocephalus in infancy. *Developmental Medicine and Child Neurology, 23,* 505–517.

Culatta, B. (1978). Language use without comprehension: A suggested methodology for the clinical evaluation of spina bifida children. *Spina Bifida Therapy, 1,* 1–6.

Culatta, B. (1980). Perceptual and linguistic performance of spina bifida hydrocephalic children. *Spina Bifida Therapy, 2,* 235–247.

Culatta, B., & Culatta, R. (1978). Spina bifida children's noncommunicative language: Examples and identification guidelines. *Allied Health and Behavioral Sciences, 1,* 22–30.

Cull, D., & Wyle, M.A. (1984). Memory functions of children with spina bifida and shunted hydrocephalus. *Developmental Medicine and Child Neurology, 26,* 177–183.

DeMol, J. (1977). Neuropsychological study of mental troubles in normal pressure hydrocephalus and their short term evolution after spinal fluid deviations. *Acta Psychiatrica Belgium, 2,* 228.

Dennis, M., Fitz, D.B., Netley, C.T., Sugar, J., Derek, D.F., Harwood-Nash, M.B., Hendrick, E.B., Hoffman, H.J., & Humphreys, R.P. (1981). The intelligence of hydrocephalic children. *Archives of Neurology, 30,* 607–613.

Dennis, M., Hendrick, E.B., Hoffman, H.J., & Humphreys, R.P. (1987). Language of hydrocephalic children and adolescents. *Journal of Clinical and Experimental Neuropsychology, 9,* 593–621.

Dorner, S. (1976). Adolescents with spina bifida: How they see their situation. *Archives of Disease in Children, 51,* 439–444.

Friedrich, W., & Shaffer, J. (1986). Adolescent psychosocial adaptation. In D. Shurtleff (Ed.), *Myelodysplasias and exstrophies: Significance, prevention and treatment* (pp. 411–420). New York: Grune & Stratton.

Hagberg, B. (1962). The sequelae of spontaneously arrested hydrocephalus. *Developmental Medicine and Child Neurology, 4,* 583–587.

Hagberg, B., & Sjorgen, I. (1966). The chronic brain syndrome of infantile hydrocephalus. *American Journal of Diseases of Children, 112,* 189–196.

Halliwell, M.D., Carr, J., & Pearson, A.M. (1980). The intellectual and educational functioning of children with neural tube defects. *Zeitschrift für Kinderchirurgie, 31,* 375–381.

Hammock, M.K. (1976). Normal pressure hydrocephalus in patients with myelomeningocele. *Developmental Medicine and Child Neurology, 18* (Suppl. 37), 55.

Hammock, M.K., Baron, I.S., & McCullough, D.C. (1983, July). *Ventriculomegaly without overt signs of increased intracranial pressure in patients with myelomeningocele; serial neuropsychological testing in 20 treated and 20 untreated cases.* Paper presented at the annual meeting of the International Society for Research in Spina Bifida and Hydrocephalus, Southampton, England.

Horn, D.G., Lorch, E.D., Lorch, R.F., & Culatta, B. (1985). Distractibility and vocabulary deficits in children with spina bifida and hydrocephalus. *Developmental Medicine and Child Neurology, 27,* 713–720.

Hurley, A.D., Dorman, C., Laatsch, L.K., Bell, S., & D'Avignon, J. (1990). Cognitive functioning in patients with spina bifida, hydrocephalus, and the cocktail party syndrome. *Developmental Neuropsychology, 6,* 151–172.

Hurley, A.D., Laatsch, L.K., & Dorman, C. (1983). Comparison of spina bifida, hydrocephalic patients and matched controls on neuropsychological tests. *Zeitschrift für Kinderchirurgie, 38,* (Suppl. 2), 116–118.

Ingram, T.T.S., & Naughton, J.A. (1962). Pediatric and psychological aspects of cerebral palsy associated with hydrocephalus. *Developmental Medicine and Child Neurology, 4,* 287–292.

Jacobs, L. (1976). "Normal pressure" hydrocephalus: Relationship of clinical and radiographic findings to improvement following shunt surgery. *Journal of the American Medical Association, 235,* 510.

Lollar, D.J. (1990). Learning patterns among spina bifida children. *Zeitschrift für Kinderchirurgie, 45* (Suppl. 1), 39.

Lonton, A.P. (1976). Hand preference in children with myelomeningocele and hydrocephalus. *Developmental Medicine and Child Neurology, 18* (Suppl. 37), 143–149.

Mazure, J.M., Aylward, G.P., Colliers, J., Stacey, J., & Menelaus, M. (1988). Impaired mental capabilities and hand function in myelomeningocele patients. *Zeitschrift für Kinderchirurgie, 43* (Suppl. 2), 24–27.

McAndrews, I. (1979). Adolescents and young people with spina bifida. *Developmental Medicine and Child Neurology, 21,* 619–629.

McLone, D.G., Czyzewski, C., Raimondi, A.J., & Sommers, R.C. (1982). Central nervous system infections as a limiting factor in intelligence of children with myelomeningocele. *Pediatrics, 70,* 338–342.

Milhorat, I.H. (1972). *Hydrocephalus and cerebral spinal fluid.* Baltimore: Williams & Wilkins.

Pearson, A.M., Carr, J., & Halliwell, M.D. (1988). The handwriting of children with spina bifida. *Zeitschrift für Kinderchirurgie, 43* (Suppl.), 40–42.

Raimondi, A.J., & Soare, P. (1974). Intellectual development in shunted hydrocephalic children. *American Journal of Diseases of Children, 127*, 664–671.

Reiss, S., Levitan, G.U., & Szyszko, J. (1982). Emotionally disturbed, mentally retarded people: An underserved population. *American Psychologist, 37*, 361–367.

Rinck, C., Berg, J., & Hafeman, C. (1989). The adolescent with myelomeningocele: A review of parent experiences and expectations. *Adolescence, 24*, 699–710.

Sattler, J.M. (1988). *The assessment of children* (3rd ed.). San Diego: Sattler.

Schwartz, E.R. (1974). Characteristics of speech and language development in the child with myelomeningocele and hydrocephalus. *Journal of Speech and Hearing Disorders, 39*, 465–468.

Semrud-Clikeman, M., & Hynd, G.W. (1990). Right hemispheric dysfunction in nonverbal learning disabilities: Social, academic, and adaptive functioning in adults and children. *Psychological Bulletin, 107*, 196–209.

Shaffer, J., Friedrich, W.N., Shurtleff, D.B., & Wolf, L. (1985). Cognitive and achievement status of children with myelomeningocele. *Journal of Pediatric Psychology, 10*, 325–336.

Shaffer, J., Wolfe, L., Friedrich, W., Shurtleff, H., Shurtleff, D., & Fay, G. (1986). Developmental expectations: Intelligence and fine motor skills. In D.B. Shurtleff (Ed.), *Myelodysplasias and exstrophies: Significance, prevention and treatment* (pp. 359–372). New York: Grune & Stratton.

Shurtleff, D.B., Folz, E.K., & Loeser, J.B. (1973). Hydrocephalus: A definition of its progression and relationship to intellectual function, diagnosis, and complications. *American Journal of Diseases of Children, 125*, 688–693.

Soare, P., & Raimondi, A.J. (1977). Intellectual and perceptual-motor characteristics of treated myelomeningocele children. *American Journal of Diseases of Children, 131*, 199–204.

Sousa, J.C., Gordon, L.H., & Shurtleff, D.B. (1976). Assessing the development of daily living skills in patients with spina bifida. *Developmental Medicine and Child Neurology, 18* (Suppl. 37), 134–142.

Sovner, R., & Hurley, A.D (1983). Do the retarded suffer from affective illness? *Archives of General Psychiatry, 40*, 61–67.

Sparrow, S.S., Balla, D.A., & Cicchetti, D.V. (1984). *Vineland Adaptive Behavior Scales.* Circle Pines, MN: American Guidance Service.

Tew, B. (1979). The "cocktail party syndrome" in children with hydrocephalus and spina bifida. *British Journal of Disorders of Communication Disorders, 14*, 89–101.

Tew, B. (1989). Spina bifida children in ordinary schools: Handicap, attainment and behavior. *Zeitgeist für Kinderchirurgie, 43* (Suppl. 2), 46–48.

Tew, B., & Laurence, K.M. (1975). The effects of hydrocephalus on intelligence, visual perception, and school attainment. *Developmental Medicine and Child Neurology, 17* (Suppl. 35), 129–134.

Tew, B., & Laurence, K.M. (1979). The clinical and psychological characteristics of children with the "cocktail party" syndrome. *Zeitschrift für Kinderchirurgie, 28* (Suppl. 1), 360–367.

Tew, B., & Laurence, K.M. (1984). The relationship between intelligence and academic achievements in spina bifida adolescents. *Zeitschrift für Kinderchirurgie, 39* (Suppl. 2), 122–124.

Tew, B., & Laurence, K.M. (1985). Possible personality problems among 10-year-old spina bifida children. *Child Care, Health and Development, 11*, 375–390.

Thompson, N.M., Fletcher, J.M., Chapieski, L., Landry, S.H., Miner, M.E., & Bixby, J.

(1991). Cognitive and motor abilities in preschool hydrocephalics. *Journal of Clinical and Experimental Neuropsychology, 13,* 245–258.

Torkelson, R.D., Leibrock, L., Gustavson, J.L., & Sundell, R.R. (1985). Neurological and neuropsychological effects of cerebral spinal fluid shunting in children with assumed ("normal pressure") hydrocephalus. *Journal of Neurology, Neurosurgery, and Psychiatry, 48,* 799–806.

Turner, A. (1985). Hand function in children with myelomeningocele. *Journal of Bone and Joint Surgery, 22,* 268–272.

Developing Abstract Concepts

Barbara Culatta

Some students with spina bifida exhibit more limited knowledge of abstract than concrete concepts. They may have difficulty with academically relevant terms such as *more than, above,* and *several.* Academic progress may be impaired when conceptual understanding is incomplete or missing. This chapter addresses the nature of abstract concept deficits that some students with spina bifida encounter and factors that influence abstract concept development for students with spina bifida. It also provides strategies for assessment and remediation.

Despite adequate knowledge of concrete words, including both nouns and verbs (Parsons, 1968; Spain, 1972), students with spina bifida may not have a fully developed understanding of abstract terms. This abstract concept deficit is evident when a student has difficulty grasping spatial, temporal, and quantitative terms and identifying abstract words in certain contexts (Agness, 1983; Fay, Shurtleff, Shurtleff, & Wolf, 1986; Horn, Lorch, Lorch, & Culatta, 1985; Stephens, 1985).

Abstract concept deficits may also be evident in the student's use of abstract words in inappropriate contexts (Culatta & Culatta, 1978). One student with spina bifida once held up a cookie and said, "This is the same," without comparing the cookie to any other object. Another student encountered an assortment of scattered objects and said, "Behind, behind, everything is behind," yet no one object was clearly in front or behind any other.

Students with spina bifida may use words in inappropriate contexts when they do not fully understand their meanings (Culatta, 1978). The inappropriate use of words may occur because words themselves are more noticeable or salient than the aspects of the environment they represent. In students with spina bifida, there may very well be a mismatch between the acquisition of a word and the student's perception of what that word means. Thus, a student with spina bifida may learn words such as *judge, suggest, still, each,* and *least* without having developed full knowledge of their meaning. Just as a toddler who plays with a screwdriver may not know how to turn a screw with it, so a student with spina bifida may use an abstract word without understanding its full and proper use. Because of this tendency, a student who uses a relational term such as *equal* cannot be automatically credited with complete knowledge of its meaning.

FACTORS INFLUENCING ABSTRACT CONCEPT DEVELOPMENT

There are several factors that may interfere with the student's abstract concept development: deficits in perception, limited experiences, and difficulty comprehending explanations.

Perceptual Deficit

The difficulty students with spina bifida have with learning abstract concepts may be related to difficulty perceptually abstracting or isolating relevant information (Culatta, 1980). (This ability to abstract a particular aspect from a whole event is often referred to as figure-ground perception, analytic perception, or selective attention.) Figures 5.1 and 5.2 are test items that illustrate figure-ground or analytic perceptual demands. Figure 5.1 is an item from the Figure-Ground subtest of the Southern California Test of Sensory Integration (Ayres, 1972). Here the student with spina bifida may have difficulty abstracting or disembedding the outline of the basket or apple from the other objects imposed upon them. Figure 5.2 is an item from the Children's Embedded Figures Test (Witkin, Oltman, Raskin, & Karp, 1971) which also relies on the ability to abstract a particular aspect of a stimulus while ignoring irrelevant stimuli. In this item the student must identify the simple form of a "tent" (triangle) which is embedded into a more complex figure.

Students with spina bifida may experience difficulty acquiring abstract concepts because abstract concept development relies on the ability to abstract relevant from irrelevant information (Bruner, 1966; Gelman, 1969). This is why an understanding of abstract words can be difficult. The meaning of an abstract word is a particular characteristic that is common to many very different events. To acquire the meaning of the word *few,* for example, the student must abstract the characteristic of "estimated small quantity" from such different events as dispersing supplies, organizing materials, and distributing snacks. Likewise, to acquire the word *equal,* the student must notice numerical equality in such different situations as calculating toys, comparing baseball cards, buying food, and counting the number of screws needed to fix a toy. It is the per-

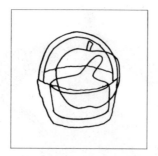

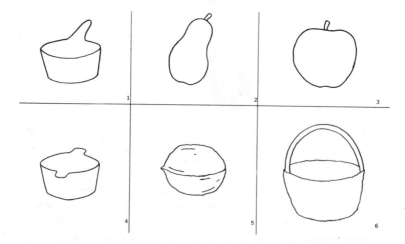

Figure 5.1. Items from the Visual Figure-Ground subtest of the Southern California Test of Sensory Integration. (From Ayres, J. [1972]. *Southern California Test of Sensory Integration*. Los Angeles: Western Psychological Services. Copyright © 1972 by Western Psychological Services. Reprinted by permission of the publisher. Western Psychological Services. 12031 Wilshire Boulevard, Los Angeles, California 90025.)

ceptual ability to recognize the characteristic of "numerical equivalence" that guides the student in learning the word *equal* and not the manner in which any given set of objects appears. In fact, the objects, their positions, and the actions applied to them are all irrelevant characteristics that must be ignored. In Figure 5.3, the equality of the dots in the two sets is the relevant or defining characteristic and the position of the dots, the size of the dots, and the length of the rows are irrelevant characteristics. The student must learn that the dots are equal even when they do not perceptually appear to be equal.

The term *same as* further illustrates the perceptual requirement

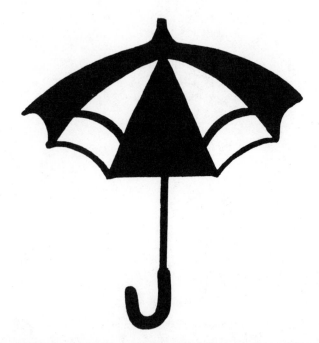

Figure 5.2.   Item from the Children's Embedded Figures Test. (Reproduced by special permission of the Publisher, Consulting Psychologists Press, Inc., Palo Alto, CA 94303 from *Children's Embedded Figures Test* by Norma Konstadt & Steven A. Karp. Copyright 1971 by Consulting Psychologists Press, Inc. All rights reserved. Further reproduction is prohibited without the Publisher's consent.)

necessary to learn abstract words. If we scan a room, we can find things or actions that are the same in some way. We could say that a pen and pencil are the same because of their shape or function, that a button on a shirt or blouse is the same shape as the knob on a slide projector, or that a legal-sized pad of paper is the same size as a briefcase. If a student is to apply the term *same as* functionally in real situations, he or she must be able to abstract similarities in a variety of different objects or actions. A student who cannot isolate those characteristics that define a word from distractions will have difficulty acquiring abstract concepts.

Students with spina bifida may have less difficulty acquiring concrete than abstract words because concrete words can be acquired with

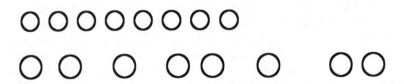

Figure 5.3.   Sets of objects in which equality of number is not perceptually clear.

concrete perceptual skills. Concrete words are more easily acquired because they can be recognized on the basis of multiple characteristics that usually occur together (Rosch, 1978). For example, if we look around a room at the various handles that we see, we note most are of a similar size and shape and, of course, all have the same purpose. Thus, a handle is always attached to something, it helps someone to move or hold things, and its size and shape conform to that of a hand. To acquire the word *handle*, the student can rely on several characteristics that are present at the same time. Concrete words such as *handle, cabinet, screw,* and *pen* are more easily acquired because they can be recognized on the basis of a set of features that occur together.

Limited Experiences

Another factor that may interfere with abstract concept development in students with spina bifida is limited experiences. Experiences provide input that feeds the development of concepts (Klausmeier, Ghatala, & Frayer, 1974). A particular history of experiences leads an individual to classify the environment in particular ways and differences in experiences are related to differences in concept attainment (Carroll, 1967; Clark, 1973). For example, to acquire the term *almost*, the student must encounter opportunities to notice such events as a milk carton that is *almost* full, shirts that are *almost* the same color, and puzzles that are *almost* complete. Similarly, knowledge of spatial and temporal terms comes from experiences with space gained, in part, from movement through space. Limited movement distorts experiences, affects perceptual development, and disrupts learning (Abercrombie, 1968; Pringle, 1971; Reynell, 1970; Werner & Burton, 1979).

In addition to a rich store of experiences, a student's experiences must follow certain conditions for concept attainment to occur. In particular, inadequate mastery of prerequisite concepts accounts for difficulty benefiting from experiences with more complex concepts (Brown, 1958; Bruner & Kenney, 1966; Owens, 1992). For example, students who do not have well established spatial concepts will have difficulty learning temporal concepts (Clark, 1973). The hierarchical sequence of basic concepts is foundational for the appreciation of more advanced conceptual growth, particularly in academics.

Difficulty Comprehending Explanations

A third factor that influences conceptual development is the ability to understand explanations. Abstract concept acquisition is aided by comprehension of verbal explanations of a word's meaning. Information about the meaning of the word *still,* for example, is presented in such explanations as:

> I wanted a horse when I was a little girl. My mom said that I couldn't have one. She said I wouldn't want one when I grew up. Now I'm all grown up but I *still* want a horse.

Clues to the meaning of the word *still* are embedded in the explanation. In some instances, verbal examples are more explicit, as in this explanation of the word *almost*:

> Your glass is almost empty. That means that your milk is not all gone yet. There's still a little bit left. You have some milk but not very much. It's almost gone. It will be all gone when you take one more drink. Not gone yet, but almost.

Students with spina bifida who currently have difficulty attending to or understanding explanations may encounter more difficulty acquiring abstract concepts. Likewise, students who have had difficulty attending to or comprehending language when they were younger are likely to have a more shallow understanding of concepts when they enter school.

Also, there may be a relationship among the factors. Limited experiences and poor attention may interfere with perceptual and comprehension skills, which, in turn, may interfere with concept development.

ASSESSING ABSTRACT CONCEPT DEFICITS

The initial assessment of word knowledge of the student with spina bifida should be done by a speech-language pathologist or another qualified person on the educational team. After this initial assessment, the classroom teacher and the speech-language pathologist can be jointly responsible for ongoing informal assessment.

Assessing a student's knowledge of abstract terminology can be tricky. First, the student with spina bifida should not be automatically credited with knowledge of the words he or she uses. In particular, if the student is using words in inappropriate contexts, one should suspect that the conceptual meaning of those words has not been acquired. Stephens (1985) cautioned against being misled by a student's use of advanced terminology. The use of words often makes the student appear academically advanced and leads to unreasonable expectations.

A second problem in assessing word knowledge is that in certain circumstances students can correctly use or identify examples of words they do not fully understand. Students with spina bifida may be able to identify an example of a word if they can rely on situational cues or prompts to let them know how to respond. Facial expressions, gestures, familiarity with routines, and the actions of others are all ways students may figure out what they are expected to say or do. For example, the student who has not learned to differentiate between the words *letter* and *sound* may be able to tell what sound the word *bear* begins with if the appropriate response has been modeled by other class members. Likewise, a student who may not be able to generalize the word *first* to all spatial arrangements may know *first* in reference to *first in line*. A student who may not fully realize that *equal* refers to parts that are equivalent to a total may use the word *equal* in reference to math problems. The student who uses words only in instances in which they have been heard or only in familiar situations may not know the full meanings of those words. In addition, one cannot assume that the student has word meaning if the student has some other way of determining how to respond.

A third assessment problem is encountered when a student may be able to recognize specific exaggerated examples of certain concepts without being able to recognize more naturalistic or less obvious examples. The meaning of the word *half* is "one of two equivalent parts." If the student sees a picture of a whole cookie clearly contrasted with a half of a cookie, the student is likely to select the half when told to find the half. However, the student might erroneously think that the word *half* means "part of." The student who thinks that *half* means "part of" can perform successfully when given the choice between a whole and a half of a cookie. However, the same student may agree that a piece of a cookie is also half and may not be able to sort a group of objects into two piles, each with half the objects. Similarly, students with spina bifida have been found to experience more difficulty identifying the meaning of words in pictures that present natural scenes than in pictures without distraction (Horn et al., 1985). Thus, some students may be able to recognize clearly depicted examples of a word without having an in-depth knowledge of the word.

In summary, the problems encountered when evaluating the conceptual knowledge of a student with spina bifida may yield a falsely inflated view of the student's knowledge of abstract concepts. The student with spina bifida can appear to have well established conceptual knowledge of abstract words, when, in reality, the knowledge is superficial. The student with spina bifida may appear to have a greater understanding of abstract words than she or he actually possesses because specific cues or prompts can let the student know how she is expected to perform. Further, shallow word knowledge interferes with academic performance, particularly in critical content areas such as reading and math (Stephens, 1985).

Assessment Strategies

Informal assessment techniques are essential when evaluating knowledge of vocabulary in the student with spina bifida. There are two reasons for relying on informal assessment procedures. First, informal assessment procedures can provide an in-depth assessment of words that may not appear on formal tests but that influence classroom performance. Second, informal assessment techniques can control factors influencing the student's performance so that the tasks reflect full knowledge, rather than mere recognition of words.

To assess vocabulary informally, the teacher should first identify words that are critical for the student to know. To identify these words, the teacher should monitor the language the student encounters in his or her texts or in classroom explanations and directions. From the sentences the student hears or sees, any words that the teacher suspects the student does not fully comprehend should be assessed.

A reasonable practice in dealing with the student with spina bifida is not to assume that the student has full or deep understanding of the abstract or relational words encountered in the classroom. A first grade student with spina bifida may not be able to benefit fully from classroom explanations because he or she may not comprehend fully the component vocabulary. Consider the explanation of the "sw" blend:

> Look at this word. (*Teacher points to the word 'swim.'*) Let's find out what this word is. You know the sounds the /s/ and /w/ stand for. When the letters /s/ and /w/ come together at the beginning of a word, the sounds they stand for are so close together that they almost seem to be just one sound.

Before the student can fully understand the explanation of the "sw" blend, he or she must know the meanings of *stand for, sound, together, almost, seem, close,* and *beginning.* The student's knowledge of such words should be specifically assessed.

Techniques for Evaluating Word Knowledge

The first and simplest way to get an indication of word knowledge is to ask the student to define a word. If the student encounters the word "protect" in a sentence, the teacher might ask the student, "What does 'protect' mean?" The student who provides several examples or describes the word's meaning may comprehend the word. It may be useful to contrast the quality and depth of a peer's definition with that of the student with spina bifida. In evaluating a student's definition, the teacher must make sure that the child is not merely repeating a statement that he or she has heard.

A second strategy that can be used to evaluate word knowledge is to ask the student to show an example of the word in a situation that does not provide any cues or prompts. Some examples are:

1. To evaluate the word *first,* the teacher could hand the student several objects such as a shoe, pen, block, and car. The teacher could then tell the student to give him or her the objects but to give the block last

and the pen first. The student must rely on knowledge of the word "first" rather than on the order in which the objects were mentioned to carry out the command.

2. To evaluate *more than*, the teacher could place a small group of objects such as pens on the table and ask the student to make it so the pens are in two piles, with one pile having two more pens than the other pile. Giving the student one group of objects to sort is better than aligning two rows of objects and asking the student to identify "more than."

3. To evaluate *almost*, the teacher could hand the student a pen and ask the student to adjust the pen cap so that it is almost on. The student should loosen the pen cap so that it could easily fall off.

4. To evaluate *same as*, the student may be handed a cup and told to "Find something that is the same size as this cup." Because alternatives are not present, the student cannot rely on recognizing one of several choices.

In each instance, the student is demonstrating word knowledge by creating novel examples.

The third strategy for assessing word knowledge is to provide the student with distracting situational information. Distracting situational information can be provided to discern true comprehension from limited knowledge. Some examples are:

1. In Piaget's standard task for assessing *equal*, the teacher could ask the student to judge the equality of two rows of equal objects that are positioned so that one row is perceptually longer than the other. The length of the rows is the distracting information.

2. Another example of this strategy can be applied to assessing the word *every*. A student could be handed 10 paper clips and told to give one to every student in a class of 25 students. The student who knows the meaning of *every* would know that 10 paper clips would not be enough to give one to every student.

3. The teacher could give the student a worksheet in which several blocks are already filled in and tell the student, "Make it so that not every space is filled in." The student must ignore the tendency to complete filling in all the spaces in order to carry out the direction.

4. To assess functional knowledge of *few*, the teacher could tell the student to pass out cookies to the entire class. Then the teacher could hand the student a full box of cookies, and tell him or her to "take a few." The situation, a class of 25 hungry students, would suggest to the student that he or she would take enough cookies for the whole class. If the student has comprehension of the word *few*, he or she will ignore the situational cues and rely on knowledge of the word. Thus,

it is the student's knowledge of the word *few* that tells him or her to remove only a small number of cookies from the box.

The fourth strategy for assessing word knowledge is to ask the student to recognize both negative and positive examples of the word and to recognize when the target word is used inappropriately. Some examples are:

1. The teacher could give the student 10 cookies and ask the student if 10 is enough for "every" member of a class of 25 students.
2. The teacher could hand the student a completely full glass and ask the student if the glass is "almost" full.
3. The teacher could hand the student an object such as a ball, that does not have an obvious front or back, and ask the student to find the "back." Or, the teacher could point to the front of a clock and ask, "Is this the back?"
4. The teacher could hand the student a handful of paper clips and ask, "Do you have a few?"

A student who has well-established comprehension of the words will recognize negative examples of words and will recognize when those words are used inaccurately.

It must be emphasized that one can never assume that a given student fully understands the vocabulary he or she hears. A teacher must not only evaluate the student's understanding of the words the student encounters, but must also ensure that knowledge of the words is well established. The student should be credited with knowledge of a word only when he or she can identify novel examples of the word, in novel contexts, without any situational cues. Gruenwald and Pollak (1990) provide useful suggestions for evaluating students' knowledge of concepts encountered in the classroom.

REMEDIATION

The strategies for teaching abstract concepts to students with spina bifida are designed to make it easy to perceive the aspect of the environment identified with the word (Fay et al., 1986). Strategies are presented that will increase the likelihood that the student will notice the word's meaning, as it occurs in the environment. The goal of these strategies is to have the child generalize word recognition to new, naturally occurring examples without reliance on cues or prompts.

The training strategies presented here can be used to train any abstract or relational words. They consist of: 1) presenting many examples, 2) exaggerating the relevant characteristics, 3) varying the types of examples, 4) providing explanations, 5) providing reasons for identifying examples, and 6) calling attention to real-world examples.

Strategy 1: Present Many Examples

By presenting many examples the teacher provides the student with opportunities to notice the word's defining characteristic. Since providing a wide variety of examples enhances the student's ability to identify the meaning of a word, the teacher's task is to maximize the number of different examples presented. In training *more than*, the teacher could present numerous examples of counting and comparing sets of objects. In training *few*, the teacher could present numerous examples by isolating a few from many objects already in the school environment. Objects used might include blocks, cards, paper clips, books, rubber bands, pennies, chips, pencils, straws, desks, rulers, and pieces of paper. The teacher must remember that the more examples presented, the easier it will be for the student to notice or to abstract the meaning of the word.

Strategy 2: Exaggerate the Defining Characteristic

In addition to providing many examples of the word, the teacher should also attempt to exaggerate the word's defining characteristic. In other words, the teacher should engage in actions that attempt to make the student "see" what the word means. In teaching the term *more than*, the teacher can exaggerate the meaning by lining up objects in two rows, counting the objects in both rows, and counting the objects in the top row that do not have a corresponding matching object in the bottom row. When demonstrating the meaning of *few*, the teacher may present a group of many objects, isolate a few, and then compare the group containing many to the group containing only a few. The contrast between groups with many objects and groups with a few objects calls the student's attention to the defining characteristic of the word *few*.

Another way of exaggerating a word's meaning is to hold irrelevant or nondefining characteristics constant. When initially training a word, the types of examples, the position of the examples, and the actions applied to them should be limited. When initially teaching *few*, examples could be limited to isolating few from many groups of identical objects. The student could be told to "give a few," "find a few," "take a few," "point to a few." Piles of objects with a few could be isolated and placed beside piles containing many so that the isolated few blocks could be clearly contrasted with the piles containing many. In teaching *more than*, nondefining characteristics such as the position of the objects can be held constant by lining up two groups of objects with equal distance between each object. The group with more than will appear larger because the position of the objects is held constant.

Figure 5.4 illustrates ways to exaggerate the word *every*. In each example, the objects are positioned so that the child can clearly see that every member of the set is being manipulated or shares a common feature. By deliberately placing identical pencils in four identical cups that are lined up, the teacher can exaggerate the meaning of *every* as she says "I put a pencil in *every* cup."

Another mechanism for exaggerating defining features is to contrast positive with negative examples. In teaching *half*, the teacher can take sets of objects and physically divide them into two parts saying, "We take this whole set and divide it into equal parts. This part is a half. Now if we put these two equal parts or halves back together again, we get the whole. Now it is not half; it is whole."

Likewise, the teacher can divide the objects into many parts and say:

> Now I divided the set into many, many parts, not just two equal parts. These are not halves. Halves are when we have two equal parts.

Strategy 3: Vary the Types of Examples

Once the child can recognize examples of concepts in an easy-to-perceive manner, the teacher should vary the types of examples presented, their positions, and the actions applied to them. When first teaching *few*, for example, the teacher selected or contrasted a few with one or many objects from large sets of identical objects. In varying the types of examples, the teacher contrasts few versus one or many objects or actions in such activities as removing pieces of tape from a continuous roll, selecting toys from a box of assorted objects, getting books from a shelf, poking holes in paper, turning cards over, jumping, saying words, tearing paper, knocking on blocks, or drawing circles. Instead of the examples being immediately visible, the student may be asked to create them. For example, instead of being provided with a pile of rubber bands, the student may be told to find a few rubber bands among a variety of objects scattered on the teacher's desk. Or, the student might be handed one paper clip and told to get a few. The student would have to retrieve a few from the supply cupboard. The goal is for the student to be able to notice that words such as *few*, *more than*, and *every* are terms that are applied to all members of a group no matter how the objects or actions are encountered.

Strategy 4: Provide Explanations of the Word's Meaning

Explanations of the word's meaning should accompany the presentation of examples. Examples of explanations include: "A few is not very many. A few can be two or three or four—not very many." Statements such as the following may help:

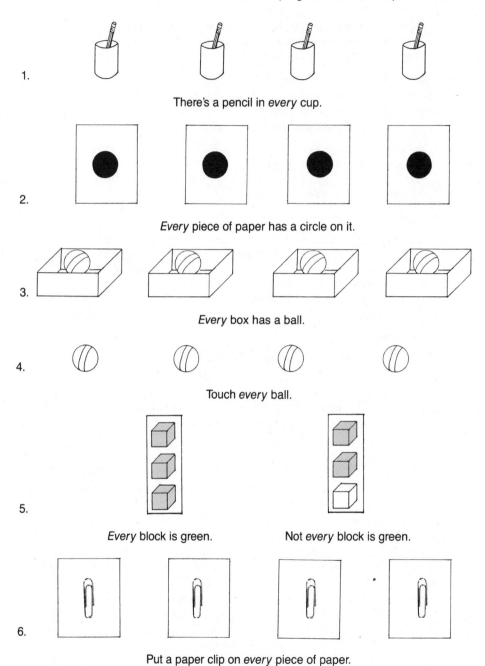

1. There's a pencil in *every* cup.

2. *Every* piece of paper has a circle on it.

3. *Every* box has a ball.

4. Touch *every* ball.

5. *Every* block is green.   Not *every* block is green.

6. Put a paper clip on *every* piece of paper.

Figure 5.4. Exaggerated examples of the word *every*.

There are a lot of paper clips here. I'll just take a *few*. Now this pile doesn't have many. There are only a *few*. A *few* is not "many." Only a *few* here. "Lots" in this pile but only a *few* in this pile.

In providing explanations, the teacher is always cautious to use words the child already knows in explaining the meaning of new words. Relating descriptions to the child's own experiences helps as well. In describing the term *more than*, the teacher can say:

We have 6 chocolate milks and 10 white milks. There are more white milks than chocolate milks. Ten is a bigger number than 6. Ten is 1–2–3–4 more than 6 (*said while pointing to the 4 white milks that do not have a corresponding chocolate milk*).

In explaining *half*, the teacher can say:

When we put all our shoes together, we get 20 shoes. Let's divide the shoes into two equal groups. We'll put 10 shoes here and 10 shoes here. Ten and 10. If we count these two groups of 10, we get 20. We took the 20 shoes and made it into two equal parts. Ten and 10 are the same number: they are equal. This group of 10 is half of the 20 shoes. And this group of 10 is half of the 20 shoes. Half is when we divide a group into 2 equal parts. Each part is a half.

Strategy 5: Provide Reasons for Noticing Examples

To make concept learning functional, the student should have a reason to focus on the examples. Mechanisms for doing this include using examples that are inherently interesting, incorporating examples into game-like tasks, providing contextual reasons for identifying examples, and ensuring that examples impact the student's own goals. Active involvement in activities such as dispersing materials, organizing the room, and creating a bulletin board can mandate the need to focus on certain aspects of the event or experience. In addition, the teacher can pose interesting problems, model curiosity, ask relevant questions, and hypothesize and predict outcomes, all of which can dictate the need to compare and contrast objects. Violating routines and calling the student's attention to unusual events are also mechanisms for calling attention to specific examples. For example, the teacher can present 10 paper cups and state in a puzzling manner that she noticed rips in them: "I wonder if there is a rip in every cup?" After thoroughly inspecting the cups, she can declare, "All cups have holes in them. We cannot use them. There is a rip in every one of these paper cups. Isn't that too bad? How did every cup get ripped?" In teaching *more than*, the teacher can compare and contrast the students' own objects, have "games" to see how many more items one student has than another, and create opportunities to guess or predict relative quantities of two sets of objects.

Strategy 6: Call Attention to Real-World Examples

It is essential that students learn to recognize and respond appropriately to the meaning of the target word in the natural environment. Consequently, the student's attention should be called to examples of the target word in real situations. Examples are pointed out, exaggerated, and explained during activities designed to teach other skills, such as art, and during routine activities, such as cleaning the room or preparing for recess. For example, while preparing for an art activity, the teacher can say: "We need the same number of pens and paper. We need to have an equal number of pens and paper. I think we have more pens than paper. How many more pens do we have?" After methodically counting and comparing, the teacher can declare, "We have five more pens than papers. That means we need five pieces of paper."

Similarly, while collecting field trip permission slips, the teacher may point out:

> We only have a *few* papers turned in. Look, there aren't many papers here. Only a couple. Only a *few* papers turned in. We will need a paper for every child. I need to get 25 papers because we have 25 students. But, I only have about three or four. I only have a *few*, not very many.

By experiencing examples during daily occurring activities, the student is able to recognize the meaning of the target word as it actually exists in the natural environment. The teacher should point out as many examples as possible during the day. For example, if *every* is the target, and the teacher notices that not all the students have their work done, the teacher could point out:

> "Not *every* one has his or her work finished. Joan and Mary do not have their work done. When Joan and Mary finish, will *every* student be done? Look, now Joan and Mary are finished. Now *every* student has his or her work done (*said while deliberately pointing to each child*).

While getting ready for lunch, it can be pointed out:

> It's time for lunch. Today let's do things differently. First, let's have *every* girl get in line. Not *every* girl is here yet. Now *every* girl is here and we don't have any boys here. There aren't any girls sitting down because *every* girl is standing in line.

EVALUATING THE EFFECTIVENESS OF TRAINING

In order to evaluate the effectiveness of training, the student's new knowledge of a target word can be evaluated. The teacher or speech-language pathologist must determine whether the student can identify new examples of the word in activities not designed to teach the word. The teacher must be careful not to be deceived by apparent knowledge of the word. Expressive use of the word in familiar situations need not indicate receptive knowledge of the word. Similarly, the ability to correctly identify examples of the word that resemble those used in training may not indicate knowledge of the word. To indicate knowledge of the word, the student must be able to identify new examples, as they exist in the natural environment, without reliance on situational support.

The objective of concept training is reached when the student can follow novel positive and negative commands containing the target word during routine, novel activities. For example, the teacher may say, "For snack today, we need a *few* straws and *many* napkins," or "Which page has a *few* apples and which does not have a few?" The other activities and objects present provide the student with naturalistic distractions.

To evaluate the effectiveness of training, the teacher can construct tasks similar to those discussed in the assessment section. Tasks without situational support should reflect the student's true knowledge of a target word. In these tasks, the student can be asked to locate examples or to manipulate objects in novel ways in order to demonstrate knowledge. For example, to evaluate knowledge of *few*, the teacher may hand the student only one block and say, "I need a few." In order to understand and respond appropriately to the message, the student must be able to focus on the meaning of the word *few*.

Evaluating word knowledge in students with spina bifida should be a continuous process. Each new term or concept that is encountered in the curriculum should be specifically assessed. Some questions or commands that can be used to evaluate a student's knowledge of the word *every* include:

1. Is there a penny in every pocket in this room? (*Student must look in every pocket.*)
2. Every person in this room has long hair. (*Student must recognize the error in the teacher's statement.*)
3. Make sure there's a reading book on every seat. (*Student must follow the command.*)
4. Find a worksheet that doesn't have a mark in every block. (*Student finds a negative example.*)
5. Knock on every block.
6. Unbutton every button on your sweater.
7. Place a piece of paper under every pen.
8. Make sure every piece of paper has writing on it.

This list shows the range of activities available for assessing knowledge of a particular word.

SUMMARY

Students with spina bifida may have shallow knowledge of abstract terms. Therefore, specific strategies for assessing and training the abstract vocabulary in students with spina bifida may need to be employed. The training strategies presented here should help students with spina bifida generalize the meaning of abstract terms to new and complex situations.

GLOSSARY

Abstract (verb)   To isolate or select a certain aspect from a whole event.

Abstract concept   Knowledge of events that is not readily available. Knowledge of the relationship between events and aspects that are difficult to perceive. Examples of abstract concepts include: *below, judge, least.*

Conceptual   Knowledge that an individual possesses of the similarities that exist in groups of objects and events. Knowledge of the functions of objects and events and of their association with each other.

Defining characteristic   Characteristics of a group of objects or events that distinguish it from other groups of objects or events (e.g., *chairs* are distinguished from *houses* on the basis of their shape and function).

Disembedding   Separating; taking apart.

Distracting situational information   Information provided in a task that competes with the correct response or that suggests a different response (e.g. a child is given 10 paper clips and told to give one to every child in a class of 25; the presence of the 25 children may interfere with the child's comprehension).

Distractions   Events in the environment that compete with the target stimulus. Examples of the target word can be pointed out during activities designed to teach other skills.

Expressive language   Ability to retrieve language rules in order to convey messages. Use of language to communicate one's perceptions, ideas, feelings, or intentions to others.

Receptive knowledge   Ability to attach meaning to language rules. Comprehension of words and grammatical rules.

Relational term   Quantity, temporal, and spatial terms or phrases such as *long, next to, ahead, several, far,* and *above.*

Situational support   Cues, prompts, or visual information that may help a child comprehend a problem or message.

Spatial concepts   Concepts that refer to space, such as *above* or *behind.*

Temporal concepts   Concepts that refer to time, such as *first* and *second.*

REFERENCES

Abercrombie, M.L. (1968). Some notes on spatial disability: Movement, intelligence quotient and attentiveness. *Developmental Medicine and Child Neurology, 10,* 200–213.

Agness, P.J. (1983). *Learning disabilities and the child with spina bifida.* Chicago: Spina Bifida Association of America.

Ayres, J. (1972). *Southern California Test of Sensory Integration*. Los Angeles: Western Psychological Services.

Brown, R. (1958). *Words and things*. New York: Free Press.

Bruner, J. (1966). On cognitive growth. In J. Bruner, R. Olver, & P. Greenfield (Eds.), *Studies in cognitive growth* (pp. 1–67). New York: John Wiley & Sons.

Bruner, J., & Kenney, H. (1966). On relational concepts. In J. Bruner, R. Olver, & P. Greenfield (Eds.), *Studies in cognitive growth* (pp. 168–182). New York: John Wiley & Sons.

Carroll, J.B. (1967). Words, meanings and concepts. In L. Jakobvits & M. Miron (Eds.), *Readings in the psychology of language* (pp. 567–586). Englewood Cliffs, NJ: Prentice Hall.

Clark, E.V. (1973). What's in a word?: On the child's acquisition of semantics in his first language. In T.E. Moore (Ed.), *Cognitive development and the acquisition of language* (pp. 65–109). New York: Academic Press.

Culatta, B. (1978). Language use without comprehension: A suggested methodology for the clinical evaluation of spina bifida children. *Spina Bifida Therapy, 1*, 1–6.

Culatta, B. (1980). Perceptual and linguistic performance of spina bifida hydrocephalic children. *Spina Bifida Therapy, 2*, 235–247.

Culatta, B., & Culatta, R. (1978). Spina bifida children's non-communicative language: Examples and identification guidelines. *Allied Health and Behavioral Sciences, 1*, 22–30.

Fay, G., Shurtleff, D., Shurtleff, H., & Wolf, L. (1986). Developmental expectations: Intelligence and fine motor skills. In D. Shurtleff (Ed.), *Myelodysplasias and exstrophies: Significance, prevention and treatment* (pp. 359–372). New York: Grune & Stratton.

Gelman, R. (1969). Conservation acquisition: A problem of learning to attend to relevant attributes. *Journal of Experimental Child Psychology, 2*, 167–187.

Gruenwald, L., & Pollak, S. (1990). *Language interaction in curriculum and instruction* (2nd ed.). Austin, TX: PRO-ED.

Horn, D., Lorch, E., Lorch, R., & Culatta, B. (1985). Distractibility and vocabulary deficits in children with spina bifida and hydrocephalus. *Developmental Medicine and Child Neurology, 27*, 713–720.

Klausmeier, H.J., Ghatala, E.S., & Frayer, D.A. (1974). *Conceptual learning and development: A cognitive view*. New York: Academic Press.

Owens, R. (1992). *Language development* (3rd ed). New York: Macmillan.

Parsons, J.G. (1968). An investigation into the verbal facility of hydrocephalic children, with special reference to vocabulary, morphology and fluency. *Developmental Medicine and Child Neurology, 13*(Supp. 17), 109.

Pringle, M. (1971). *Deprivation and education* (2nd ed). New York: Longman.

Reynell, J. (1970). Children with physical handicaps. In P. Mittler (Ed.), *The psychological assessment of mental and physical handicaps* (pp. 443–467). London: Methuen.

Rosch, E. (1978). Principles of categorization. In E. Rosch & B. Lloyd (Eds.), *Cognition and categorization* (pp. 27–48). Hillsdale, NJ: Lawrence Erlbaum Associates.

Spain, B. (1972). Verbal and performance ability in pre-school spina bifida children. *Developmental Medicine and Child Neurology, 14*, 155, 527.

Stephens, S. (1985). *Educating the student with spina bifida*. Austin: Spina Bifida Association of Texas.

Werner, P., & Burton, E. (1979). *Learning through movement*. St. Louis: C.V. Mosby.

Williamson, G.G. (Ed.). (1987). *Children with spina bifida: Early intervention and preschool programming.* Baltimore: Paul H. Brookes Publishing Co.

Witkin, H., Oltman, P., Raskin, E., & Karp, S. (1971). *Children's Embedded Figures Test.* Palo Alto, CA: Consulting Psychologists Press.

Building Mathematic Skills

Barbara Culatta

Some students with spina bifida are prone to difficulty developing in mathematics (Badell-Ribera, Shulman, & Paddock, 1966; Diller, Gordon, Swinyard, & Kastner, 1969; Hurley, Dorman, Laatsch, Bell, & D'Avignon, 1990; Shaffer et al., 1986; Spain, 1974). They tend to perform below their mental age peers in mathematics achievement (Tew & Laurence, 1972, 1975, 1984).

The mathematic deficits that students with spina bifida experience are felt to be similar to the deficits that other students with learning disabilities experience (Stephens, 1985). The rote calculation aspect of mathematics may be less involved than the conceptual and problem-solving components (Agness, 1983; Mattson, 1982).

While much is yet to be learned about the mathematic skill development in students with spina bifida, it is essential for educators to have a framework with which to view the functioning of individual students. Emphasis in this chapter is placed on the assessment and facilitation of each component of mathematics: calculation, conceptual knowledge, and problem-solving. Individual students with spina bifida may exhibit deficits in each of these component skill areas. The deficits they exhibit are likely to be influenced greatly by conceptual and linguistic factors. Students with spina bifida who have difficulty with conceptual or linguistic demands may exhibit a performance variance between calculation and problem-solving skills.

CALCULATION

A common problem among students with learning disabilities is better calculation than problem-solving performance (Blankenship & Lovitt 1976; Levy & Schenck, 1981). This gap between calculation and problem-solving, suspected to exist as well in students with spina bifida, may be reflected in a tendency to "rotely calculate" the numbers encountered in word problems. Rote calculation refers to the impulsive adding or subtracting of numbers without determining which operation should be used or which numbers should be included in the calculation process. Students who rotely calculate often do so without an understanding of how numbers are related or verbally manipulated to derive correct solutions.

Even though calculation may be better than problem-solving, students with spina bifida may not acquire all calculation procedures with equal proficiency. The calculation deficits that are likely to exist are those that require more advanced conceptual skill (Agness, 1983). The procedures that students with spina bifida may have difficulty with include: borrowing and carrying (most likely due to an incomplete knowledge of the tens-and-ones concept); calculating missing subset quantities, as in "___ + 9 = 16" (most likely due to an incomplete knowledge of the part/ whole concept); recognition that multiplication is repeated addition; recognition that addition and subtraction are converse operations (possibly due to limited grasp of the part/whole concept); converting fractions to whole numbers; and recognizing the relationship among fractions, decimals, and whole numbers. Calculation problems often result from an inadequate knowledge of underlying concepts (Greeno, 1987b; Resnick, 1983).

The perceptual and motor deficits that some students with spina bifida exhibit may also affect their calculation performance. Visual motor deficits reduce copying speed and may create difficulties in lining up work correctly. These visual motor deficits are discussed in greater detail in Chapter 8.

CONCEPTUAL KNOWLEDGE

In addition to deficits in performing certain calculation procedures, conceptual deficits may also be manifested in other ways. Conceptual deficits may be apparent in incomplete knowledge of quantifier terms, differential performance on types of word problems, and failure to explain the rationale underlying operations. Visual perceptual deficits may interfere with the acquisition of mathematic concepts as they may reduce the child's ability to recognize relevant attributes of sets of objects. These perceptual deficits are discussed in greater detail in Chapters 5 and 8.

Incomplete Knowledge of Quantifier Terms

Incomplete knowledge of quantifier terms such as *equal*, *greater than*, and *least*, may interfere with mathematic performance in students with spina bifida. Incomplete knowledge of indefinite quantifier terms such as *some*, *each*, and *another* may also interfere with mathematic performance. Indefinite quantifier terms are words that have an unspecified quantity. The indefinite quantifier can refer to an additional member of a set (as with the terms *a* and *another*), can direct the student to the totality of the set (as with the words *all*, *each*, *every*, and *both*), or can direct the student to a subset that needs to be determined (as with the word *some*).

Students with spina bifida may be able to comprehend quantifier or indefinite quantifier terms under conditions where situational support is provided but not when it is eliminated. For example, the student may be able to comprehend the statement "Give a cookie to each of the students" if the teacher glances toward the students who are to receive the cookies. This same student may not know that the word *each* refers to every member of the set when encountered in a word problem such as:

> There are five boys waiting in the lunch line. Each of the boys wants to buy a carton of milk. How many cartons of milk will be sold to the boys?

To function in math, the student must process the meaning of quantifier and indefinite quantifier terms and affix values to those terms without any perceptual or situational cues. (Chapter 5 of this volume provides additional information on the conditions in which students with spina bifida can be credited with complete knowledge of a concept.)

Differential Performance on Word Problems

Conceptual knowledge influences the types of word problems students can readily solve, and therefore conceptual deficits may be manifested in differential performance on various word problems (Carpenter & Moser, 1983; De Corte & Verschaffel, 1981; Greeno, 1987a; Riley, Greeno, & Heller, 1983). The conceptual demands of word problems vary depending on the quantitative relationship that exists among the sets of objects in the problem. Children must recognize these quantitative concepts prior to selecting the appropriate problem-solving strategy (Carpenter & Moser, 1983; Riley et al., 1983). The most common conceptual relations that are coded in addition and subtraction word problems are: *change*, *compare*, and *combine*.

Change problems incorporate an action that results in an increase or decrease in the total number of objects in a set. An example of a change problem is:

> Mary had seven cookies. She gave two away. How many does she have left?

Students may not experience significant difficulty with change problems if the change is signaled with key words or phrases such as *left out* or *altogether.* However, if they are relying on key words, the students may actually not be understanding the numerical relationship coded (Cawley & Vitello, 1972).

Compare problems contain two sets of objects that are compared in number. An example of a compare problem is:

> Sally had seven blocks. Jody had two blocks. How many more blocks did Sally have than Jody?

Compare problems may be more difficult for students with spina bifida than *change* problems because the phrase *more than* connotes addition, even though the problem is solved by subtraction (Nesher & Teubal, 1975). To select the correct operation, the student must realize that the solution is dependent upon comparing quantities in two sets. Students will have difficulty with *compare* problems if they fail to grasp fully the meaning of "more than."

Combine problems require a conceptual understanding of how subsets are classified. In *combine* problems, subsets of objects are combined into generic categories. For example:

> Mary works in a pet store. One day Mary sold two parakeets, one canary, and three kittens. How many birds did Mary sell? How many animals did Mary sell?

In the above problem, the ability to classify subsets into the generic categories of *birds* and *animals* influences the problem-solving process. Problem-solving may become difficult when classification requirements become demanding (Goodstein, 1981).

Difficulty Selecting the Appropriate Operation

Students may have difficulty understanding the conceptual relationship underlying operations (Lindquist, 1989). The students may not be able to select appropriate operations if they don't have conceptual knowledge of those operations. A student who does not understand that multiplication is the same as repeated addition will have difficulty knowing when to use multiplication to solve problems. Failure to understand fully the conceptual nature of operations may be detected in an inability to select the appropriate operations in a problem such as:

> John took a job raking leaves. He charged $3.00 an hour for leaf raking. On the first day John worked 2 hours, 1 hour on the second day, and 3 hours on the third. How much money did John make in the three days that he worked?

In such a problem the student must know when to use addition and when to use multiplication.

Difficulty with Start- or Subset-Unknown Problems

Another conceptual dimension is what item of information is unknown. The unknown information can be the *start*, *subset*, or *result* quantity (Riley et al., 1983). In problems in which the *start* quantity is unknown, the initial number is not provided. The *start* quantity is unknown in the following problem:

> Mark bought some cookies. He ate two of them. Then he had seven. How many cookies did Mark buy?

In problems in which the *subset* quantity is unknown, one of the parts of the whole is missing. The subset quantity is unknown in the following problem:

> Mark bought nine cookies. He gave some away. Then he had seven. How many did he give away?

In contrast, the *result* quantity is unknown in a problem such as:

> Mark bought nine cookies. He ate two of them. How many did he have left?

Problems in which the *start* or *subset* quantity is unknown may be more difficult for individual students with spina bifida than problems in which the *result* quantity is unknown. Problems in which the result quantity is known are easier because the student may not need a fully developed knowledge of the part/whole concept in order to solve the problem. The student can often solve *result*-unknown problems by rotely calculating, without knowing which number represents the part and which represents the whole. A student's successful performance on some *result*-unknown problems does not necessarily imply underlying conceptual knowledge (Dean, Chabaud, & Bridges, 1981).

Conceptual deficits may be manifested in problem-solving difficulties. Problems that code more complex quantitative relationships (e.g., *compare* problems), problems that require a knowledge of the part/whole concept (*start*- or *subset*-unknown problems), and problems that incorporate indefinite quantifiers may be particularly difficult for students who have limited conceptual knowledge.

PROBLEM-SOLVING

In addition to conceptual knowledge, linguistic factors may also influence problem-solving performance. The student must comprehend the problem before being able to select the appropriate problem-solving strategies. Comprehending the problem entails determining "who has what and who is doing what to whom." Consider the processes involved in solving the following problem:

> Mary and Susan were playing a game of cards. Some of the cards had marks on them and some didn't. The girls wanted to see who could get the most cards with marks. The girls took turns picking cards from a pile. At the end of the game, Mary had five cards with marks and one plain card. Susan had two plain cards and three with marks. How many more cards with marks did Mary have than Susan? Who was the winner?

To solve the problem, the student must first comprehend the language in the problem statements. The student must understand the problem in order to identify the quantitative relationship coded in the problem and make the correct problem-solving decisions. Rote computation can occur when a student fails to comprehend the problem.

Several linguistic factors influence comprehension of math word problems and thus impede problem-solving performance. These include the use of: extraneous information, natural language, and missing information (Goodstein, 1981). These difficulties in remembering and organizing the components of the problem situation make it difficult to determine "who has what and who is doing what to whom." This may account for higher levels of performance in calculation than problem-solving in some students with spina bifida.

Extraneous Information

Extraneous information refers to content that is not needed to solve the problem. The extraneous information can consist of distracting facts or distracting numbers (Goodstein, 1981). The following is an example of a problem containing extraneous facts:

> Mary and Sue decided to go to a bakery. On the way to the bakery they met Sara, and Sara went along. When they got to the bakery, Mary ordered a cupcake. Sara wasn't hungry. Sue was very hungry. She wanted two cupcakes with chocolate icing. How many cupcakes did the girls buy? Which of the girls didn't buy a cupcake?

Extraneous facts can interfere with problem-solving because they increase attention and memory demands, and because they require the student to connect pronouns with the nouns to which they refer.

An example of a problem that contains an extraneous or irrelevant number is the following:

> Mary bought three cookies and two cupcakes. Joan bought one cookie. How many cookies did the girls buy?

Problems with extraneous numbers will be solved by rote calculation if the student doesn't comprehend the problem. Students who use all of the numbers in problems that contain irrelevant quantities are not processing the language in order to determine which subsets should be included in the calculation (Blankenship & Lovitt, 1976; Englert, Culatta, & Horn, 1987).

Natural Language

Students with spina bifida may experience difficulty solving problems that are presented in natural language. Natural language or "nonroutine" problems use neutral questions to present the problem situation. Neutral questions are questions in which key words and phrases such as *all together, left out, remain,* and *take away* are eliminated (Goodstein, 1981). Thus, in "natural language" problems, the selection of the appropriate procedure is not specified by the presence of key words (Carpenter, Corbitt, Kepner, Lindquist, & Reys, 1980). Here are two examples of problems presented in natural language:

> We all want to eat in the lunchroom but there won't be enough room for us to eat together. There are seven of us here. Two of us will have to eat in Mrs. Smith's room. How many of us will get to go to the lunchroom?

> A teacher asked Mary and John to put the things that they had in their pockets on her desk. Mary had two balls and one stick. John had the same things in his pocket. What did the teacher find on her desk?

Problems presented in natural language often require the student to know that the same meaning can be signaled in several different ways. For example, the concept of equality can be coded linguistically in such alternative ways as *as many as, equal,* and *same number as.* In addition, problems presented in natural language often require the student to make linguistic inferences. A student must comprehend that there is an implied loss in problems that use such words as *borrow, rotten, chapped,* and *crumbled.*

Missing Information

The third linguistic demand that can impede problem-solving in students with spina bifida is the absence of essential information. Students who cannot understand a problem well enough to identify essential yet missing information will most likely resort to guessing. An example of a missing information problem is:

> The janitor was asked to set up the auditorium so that a movie could be shown to the students. The janitor placed 16 chairs in each row. How many students will be able to watch the movie in the auditorium?

The student with spina bifida may not realize that the total number of rows is an essential piece of information.

In summary, students with spina bifida may be prone to deficits in each component skill area: calculation, conceptual knowledge, and language processing. There may be, however, a trend toward greater difficulty in the areas of conceptual knowledge and language processing. Word problems that are more demanding in conceptual knowledge and language processing may be more difficult for the students with spina bifida than for their mental age–peers.

ASSESSMENT STRATEGIES

Even though students with spina bifida may be susceptible to common weaknesses in mathematic performance, the specific performance patterns of individual students will vary. Because of variability among students, an individualized approach to the assessment of students with spina bifida is recommended. The assessment strategies to be presented here serve to isolate the individual student's strengths and weaknesses in each component of mathematics: calculation, conceptual knowledge, and problem-solving.

Calculation

Calculation skills can easily be assessed using formal measures such as the Key Math Test—Revised (Connolly, 1985), the Test of Math Abilities (Brown & McEntire, 1984), or the Wide Range Achievement Test—Revised (Jastak & Wilkinson, 1984), which are widely available to teachers through major test distributors. The efficiency of the student's calculation strategies may also be assessed by requiring the child to demonstrate knowledge with blocks or manipulatives. Observation of the child's calculation in the presence of manipulatives reflects his or her understanding of the operation (Carpenter & Moser, 1983).

Calculation skills should be assessed before assessing problem-solving so that decisions can be made as to which operations should be included in problem-solving tasks. It is best to assess and train problem-solving skills using number facts and operations that are well established. By using well-known operations, the teacher can be assured that deficits in problem-solving are not being caused by deficits in calculation.

Conceptual Knowledge

There are several ways to assess a student's conceptual knowledge. One is to determine the student's knowledge of mathematic concepts directly. Tasks can be presented to assess such concepts as conservation (knowledge of equality in sets of objects despite the perceptual appearance of inequality), ordination (knowledge of how numbers are ordered in terms of greater and lesser values), cardination (knowledge of the relationship between number words and their numerical equivalences), and of spe-

Table 6.1. Common mathematic terms and concepts

a	further from	one half
add	goes into	order
after	greater than	ordinal
ahead of	group	numbers
all	half	other
almost	height	pair
another	high number	part
apart	highest	product
before	in back of	rest of
beginning	in front of	right
behind	include	round
below	last	row
between	left	same number
bigger than	left out	as
borrow	less than	set
both	like terms	shallow
bottom	low number	size
bottom number	lowest	smaller number
cardinal numbers	measure	smaller than
carry	member	smallest
column	middle number	some
combine	minus	subtract
count	missing number	sum
deep	more than	times
difference	most	together
different	multiply	top
divide	narrow	total
each	nearer to	unequal
empty set	nearest	unlike terms
end	next to	value
equal	none	whole
every	number line	wide
except	number words	zero
fewer	numbers	
first, second, etc.	numerals	

cific terms (*every*, *equal*, *less than*, *least*, *more than*, and *fraction*). To be credited with knowledge of a mathematic term or concept (Table 6.1), the student must be able to create or identify novel examples without the presence of situational support. For example, if the child is expected to identify the equality of two equal rows of objects with one row spread out and the other condensed, the child is not being presented with any situational support. Situational support can falsely inflate a student's knowledge. (Information on how to assess concepts appears in Chapter 5; in Carlson, Gruenewald, & Nyberg, 1980; and in Gruenewald & Pollak, 1990.) In addition to assessing the student's knowledge of mathematic concepts directly, conceptual deficits can be inferred if the student exhibits certain calculation and problem-solving difficulties. Conceptual deficits should be suspected in the student with spina bifida if any of the following is observed:

1. The student has difficulty borrowing, carrying, or calculating missing subsets (7 minus_____equals 4); making fraction and measurement conversions; telling time; and making change.
2. The student cannot identify alternate ways of expressing the same quantity terms (i.e., *equal, same number as, as many as.*)
3. The student cannot explain the relationship between addition and subtraction, multiplication and division, addition and multiplication, tens and ones, and whole numbers and fractions. Conceptual knowledge is reflected in the student's ability to explain how and why certain operations should be used and how they operate (Ginsberg, 1989). For example, students should be able to explain why a single digit number, for example 6, cannot be written in the tens column.
4. The student does not select the right operation.
5. The student fails to solve *start-* and *subset-*unknown problems.
6. The student engages in rote computation.

The presence of any of the above deficits in a student with spina bifida should lead to a deeper inspection of the mathematic concepts that underlie the particular task. Carlson et al. (1980) and Gruenewald and Pollak (1990) provide suggestions for assessing concepts that underlie functional mathematics.

Problem-Solving

Since problem-solving deficits are felt to stem from failure to comprehend the problem, it is essential to assess a student's processing of the language in the problem's statements. Approaches for assessing language-related problem-solving deficits have been proposed by Cawley, Fitzmaurice, Shaw, Kahn, and Bates (1979) and Goodstein (1981). Of these approaches, the examiner might try:

1. *Asking the student to retell word problems in his or her own words.* A student's version of a word problem can reflect his or her comprehension of the problem situation. The student's retold version can be analyzed for inclusion of the relevant numbers, specification of missing information, and inclusion of critical problem elements. A student who tries to recite a memorized version of a problem probably does not have as much understanding as the student who can convey the problem in his or her own words. Silver (1981) has shown that good and poor problem-solvers differ in their recall of problem information. Good problem-solvers recall the structural features of a problem, whereas poor problem-solvers tend to recall the specific details of a problem. Students who try

to memorize problems verbatim may experience difficulty learning mathematics (Davis, 1984).

2. *Asking the student to re-create or represent the problem situation.* Asking the student with spina bifida to re-create the problem with toys, blocks, or drawings also provides a way to inspect the student's understanding of the problem situation. A student can be handed toy dolls, trucks, and blocks and told:

> This mother and father will be building a sidewalk with bricks. The mother and father will take the bricks home in two trucks. Mother will take three more bricks than father in the yellow truck. The father will follow her in the green truck with 10 bricks.

A more developmentally advanced student can be asked to represent fractions in the following way:

> This couple wants to build a walkway to their house. They will need 20 bricks. The mother and father will take the load of bricks in two separate vehicles. The mother will take ¾ of the load in her yellow car. The father will take ¼ of the load home in his blue truck.

Real objects, toy replicas, or symbolically abstract objects such as counters, chips, or pennies may be used to evaluate the student's ability to represent the problem (Carpenter & Moser, 1983). In addition, asking students to explain their solutions reflects students' understanding (DeVincenzo-Gavioli, 1983; Ginsberg, 1989; VanDevender & Harris, 1987).

3. *Presenting problems with missing information.* While the Key Math Test (Connolly, Nachtman, & Pritchett, 1971) includes a missing information subtest, the teacher may also assess a student's ability to identify missing information in informal ways. The student with spina bifida may be given such problems as:

> I'd like to figure out how many keys the janitor has on his key ring. He has a key for every room in his house, a key for his truck, and two keys for his car. How many keys does he have on his key ring? What do we need to know in order to figure out how many keys he has?

4. *Presenting problems with irrelevant numbers.* The inclusion of irrelevant numbers gives the teacher a strategy for detecting a "rote calculation" set. Students who include irrelevant numbers are engaging in habitual and automatic calculation without implementing problem solving strategies (Goodstein, 1981).

5. *Asking questions about the problem situation.* A student's ability to answer both factual and inferencing questions reflects comprehension of the problem. Factual questions can be asked about the relevant actors, quantities, missing information, and how the sets of objects are related. Examples of questions are:

Which of the girls will buy the cookies?
If I want to keep ¼ of this pie and give ¾ away, how many pieces will I need?
Do we know how many socks Jack already has?
Will John lose marbles or will he get some extra ones?

Inferencing questions can be used to ask the student to predict outcomes. For example:

Steve and Holly are playing a game of marbles. Steve wants to win. The winner has to get five more marbles than the loser. Steve got six marbles. Holly got three marbles. Why might Steve be disappointed?

The teacher may elect to ask the student questions about the problem situation without requiring the student to solve the problem. For example:

John wanted to build a puzzle with at least 15 pieces. He bought a puzzle that had 17 pieces. Did John get what he wanted?

Such questions require the student with spina bifida to recognize essential aspects of the problem situation.

6. *Presenting problems in natural language.* Problems presented in natural language, with key words eliminated, demand processing the information in the problem situation (Lappan & Schram, 1989). Consider the following example:

I have 20 pens and there are 20 children in our class. Some of the pens write well, but some don't work well and can't be used. Six of the pens won't write at all and two leak. How many students will have trouble getting their work sheets done? How many students are likely to get ink on their hands?

In evaluating problem-solving, it must be remembered that certain word problems do not actually tap the problem-solving process. Problems that are printed or spoken in word statements may not place any more of a problem-solving demand on the student than actual computational practice (Cawley & Vitello, 1972). Word problems must require the child to process mathematical information before they can actually be considered problems. Some students with spina bifida who have conceptual or linguistic deficits may be able to handle problems that can be solved with rote computation but not be able to perform problems that demand conceptual and linguistic processing.

Concluding Remarks

The assessment of the mathematic capacities in students with spina bifida must address performance in calculation, conceptual knowledge, and problem-solving. The complexity of the problems the student encounters can be controlled by manipulating conceptual and linguistic factors. Those factors include: the quantitative relationships coded, the unknown quantity, extraneous information, missing information, and natural language. How these factors interrelate should also be determined. The teacher may find that a particular student can handle irrelevant language in a *change* problem with the result-quantity missing, but not in a *compare* problem with a missing start-quantity. Thus, the teacher needs to determine the particular concepts and linguistic skills the student with spina bifida has not yet acquired and how these various factors interrelate.

GOALS

Facilitating mathematic skills for the student with spina bifida entails setting objectives in each component skill area: calculation, conceptual knowledge, and problem-solving. Calculation objectives should include the automatization of known number facts and the development of efficient counting strategies (Carpenter & Moser, 1983). An important goal is to ensure that calculations are not performed without conceptual understanding.

Conceptual objectives should include knowledge of basic number terms, knowledge that certain numerical terms have equivalent meanings, and knowledge of the concepts that underlie operations. Students should also be expected to identify the quantitative relationships coded in word problems.

Problem-solving objectives should be individualized and should emphasize comprehension of the conceptual and linguistic structure of the problem. Students should eventually be helped to recognize the conceptual structure underlying problems so that the correct operation can be selected. They should also be helped to solve problems presented in natural language, in the presence of distracting information, and to identify missing information. Cawley et al. (1979) suggested a method of individualized goal setting in what they refer to as "matrix programming." In matrix programming, specific goals are developed by selecting the conceptual and linguistic factors that will be introduced and how they will be combined. Silbert, Carnine, and Stein (1981) also based programming on identifying and integrating factors that influence problem-solving performance. Establishing goals that eliminate or reduce conceptual and linguistic factors would actually serve to eliminate problem-solving demands (Goodstein, 1981).

In addition to deciding which conceptual and linguistic factors should be controlled for the individual student with spina bifida, the teacher must also decide which operations will be required during the problem-solving process. Well-established number facts and calculation

Table 6.2. Individualized mathematic objectives

Karen	Mark
Conceptual goals	
Part-whole concept	Quantifier terms *some, every, each,* and
Classification skills	*half*
Tens and ones concept	Multiplication is repeated addition
Term *more than*	Division is the converse of addition
Indefinite quantifiers *a, both,* and *another*	
Problem-solving goals	
Change problems:	
addition operation	subtraction and addition
neutral questions	start unknown
result unknown	distracting numbers
Combine problems	
addition operation	two-part classification
no extraneous information	neutral questions
one extraneous number	subtraction and addition
Compare problems	no distracting language or numbers
	subtraction and addition

operations should be used when initially increasing the conceptual and linguistic demands.

The best way to illustrate the process of individualizing objectives is to compare two different assessment profiles. As can be seen in Table 6.2, Karen's math skills are less developed than Mark's. Karen is learning how to solve *change* and *combine* problems without reliance on key words. Mark, on the other hand, is learning to solve *change* problems with irrelevant information presented and with unknown start quantities. Mark is also beginning to solve more complex *compare* problems and will not be encountering them with distracting information or distracting numbers. Individualized objectives can be set for each student with spina bifida by identifying the factors that interfere with the student's performance.

REMEDIATION ACTIVITIES

Remediating mathematic deficits in students with spina bifida entails placing heavy emphasis on activities designed to improve conceptual knowledge and problem-solving. When instruction focuses on mastery of facts and procedures, students are not likely to develop the needed higher level skills necessary for functioning in the real world (Schoenfeld, 1985).

The suggestions for remediating conceptual deficits presented in Chapter 5 can also be applied to the training of math concepts. Additional strategies for remediating conceptual and problem-solving deficits in students with spina bifida will be presented here. The remediation strategies include: calculating with manipulatives, reducing time constraints, increasing problem-solving opportunities, motivating problem-solving, and modeling problem-solving.

Calculating with Manipulatives

Manipulatives such as objects, counters, chips, blocks, or fingers help the child to visualize the mathematic process. The use of manipulatives when calculating gives the child perceptual data with which to form concepts. Purposeful, functional counting, comparing and contrasting sets of objects, and efficient counting strategies serve to establish numerical concepts (Baretta-Lorton, 1985; Ginsberg, 1989; Greeno, Riley, & Gelman, 1984; Groen & Resnick, 1977; Riley et al., 1983).

Reducing Time Constraints

Some students with spina bifida experience difficulty completing work under timed conditions (Stephens, 1985). Reducing the quantity and complexity of assignments is a suggested strategy for mainstreaming the student with spina bifida (Fay, Shurtleff, Shurtleff, & Wolf, 1985). In the area of math, rote calculation rather than true problem-solving is likely when time constraints are provided.

While mathematics instruction does include an area where speed of recall may be important (i.e., mastery of addition, subtraction, and multiplication facts) it must be remembered that memorization of facts is of no value if not combined with full conceptual knowledge. In addition, there is often a speed accuracy trade-off, with accuracy suffering at the expense of increased speed. And, in problem-solving, accurate comprehension of the problem is of far greater practical value than speed of calculation. Students with spina bifida, as well as adults, are likely to be at a greater disadvantage if they cannot solve real world problems than if they solve problems slowly.

Increasing Problem-Solving Opportunities

The teacher can improve problem-solving in the student with spina bifida by presenting many opportunities to engage in functional problem-solving throughout the day. Instructional activities that emphasize problem-solving are more important to the student's ability to function than activities that are based upon mastery of calculation facts and operations (Schoenfeld, 1985). Problem-solving can be tied to such naturally occurring events as organizing supplies, dispersing materials, preparing snacks, distributing papers, and creating craft projects (Van Brackle, 1989). Problem-solving can also be integrated into academic subjects such as reading and social studies. A dramatic increase in problem-solving opportunities can occur without sacrificing existing programs. The teacher can incorporate problem-solving into every event the student encounters. The following task options provide the teacher with a variety of mechanisms for increasing problem-solving opportunities:

1. *Estimating and predicting outcomes* Estimating and predicting outcomes permits the student to think about the problem and establish concepts without the pressure to calculate. An example of a problem that requires a student to predict an outcome is:

> We have 17 cups. Two of the cups leak. Will we have enough cups that won't leak for every member of our class?

2. *Representing problem situations* A task that facilitates problem-solving is the representation of a problem situation with drawings or manipulatives. Given a set of blocks or tokens, the student can be presented with such directions as:

> Mary and Susan are building with blocks. Mary made a tower that is half as tall as Susan's tower. Susan's tower was made with ten blocks. Show me with these blocks what Mary's and Susan's towers look like.

Many remediation programs advocate giving students experience representing problem situations (Cawley et al., 1979; Fuson & Willis, 1989; Goodstein, 1974, 1981; Silbert et al., 1981). Manipulatives, drawings, graphs, and schematic representations all aid the problem-solving process (Montague, 1991; Pea, 1987). Dunlap and Brennan (1979) specified a set of guidelines for using manipulatives in teaching students with learning disabilities. These guidelines may also be used to help the student with spina bifida progress from concrete to abstract levels of representation. Mechanisms to represent problems are illustrated in Figure 6.1 and in Greeno (1987a), Rathnell and Huinker (1989), and Resnick and Ford (1981).

3. *Identifying missing, irrelevant, or erroneous information* Asking the student with spina bifida questions about the problem situation will activate decision-making. Consider the types of questions that can be asked about the following problem:

> Jeff and Mary were drawing pictures. They were using two pieces of paper. They both drew a tree and some houses. How many trees did they draw? How many objects did they draw? Do we know how many houses the children drew? Do we need to know how many pieces of paper the clinician used?

Teaching children to ignore irrelevant information ensures that students are engaged in the analysis of the problem (De Corte & Verschaffel, 1981; Greeno, 1987b). Programs such as those advocated by Cawley et al. (1979) and Goodstein (1974, 1981) advocate alerting students to the presence of

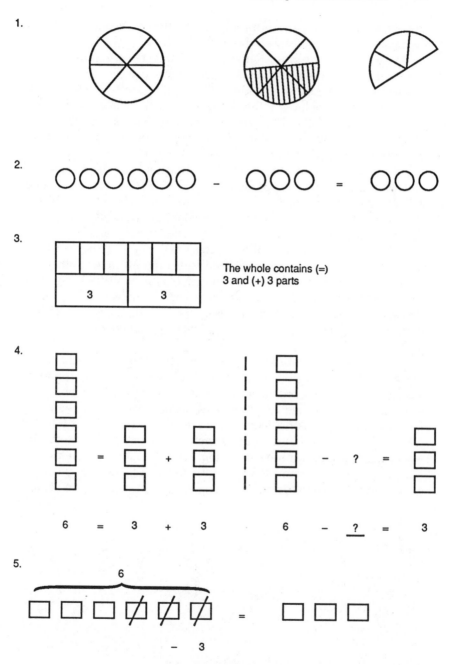

Figure 6.1. Examples representing the problem 6 − 3 = 3.

irrelevant information and providing them with practice in identifying pertinent objects and events in problem situations.

4. *Retelling problems* Requesting the student with spina bifida to paraphrase problems will place a demand on active processing of the problem situation. Learning mathematics requires an understanding of concepts and procedures rather than a verbatim repeating of verbal statements (Davis, 1984). The more experience a child has in conveying a problem in his or her own words, the less likely he or she will be to calculate rotely (Montague, 1991).

5. *Solving real-world problems* Throughout the day, real-world problems can be presented or created (Lappan & Schram, 1989). Before going to the lunchroom, the teacher may want to know which students already know what they are going to have for lunch and which students buy their lunch versus bring their lunch. The teacher can use the students themselves to compare the students who know what they will have with the students who have not yet decided. For more advanced students, the teacher can determine the percentage of students who bring their lunch. Real problem-solving events can serve to activate the learning process in the student with spina bifida. The cartoon in Figure 6.2 illustrates the importance of providing students with functional reasons to problem solve.

6. *Solving story problems* Story problems can be created to meet the needs of each individual student. A file of developmentally appropriate and relevant story problems can be kept on hand or story problems can be made up spontaneously. Problems can be created from interesting pictures, story books, or objects that are readily on hand (Irons & Irons, 1989). Minor modifications in the structure of story problems can be made to individualize problem-solving demands. Story problems can easily be generated from such relevant stimuli as interesting pictures, stories from the student's texts, cartoons, bulletin boards, and school

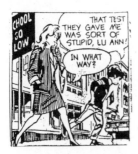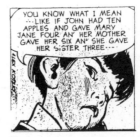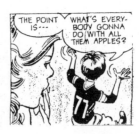

Figure 6.2.   Illustration of why word problems should be relevant to the student.(Copyright © 1992 by North America Syndicate, Inc. World rights reserved. Reprinted with special permission of North America Syndicate.)

events. A critical review of commercially available tools will also yield some useful resources. Cawley et al. (1979) provided examples of story problems that place heavy emphasis on comprehension of the problem situation.

Modeling Problem-Solving

Modeling problem-solving entails demonstrating decision-making, representation of the problem, and active rehearsal. Modeling techniques are designed to improve the student's ability to comprehend the problem situation and to keep relevant problem information active in working memory.

1. *Decision making* To model active decision making, the teacher should verbally direct the student through the problem-solving process. The teacher should prompt the student to identify relevant information and to identify the conceptual structure of the problem (Hyde & Hyde, 1991). Consider the following *change* problem with a subset of unknown quantity:

> John was playing a game with marbles. John had six marbles in his game. Some of John's marbles rolled under the couch. Then he had three marbles. How many marbles rolled away?

With the supplement of visual aids, the teacher could explain the problem-solving process in the following manner:

> John started with six marbles. Six marbles is all the marbles John had. The six marbles is the whole group of marbles that John had. Then John lost some of his marbles. A part of his marbles rolled under the couch. We don't know yet how many marbles rolled under the couch, but we do know that John had three marbles left. Part of John's marbles are under the couch and three of his marbles are still with his game. The marbles under the couch and the marbles that he still has would make up the entire six marbles that he started with. If we subtract the three that he still has from the number in the whole group, we can find out how many are missing. The part under the couch and the part he still has would make up the entire six marbles.

Questions can be used to aid the child in deciding what information is relevant, how the sets of objects are related, and what information is missing (Nuzum, 1987).

2. *Representation of the problem* To aid in the representation of the problem, the teacher can demonstrate the use of symbols to re-create the problem situation. Many possibilities are available. These include: drawing pictures; creating the problem situation with blocks, toys, or other manipulatives; having the students themselves enact problem situations, and referring to the numerical equations (Hyde & Hyde, 1991).

Representation is important because it provides the student with the structure of the problem so that the appropriate problem-solving strategy can be selected (Resnick & Ford, 1981). Merely observing another person's representation of the problem has been shown to improve problem-solving performance (Ibarra & Lindvall, 1979). Lewis (1989) found that teaching students to represent problems was more effective than teaching students to focus on relevant statements within a problem.

3. *Active rehearsal*   To aid the memory and rehearsal process, the teacher should slow his or her speech and frequently repeat the problem situation. Frequent repetition keeps the problem active in the student's working memory. The teacher should present the problem in several alternative ways, always being alert to adjust the complexity of the language he or she uses in order to ensure comprehension.

It may be of interest to note that the teacher can model decision-making, representation, and rehearsal without requiring the student to solve the problem. It may not be essential for the student to solve the problem as long as he or she is actively attending to and comprehending the problem-solving process. The teacher could present a problem such as the following:

> We usually have more students who want chocolate milk than white milk. I have a feeling that today will be different. Let's see if I'm right. We have seven students who want white milk and the rest want chocolate milk. There are 18 students in the class. Let's figure out if today we have more students who want white milk.

The teacher proceeds to repeat the problem while altering the language, drawing pictures, representing the situation with blocks, and asking questions to guide the process.

Motivating Problem-Solving

Techniques for motivating students to problem-solve include: personalizing the problem, modeling interest in problem-solving, and using a variety of novel objects.

1. *Personalizing and communicating about problems*   The best technique for motivating problem-solving is to tie problem-solving to the student's own needs, desires, experiences, and possessions. Often problem-solving cannot occur unless or until the student perceives the problem as being relevant. Personalizing problem-solving can also occur when the teacher shares his or her own problems. Students are often interested in the lives of their teachers. Students' active identification and discussing problems and solutions with their teachers is critical to meaningful problem-solving (Ginsberg, 1989; Irons & Irons, 1989; Lappan & Schram, 1989; Steffe & Wood, 1990).

2. *Modeling interest in problem-solving* When a teacher models interest in the problem-solving process, he or she becomes emotionally involved in the problem. He or she could be curious to find out how many baseball cards the students have or eager to know if there are enough nuts to be divided equally among the students. The teacher could also be worried that there will not be enough cookies for the class and disappointed upon discovering that one-fourth of the pieces of chalk in a new box are broken. The teacher could also provide a verbal explanation for why the problem is interesting or important to solve. For example, the teacher could state that he or she would not want to have to carry around the janitor's keys because he has so many. The teacher could proceed to wonder how many keys the janitor has on his key ring and how many keys he could eliminate. The teacher could wonder how much each key weighs and how much the key ring would weigh if he eliminated all non-essential keys.

3. *Presenting novel objects* Novel objects are often inherently reinforcing. Available options for functionally relevant and desirable objects include: toys, personal belongings, school materials, things on the teacher's desk, refreshments, stones in the school yard, and steps in the school. The objects being calculated should change frequently so that novelty and variety are maintained.

Facilitating math development in the student with spina bifida entails manipulating conceptual and linguistic demands of the problems the student encounters. Activities to improve math include: increasing the frequency with which the student encounters real-world problems to solve, motivating problem-solving, and demonstrating problem-solving strategies. This remediation process will be most effective if members of the educational team engage in a concerted coordinated effort to improve the problem-solving skills of the student with spina bifida. The speech-language pathologist may be helpful in dealing with the conceptual and linguistic factors that may influence performance in individual students with spina bifida.

SUMMARY AND CONCLUSION

This chapter outlined variables that influence mathematic performance in students with spina bifida. Each of the variables can be manipulated in assessing and facilitating problem-solving skills. The student's educational program should place heavy emphasis on teaching concepts and facilitating problem-solving. The educational team should specifically structure an individualized program for the student with spina bifida with coordinated objectives and strategies. Every effort should be made to involve the parents in the remediational process. Most important, problem-solving should be made functional and relevant to the student. The primary objective in developing an education program is to ensure that mathematic skills can be used to meet functional real-world demands.

GLOSSARY

Calculation   Process of obtaining a result by using mathematical procedures.

Cardination   Correspondence between numbers and their numerical equivalences. The set value of numerals (e.g., the cardinal number 5 refers to five objects in a set.

Change problem   Problem that incorporates an action that results in an increase or decrease in the total number of objects in a set.

Coded: Put in the form of symbols.

Combine problem   Problem in which subsets of objects are combined into generic categories.

Compare problem   Problem that contains two sets of objects that are compared in number.

Conceptual knowledge   Knowledge of the similarities that exist in groups of objects and events in the environment. Knowledge of the functions of objects and events and of their associations.

Conservation   Concept that two equal quantities stay the same regardless of changes in shape or position.

Deficit   Lack or deficiency in abilities in a particular area.

Differential performance   Performing different tasks with different ability levels: for example, a child's performance on one type of math problem may be different (better or worse) than his performance on another type of math problem.

Extraneous information   Content that is not needed to solve a math problem.

Generic categories   Categories that are inclusive. Referring to a whole kind, class, or group; general, for example, birds, animals.

Indefinite quantifier   Refers to an unspecified quantity (e.g., each, every, both, and all).

Irrelevant language   Language in a word problem that is not necessary to understand or solve the problem.

Irrelevant quantities   Amounts presented in a word problem that are not needed to derive the answer to the problem.

Linguistic factors   Aspects of language that are used to form word problems. Word problems vary in complexity of syntax, vocabulary, and sentence length. Problems are more or less difficult depending on the complexity of the language they use.

Linguistic inferences   Drawing conclusions about information that is not explicitly stated. In a word problem, a child must infer that words such as "borrow," "crumbled," or "ripped" can imply a decrease in number.

Manipulatives   Perceptual cues that give the child visual information when solving word problems. Examples are: fingers, chips, blocks, or counters.

Matrix programming   Strategy for the remediation of math difficulties. Specific goals are developed by determining how conceptual and linguistic factors will be combined.

Missing information   Information essential to solving a problem that is not specified in the problem.

Modeling   Procedure for inducing a student to develop a behavior through imitation.

Natural language   Word problems that present information in a variety of ways. Natural language problems use everyday descriptions rather than relying on a few standard mathematical expressions. To comprehend problems presented in natural language, a child must know that the same meaning can be signaled in several different ways.

Neutral questions   Questions used in word problems that eliminate key words or phrases such as "remain," "all together," or "take away." In problems with neutral questions the selection of the appropriate procedure is not specified.

Numerical relationship   Relationship expressed by numbers.

Ordination   Showing the order of anything in a series (e.g., first, second, third, fourth). Knowledge of the ordered values of numbers (e.g., 4 is larger than 3 and smaller than 5).

Perceptual cues   Support, prompts, or visual clues that aid the student in identifying the meaning of a word.

Problem-solving   Act of finding a solution to a proposed question.

Quantifier terms   Words expressing amounts (e.g., *five, twenty, a few, more*).

Quantitative relationship   Relationship in a word problem that is expressed by numbers or symbols.

Quantities   Thing that has the property of being measurable in dimension or amount.

Result quantity   In a word problem, the end result or amount.

Rote calculation   Impulsive adding or subtracting of numbers without determining which operation should be used or which numbers should be included in the calculation process.

Start quantity   In a word problem, the initial number provided.

Subset quantity   In a word problem, each part of the whole quantity is labeled a subset quantity.

Unknown quantity   Information in a word problem that is not known.

Word problem   In math, a proposition requiring a solution by mathematical operations that is expressed in narrative or word form, rather than numbers.

REFERENCES

Agness, P.J. (1983). *Learning disabilities and the child with spina bifida.* Chicago: Spina Bifida Association of America.

Andrews, M., & Brabson, C. (1977). Preparing the language-impaired child for classroom mathematics. *Language Speech and Hearing Services in the Schools, 8,* 44–53.

Badell-Ribera, A., Shulman, K., & Paddock, N. (1966). The relationship of nonprogressive hydrocephalus to intellectual functioning in children with spina bifida cystica. *Pediatrics, 37*(5), 787–793.

Baretta-Lorton, M. (1985). *Mathematics their way.* Menlo Park, CA: Addison-Wesley.

Blankenship, C.S., & Lovitt, T.C. (1976). Story problems: Merely confusing or downright befuddling? *Journal of Research in Mathematics Education, 7,* 290–298.

Brown, V.L., & McEntire, E. (1984). *Test of Mathematical Abilities*. Austin, TX: PRO-ED.

Carlson, J., Gruenewald, L., & Nyberg, B. (1980). Everyday math is a story problem: The language of the curriculum. *Topics in Language Disorders and Learning Disabilities, 1*, 59–70.

Carpenter, T.P., Corbitt, M.K., Kepner, H.S., Lindquist, M.M., & Reys, R.E. (1980). Solving verbal problems: Results and implications from national assessment. *Arithmetic Teacher, 28*, 8–12.

Carpenter, T., & Moser, J. (1982). The development of addition and subtraction problem-solving skills. In T.P. Carpenter, J.M. Moser, & T.A. Romberg (Eds.), *Addition and subtraction: A cognitive perspective* (pp. 9–24). Hillsdale, NJ: Lawrence Erlbaum Associates.

Carpenter, T., & Moser, J. (1983). The acquisition of addition and subtraction concepts. In R. Lesh & M. Landau (Eds.) *Acquisition of mathematic concepts and processes* (pp. 7–44). New York: Academic Press.

Cawley, J.F., Fitzmaurice, A.M., Shaw, R.A., Kahn, H., & Bates, H. (1979). Math word problems: Suggestions for LD students. *Learning Disability Quarterly, 2*, 25–41.

Cawley, J., & Vitello, S. (1972). Model for arithematical programming for handicapped children. *Exceptional Children, 39*, 101–110.

Connolly, A.J. (1985). *Key Math Diagnostic Arithmetic Test*. Circle Pines, MN: American Guidance Services.

Connolly, A.J., Nachtman, W., & Pritchett, E. (1971). *Key Math Diagnostic Arithmetic Test*. Circle Pines, MN: American Guidance Services.

Davis, R. (1984). *Learning mathematics: The cognitive science approach to mathematics education*. Norwood, NJ: Ablex.

Dean, A.L., Chabaud, S., & Bridges, E. (1981). Classes, collections, and distinctive features: Alternative strategies for solving inclusion problems. *Cognitive Psychology, 12*, 84–112.

De Corte, E., & Verschaffel, L. (1981). Children's solution process in elementary arithmetic problems. *Journal of Educational Psychology, 73*, 765–779.

DeVincenzo-Gavioli, M. (1983). Diagnosing student error patterns. In G. Shufelt (Ed.). *Agenda in action* (pp. 163–168). Reston, VA: National Council of Teachers of Mathematics.

Diller, L., Gordon, W.A., Swinyard, C.A., & Kastner, S. (1969). *Psychological and educational studies in spina bifida children* (Project No. 5–0412). Washington, DC: United States Department of Health, Education and Welfare (Office of Education).

Dunlap, W., & Brennan, A. (1979). Developing mental images of mathematical processes. *Learning Disabilities Quarterly, 2*, 89–96.

Englert, C. S., Culatta, B., & Horn, D. (1987). Mathematic problem solving in children with learning disabilities. *Learning Disabilities Quarterly, 1*, 29–36.

Fay, G., Shurtleff, D., Shurtleff, H., & Wolf, L. (1985). Developmental expectations: Intelligence and fine motor skills. In D. Shurtleff (Ed.), *Myelodysplasias and exstrophies: Significance, prevention and treatment* (pp. 373–396). New York: Grune & Stratton.

Fuson, K.C., & Willis, G.B. (1989). Second grader's use of schematic drawings in solving addition and subtraction word problems. *Journal of Educational Psychology, 4*, 514–520.

Ginsberg, H.P. (1989). *Need for concrete experiences. Children's Arithmetic: How they learn it and how you teach it*. Austin, TX: PRO-ED.

Goodstein, H. (1981). Are the errors we see the true errors? Error analysis in verbal problem solving. *Topics in Learning & Learning Disabilities, 13*, 31–45.

Goodstein, H.A. (1974). Solving the verbal mathematics problem: Visual aids + teacher planning = the answer. *Teaching Exceptional Children, 6*, 178–184.

Greeno, J. (1987a). Instructional representations based on research about understanding. In A. Schoenfeld (Ed.), *Cognitive science and mathematics education* (pp. 69–98). Hillsdale, NJ: Lawrence Erlbaum Associates.

Greeno, J. (1987b). A study of problem solving. In R. Glasser (Ed.), *Advances in instructional psychology*. Hillsdale, NJ: Lawrence Erlbaum Associates.

Greeno, J.G. (1991). A view of mathematical problem solving in school. In M. Smith (Ed.), *Toward a unified theory of problem solving* (pp. 69–98). Hillsdale, NJ: Lawrence Erlbaum Associates.

Greeno, J., Riley, M., & Gelman, R. (1984). Conceptual competence and children's counting. *Cognitive Psychology, 16*, 94–143.

Groen, G., & Resnick, L. (1977). Can preschool children invent addition algorithms? *Journal of Educational Psychology, 69*, 645–652.

Gruenewald, L., & Pollak, S. (1984). *Language interaction in teaching and learning*. Baltimore: University Park Press.

Gruenewald, L., & Pollak, S. (1990). *Language interaction in curriculum and instruction* (2nd ed.). Austin, TX: PRO-ED.

Hurley, A., Dorman, C., Laatsch, L., Bell, S., & D'Avignon, J. (1990). Cognitive functioning in patients with spina bifida, hydrocephalus, and the "cocktail party" syndrome. *Developmental Neuropsychology, 6*, 151–172.

Hyde, A.A., & Hyde, P.R. (1991). *Mathwise: Teaching mathematical thinking and problem solving*. Portsmouth, NH: Heinemann.

Ibarra, C., & Lindvall, C. (1979, April). *An investigation of factors associated with children's comprehension of simple story problems involving addition and subtraction prior to formal instruction on these operations*. Paper presented at the annual meeting of the National Council of Teachers of Mathematics, Boston.

Irons, R.R., & Irons, C.J. (1989). Language experiences: A base for problem solving. In P.R. Trafton & A.P. Shulte (Eds.), *New directions for elementary school mathematics* (pp. 85–98). Reston, VA: National Council of Teachers of Mathematics.

Jastak, S., & Wilkinson, G.S. (1984). *Wide Range Achievement Test—Revised*. Wilmington, DE: Jastak Associates.

Lappan, G., & Schram, P.W. (1989). Communication and reasoning: Critical dimensions of sense making in mathematics. In P.R. Trafton & A.P. Shulte (Eds.), *New directions for elementary school mathematics* (pp. 14–30). Reston, VA: National Council of Teachers of Mathematics.

Levy, W., & Schenck, S. (1981). The interactive effect of arithmetic and various reading formats upon the verbal problem solving performance of learning disabled children. *Focus on Learning Problems in Mathematics, 3*, 5–10.

Lewis, A.B. (1989). Training students to represent arithmetic word problems. *Journal of Educational Psychology, 81*, 521–531.

Lindquist, M.M. (1989). It's time to change. In P.R. Trafton & A.P. Shulte (Eds.), *New directions for elementary school mathematics* (pp. 1–13). Reston, VA: The National Council of Teachers of Mathematics.

Mattson, B. (1982). Learning problems of children with spina bifida. *Clinical Proceedings: Children's Hospital National Medical Center, 8*, 225–230.

Montague, M. (1991). Teaching verbal mathematical problem solving skills to students. In C. Simon (Ed.), *Communication skills and classroom success* (pp. 434–442). Eau Claire, WI: Thinking Publications.

Nesher, P., & Teubal, E. (1975). Verbal cues and an interfering factor in verbal problem solving. *Educational Studies, 6*, 41–51.

Nuzum, M. (1987). Cognitive technologies for mathematics education. In A.

Schoenfeld (Ed.), *Cognitive science and mathematics education*. Hillsdale, NJ: Lawrence Erlbaum Associates.

Pea, R. (1987). Cognitive technologies for mathematics education. In A. Schoenfeld (Ed.), *Cognitive science and mathematics education* (pp. 89–122) Hillsdale, NJ: Lawrence Erlbaum.

Rathnell, E.C., & Huinker, D.M. (1989). Using "part-whole" language to help children represent and solve word problems. In P.R. Trafton & A.P. Shulte (Eds.), *New directions for elementary school mathematics* (pp. 99–110). Reston, VA: National Council of Teachers of Mathematics.

Resnick, L. (1983). A developmental theory of number understanding. In H. Ginsburg (Ed.), *The development of mathematical thinking* (pp. 109–151). New York: Academic Press.

Resnick, L., & Ford, W. (1981). *The psychology of mathematics instruction*. Hillsdale, NJ: Lawrence Erlbaum Associates.

Riley, M., Greeno, J., & Heller, J. (1983). Development of children's problem solving ability in arithmetic. In H. Ginsberg (Ed.), *The development of mathematical thinking* (pp 153–196). New York: Academic Press.

Shaffer, J., Wolf, L., Friedrich, W., Shurtleff, H., Shurtleff, D., & Fay, G. (1986). Developmental expectations: Intelligence and fine motor skills. In D. Shurtleff (Ed.), *Myelodysplasias and exstrophies: Significance, prevention, and treatment*. New York: Grune & Stratton.

Schoenfeld, A. (1985). *Mathematical problem solving*. New York: Academic Press.

Silbert, J., Carnine, D., & Stein, M. (1981). *Direct instruction mathematics*. Columbus, OH: Charles E. Merrill.

Silver, E. (1981). Recall of mathematical problem information: Solving related problems. *Journal of Research in Mathematics Education, 12*, 54–64.

Spain, B. (1974). Verbal and performance ability in preschool children with spina bifida. *Developmental Medicine and Child Neurology, 16*, 773–780.

Steffe, L.P., & Wood, T. (1990). An analysis of first-grade children's writing number sentences in solving word problems. *Transforming Children's Mathematics Education*. Hillsdale, NJ: Lawrence Erlbaum Associates, 143–155.

Stephens, S. (1985). *Educating the student with spina bifida*. Austin, TX: Spina Bifida Association of Texas.

Tew, B., & Laurence, K.M. (1972). The ability and attainment of spina bifida patients born in South Wales between 1956–1962. *Developmental Medicine and Child Neurology, 15*, 124.

Tew, B., & Laurence, K.M. (1975). The effects of hydrocephalus on intelligence, visual perception and school attainment. *Developmental Medicine and Child Neurology, 17* (Suppl. 35), 129–134.

Tew, B., & Laurence, K.M. (1984). The relationship between intelligence and academic achievements in spina bifida adolescents. *Zeitschrift fur Kinderchirurgie, 39* (Suppl. 2), 122–124.

VanBrackle, A.S. (1989). Hidden mathematics lessons. In P.R. Trafton & A.P. Shulte (Eds.), *New directions for elementary school mathematics* (pp. 191–198). Reston, VA: National Council of Teachers of Mathematics.

VanDevender, E.M., & Harris, M.J. (1987). Why students make math errors. *Academic Therapy, 23*, 79–85.

Intervening for Language-Learning Disabilities

Barbara Culatta

Students with spina bifida are highly susceptible to learning disabilities (Agness, 1983; Mattson, 1982; Stephens, 1982; Tew, 1979; Tew & Laurence, 1975, 1984). Learning disabilities in students with spina bifida are evidenced by low achievement scores (Diller, Gordon, Swinyard, & Kastner, 1969; Tew & Laurence, 1972) and greater verbal than performance measures on intelligence tests (Badell-Ribera, Shulman, & Paddock, 1966; Halliwell, Carr, & Pearson, 1980; Lonton, 1979; Powers & Range, 1990; Shaffer, Friedrich, Shurtleff, & Wolf, 1985; Tew & Laurence, 1975). In addition, learning disabilities in students with spina bifida are evidenced by specific deficits in attention, perception, and language.

The particular pattern of learning problems in students with spina bifida presents educators with a paradox. Even though students with spina bifida perform better on verbal than performance measures of intelligence, deficits in verbal processes still exist (Shaffer et al., 1986). Concern has been expressed that certain verbal strengths actually mask significant verbal and perceptual deficits (Agness, 1983; Mattson, 1982; Stephens, 1985).

This chapter intends to lead educators to a better understanding of the language and learning deficits in students with spina bifida. It will provide mechanisms for identifying and assessing attentional, perceptual, and language processes.

ATTENTIONAL AND PERCEPTUAL DEFICITS

Attentional and perceptual deficits have been implicated in the learning problems of students with spina bifida (Laurence, 1971; Lollar, 1990; Mattson, 1982; Stephens, 1982; Williamson, 1987). Deficits lie primarily in the ability to maintain attention (attention span) and in the ability to focus on or isolate relevant from irrelevant stimuli (selective attention, figure/ground perception, or analytic perception).

Evidence of attentional and perceptual deficits in students with spina bifida comes from better verbal than performance intelligence test scores, significantly different performance on tests of attention and perception, and distractibility. Students with spina bifida have repeatedly performed below matched controls on selective attention, figure/ground, or embedded figures tests that require the student to focus on a particular target while ignoring irrelevant background stimuli (Hurley, Laatsch, & Dorman, 1983; Miller & Sethi, 1971; Sands, Taylor, Rawlings, & Chitnis, 1973; Willoughby & Hoffman, 1979). Culatta (1980) found that figure-ground perception served to differentiate students with spina bifida from mental age controls more than other measures of cognitive or language performance. Horn, Lorch, Lorch, and Culatta (1985) found that the presence of irrelevant background information interfered with attention to a relevant stimulus more in a spina bifida group than in mental age controls. These findings indicate that students with spina bifida exhibit difficulty attending to relevant stimuli or perceptually abstracting relevant from irrelevant stimuli.

While attentional and perceptual deficits are most notably identified by off-task behavior, short attention spans, and distractibility in the classroom (Hunt, 1981; Lollar, 1990; Stephens, 1982), formal tools for assessment are available. Tools for assessing attention and perception include:

Bender-Gestalt Test (Koppitz, 1960)
Children's Embedded Figures Test (Karp & Konstand, 1971)
Developmental Test of Visual-Motor Integration (Beery, 1967)
Gordon Diagnostic System (a computerized version of the Continuous Performance Test) (Gordon, 1983)
Marianne Frostig Developmental Test of Visual Perception (Frostig, Lefever, & Whittlesey, 1966)
Matching Familiar Figures (Kagan, Rosman, Day, Albert, & Philips, 1964)
Motor Free Visual Perception Test (Colarusso & Hammill, 1972)
Test of Visual Perceptual Skills (Gardner, 1982)
Visual Closure Subtest of the Illinois Test of Psycholinguistic Abilities (Kirk, McCarthy, & Kirk, 1968)
Visual Figure/Ground Subtest of Southern California Integration Test (Ayres, 1972)

In addition to using formal measures, observations are useful for identifying attentional and perceptual deficits. In particular, the *Diagnos-*

tic and Statistical Manual of Mental Disorders (3rd ed.) (*DSM— III*, 1980) of the American Psychiatric Association specifies behavioral characteristics of inattention, distractibility, and impulsivity that are useful in identifying attention deficit disorders. Chief among these are off-task behavior, greater need for supervision, and talking out of turn. The specific *DSM— III* criteria for diagnosing an attention deficit are:

1. Inattention (at least three of the following)—Often fails to do things he or she starts, often doesn't seem to listen, easily distracted, has difficulty concentrating on school or other tasks requiring sustained attention, has difficulty sticking to a play activity
2. Impulsivity (at least three of the following)—Often acts before thinking, shifts excessively from one activity to another, has difficulty organizing work, needs a lot of supervision, frequently calls out in class, has difficulty awaiting turn in games or group
3. Onset before age 7
4. Duration of at least 6 months
5. Not due to schizophrenia, affective disorder, or severe or profound retardation

It may be noted that the characteristics listed above often match teachers' descriptions of the classroom behavior of students with spina bifida.

To identify attention deficits in students with spina bifida, behavioral checklists may supplement the *DSM— III* criteria. These published checklists serve to behaviorialize inattention, impulsivity, and distractibility. While some of these checklists also include observations of hyperactivity, which are not applicable to the student with spina bifida, the components dealing with impulsivity, inattention, and distractibility are useful. Descriptions of rating scales found in Barkley (1990, 1991) and Kirby and Grimley (1987) are useful. These include:

Home Situations Questionnaire—Revised (DuPaul, 1990b)
School Situations Questionnaire—Revised (DuPaul, 1990b)
Child Attention Problems (Edelbrock, 1989)
Academic Performance Rating Scale (DuPaul, Rapport, & Perriello, 1990).
ADHD Rating Scale (DuPaul, 1990a)

In the absence of hyperactivity in the student with spina bifida, the diagnostic team may be able to rely on the presence of irrelevant, content-free speech as an additional indication of attention difficulty. Perhaps a high frequency of superficial talking, often referred to as "cocktail party syndrome," replaces hyperactivity as a reflection of an attention deficit. Students who have difficulty attending to or perceptually abstracting key aspects of events will have difficulty verbally relating those events. As a result, their communication may be shallow. In addition, superficial communicative interchanges may be used to avoid tasks that demand focused attention.

In summary, educators should be alerted to the possibility of a specific deficit in attention and/or analytic perception in students with spina bifida. The presence of distractibility, impulsivity, and hyperverbal speech may all be used as diagnostic indicators of cognitive deficits. In the case of suspected deficits, referrals should be made to the school psychologist or occupational therapist for a more extensive evaluation.

LANGUAGE DEFICITS

The language of students with spina bifida usually appears adequate upon initial inspection. Students with spina bifida tend to produce grammatically well-formed sentences, score well on tests of concrete vocabulary, and comprehend simple directions and statements (Parsons, 1968; Spain, 1974; Swisher & Pinsker, 1971). Despite these apparently good language skills, language deficits in students with spina bifida do exist. The particular pattern of verbal expression that appears in some students with spina bifida which was noted earlier has been referred to as the "cocktail party syndrome." The "cocktail party syndrome" consists of utterances that are frequently not related to the topic or context, expressions that are overused, and content that is superficial (Culatta, 1980; Fleming, 1968; Hagberg, 1962; Hagberg & Sjorgen, 1966; Ingram & Naughton, 1962; Schwartz, 1974; Stough, Nettelbeck, & Ireland, 1988; Swisher & Pinsker, 1971; Tew & Laurence, 1972). In addition to a unique pattern of verbal expression, students with spina bifida also exhibit deficits in abstract vocabulary and language comprehension (Williamson, 1987).

Because the language of students with spina bifida may appear to be adequate, an in-depth assessment of subtle language processes is essential (Dennis, Hendrick, Hoffman, & Humphreys, 1987). It is important to evaluate listening and reading comprehension, abstract concept knowledge, and narrative, conversational, metalinguistic, and problem-solving skills.

Listening Comprehension

While the student with spina bifida may have adequate comprehension of sentences, processing of connected passages and verbal problem-solving may pose some problems (Swisher & Pinsker, 1971). To evaluate comprehension of paragraphs and passages, tasks should be used that require the student to build meaning beyond the sentence level. The most commonly used tests for assessing language processing are those that require the student to comprehend stories. For example, in the Informal

Reading Inventory (Burns & Roe, 1989), stories are read to the student and he or she is required to answer questions about the information presented. The stories are presented in passages of increasing length and complexity. The student is asked questions about the events and is asked to make inferences about the information. One caution in evaluating story comprehension is that a student's performance on a story comprehension task, when the passages are presented orally, should be several grade levels above reading comprehension. Thus, a third grader who can comprehend only orally presented third-grade–level passages exhibits a delay in language comprehension. Another caution is that simple recognition of details may not be a sensitive indicator of story comprehension. Inference questions, however, that require the student to speculate how the information presented in the passage relates to real world experiences more directly address comprehension of the relationship among ideas.

Additional examples of tools for assessing story comprehension include: Classroom Reading Inventory (Silvaroli, 1986), Diagnostic Reading Scales (Spache, 1981), Basic Reading Inventory (Johns, 1981), Gray Oral Reading Test (Wiederholt & Bryant, 1986).

A student's ability to comprehend language can also be evaluated informally by using the language the student encounters in the classroom as stimuli. The student's comprehension of his or her own texts and of the teacher's explanations and directions can be assessed by asking the student to restate the message or by asking the student questions about the information. Several sources exist that provide mechanisms for assessing the demands of texts and materials relative to the comprehension skills of the child (Gruenewald & Pollak, 1990; Nelson, 1991; Wallach & Miller, 1988).

In addition to structuring informal tasks to assess the student's ability to process language, the teacher must be prepared to observe how the student responds to naturally presented language. The student with spina bifida may understand language more efficiently when the topic refers to a task at hand and when the complexity of the language is reduced (Williamson, 1987). Students with spina bifida may also perform better when demonstrations are provided, when repetitions are provided, and when speed of talking is reduced. An abnormal delay in responding to a message may indicate processing difficulty. In addition, the student who begins to respond before the message is completed may have learned to ignore verbal messages that are demanding to process. Impulsivity may be observed in response to complex verbal tasks and may signal comprehension difficulty.

Another clue that might signal a language comprehension deficit is what the student says in response to a preceding utterance. If a student has trouble understanding a message, he or she may agree with whatever the speaker says or may produce sentences that are not related to the topic at hand. A student who produces irrelevant remarks or changes the topic of conversation may be experiencing comprehension difficulty (Blank, Rose, & Berlin, 1978; Williamson, 1987).

When observing the student with spina bifida, note whether the student watches other students for performance cues. If the student is using contextual information to determine how to respond, he or she may not actually be comprehending the language. Care must be taken also not to attribute language abilities to the student who responds correctly to commands that he or she has heard in the past. Responses to commands such as "Raise your hand if you want white milk" can be made without processing the language. The student may be conditioned to respond to statements he or she has heard used in particular contexts. One teacher familiar to the author noted that a mainstreamed student with spina bifida, who was not making academic progress, had good language abilities. She observed that the student talked a lot and that he followed commands such as "Open your books to the story that we were reading yesterday" and "Sharpen your pencil." The teacher failed to notice, however, that he became confused when she presented more complex explanations or novel directions and that he had difficulty comprehending stories.

Reading Comprehension

Success in reading is tied to language comprehension because comprehension of written material also entails the ability to connect components of a passage, to make inferences, and to differentiate main ideas from supportive details. As with oral comprehension, students with spina bifida may have less difficulty comprehending isolated sentences than comprehending the relationship among elements in a passage. Many of the tests identified as being appropriate to assess oral comprehension are appropriate for assessing reading comprehension as well. One additional and particularly useful tool for evaluating the reading comprehension in students with spina bifida is the Analytical Reading Inventory (Woods & Moe, 1985). The Analytical Reading Inventory is useful because in addition to asking factual questions, it also asks inferential, cause-and-effect, and main idea questions.

Informal measures can also be used to assess comprehension more directly (Baker & Stein, 1981). The student's retelling of a story he or she has read may permit the teacher to determine whether the student identifies the main idea or presents relevant supporting detail. Stories presented in illogical order can be used to determine if the student can impose order and if the student recognizes incongruities in the passages. Inferential questions can always be devised by the teacher. If standardized materials do not ask inferencing questions, the teacher should be particularly alert to the need to make up his or her own.

In addition to formal measures of reading, an informal analysis of phonetic decoding skills can yield information that may be relevant to comprehension. Phonetic decoding that is particularly slow or laborious may impede comprehension. When the student's cognitive processes are tied up at the sound or word level, there may be limited resources available for identifying the connections among ideas or making inferences. Fey, Shurtleff, Shurtleff, and Wolf (1986) provided suggestions for informally evaluating the reading skills of students with spina bifida.

Metalinguistic, Metaphoric, and Problem-Solving Tasks

Metalinguistic, metaphoric, and problem-solving tasks require the student to reflect on or apply his or her knowledge of language. These tasks may be used to evaluate higher level language skills and include such items as identifying missing information, making judgments about correctness, and identifying absurdities. Some available tests include: Test of Problem Solving (Zachman, Jorgensen, Huisingh, & Barrett, 1984), Analysis of the Language of Learning (Blodgett & Cooper, 1987), Missing Elements Subtest of the Key Math (Connolly, Nachtman, & Pritchett, 1976), the Ross Test of Higher Cognitive Processes (Ross & Ross, 1976), Metaphoric Language Test (Burns, Halper, & Mogil, 1985), The Language Processing Test (Richard & Hanner, 1985), and the Word Test (Jorgensen, Barrett, Huisingh, & Zachman, 1981). Dennis et al. (1987) found that students with hydrocephalus performed less well than controls on metalinguistic tasks that require identification of anomalies. Hurley, Dorman, Laatsch, Bell, and D'Avignon (1990) found that children with spina bifida exhibited difficulty comprehending meanings that underlie metaphorical expressions such as "it's raining cats and dogs."

Narrative Skills

Narrative skills entail the ability to relate stories and to convey experiences, either in oral or written form. Narrative skills require the student to retrieve appropriate ideas from memory, organize them into themes, and sequence them in a logical manner. The student with spina bifida may have difficulty retrieving words and sentences and organizing them, particularly if the information being conveyed is removed in time and space. Observations of the student's spontaneous attempts to relate specific events can reveal a great deal about the student's narrative skills.

While it is possible to hazard a guess as to the appropriateness of a student's attempts to convey experiences, the best way to evaluate narrative ability is to know the event to which the student is referring. If the student is provided with an experience to relate, the teacher is provided with a way to evaluate the accuracy of the student's language. Ways of evaluating narrative skills include structuring novel experiences for the student to retell, asking the student to retell stories, asking the student to generate stories from sequenced pictures, and asking the student to create stories. The teacher can have the student participate in an unusual event and relate it to a listener who was not present. The experience can consist of teaching the student a magic trick, pretending to try out a new product, trading clothes, cleaning out a cupboard, creating a new game, and making Kool-Aid. While making Kool-Aid, the teacher can forget an ingredient, hide the needed container, stir with a ruler, taste the Kool-Aid without sugar, and pour it into a cup that leaks. In evaluating the student's version of the story or experience, the teacher should note if the student:

1. Includes all essential details and story components (describes the setting, the characters, the main events, the characters' reactions to the main events, the goals, and the outcome).
2. Organizes the information (places the events in the correct order).
3. Erroneously includes events that did not occur or repeats the same content (makes up things to say or relates only events that are routine).
4. Connects ideas (attaches pronouns to the appropriate nouns and uses connective words such as *but, since, if, then, so,* and *because*).

Furthermore, a speech-language clinician can conduct detailed analyses of student's narrative skills by applying story structure analyses and narrative analysis systems such as those described in Owens (1991) and Wallach and Miller (1988).

Conversational Skills

The best way to evaluate conversational skills is to observe the student participating in a variety of conversational exchanges with a variety of partners. Conversational analyses can then be applied to samples of actual conversations. While it should be within the realm of the speech/language clinician to actually perform such analyses, members of the educational team should be aware of the dimensions that constitute adequate conversational exchanges. Students with spina bifida have been observed to exhibit deficits in conversational skills, including:

1. *Frequently repeating the same content*   Topics discussed by students with spina bifida may be limited. The student with spina bifida may frequently repeat the same information (Schwartz, 1974). Relevant conversational exchanges may occur more frequently when the student is familiar with the topic.

2. *Difficulty maintaining exchanges about unfamiliar or remote events*   Students with spina bifida may maintain conversations by asking and answering questions. However, the number of back-and-forth

turns per topic may be limited. Conversational exchanges are also more limited when the topic is not familiar to the student. The more removed the topic is from immediate or personal experience, the more difficulty the student will have in maintaining the conversational exchange (Williamson, 1987).

3. *Difficulty elaborating or expanding the topic* The student with spina bifida may have difficulty extending topics. The student may have difficulty producing utterances that are related to the conversational partner's preceding statements. The student with spina bifida may not extend the established topic by adding new information (Williamson, 1987).

4. *Dominating the conversation* Students with spina bifida are likely to dominate the conversation and, therefore, adults may be impressed with their language facility. It is often easier to dominate the conversation than it is to respond relevantly and appropriately to the information provided by the partner. It is easier to control the topic than it is to follow the lead of a partner. The student with spina bifida may attempt to distract the teacher from a required task by maintaining a flow of inappropriate speech (Mattson, 1982).

5. *Changing the topic and introducing irrelevant statements* It is less demanding to introduce new information than it is to relate one's own statement to a prior remark. Because of the tendency to initiate conversations without addressing the information in the partner's preceding utterance, students with spina bifida have been described as "verbal noncommunicators" (Fey, 1986). The student may change the topic rather than comment on the partner's message. If a student does not know an answer or is presented with a difficult task, he or she is more likely to make irrelevant remarks (Mattson, 1982; Williamson, 1987).

It must be pointed out that an evaluation of conversational skills can be conducted only when considering the familiarity of the topic and context. Students with spina bifida have an easier time engaging in conversations about immediately present situations, about topics that are familiar, and about topics that they introduce.

Teachers may reflect on whether individual students with spina bifida present conversational deficits. Additional guidelines for identifying verbal deficits in students with spina bifida are found in Damico (1991) and in the appendix at the end of this chapter.

RELATIONSHIP BETWEEN
ATTENTIONAL, PERCEPTUAL, AND LANGUAGE DEFICITS

Attentional and perceptual deficits have been associated with the irrelevant/inappropriate use of language in students with spina bifida (Hurley et al., 1990; Shaffer et al., 1986). There are three possible explanations for related attentional, perceptual, and verbal deficits. The first explanation assumes that students with spina bifida use their expressive language to avoid perceptually complex tasks. When perceptual task demands are complex, the student may change the topic of conversation to terminate the activity. Kozbelt-Culatta (1975) observed that students with spina bifida changed the topic of conversation more frequently when perceptual task demands were difficult.

The second explanation for the inappropriate language in students with spina bifida pertains to their use of words without relation to their usual meanings. Culatta and Culatta (1978) proposed that for students with spina bifida the word itself is often more salient than the aspect of the environment it represents. The words used in inappropriate contexts were those that the students failed to identify on a subsequent comprehension test. Although particular classes of experience are usually learned in association with particular words, students with spina bifida may acquire the word without having a fully developed understanding of what the word means.

The third explanation assumes that relevant conversation is attentionally demanding and thus is beyond the capacity of some students with spina bifida (Foster, 1985; Williamson, 1987). Blank and Franklin (1980) suggested that a student who has difficulty maintaining attention will have difficulty following a topic and consequently will produce irrelevant responses rather than extending the topic. In addressing related perceptual and linguistic deficits in students with spina bifida, Culatta (1980) found a significant negative correlation between irrelevant utterances and performance on a test of attention and perception. As irrelevant utterances increased, attentional/perceptual performance decreased in a group of students with spina bifida.

A full understanding of how attention, perception, and language are related in students with spina bifida is not yet available. It seems, however, that language and attentional and perceptual remediation efforts should be tied together whenever possible. Educational programs should ensure that the student integrates language with sensorimotor experiences and that the student's attachment of words to perceptions is accurate. Language should be presented in direct, clear, one-to-one association with the perceptual array it represents.

INTERVENTION IMPLICATIONS

As noted in this chapter, the student with spina bifida is likely to exhibit specific learning problems in the areas of attention, perception, and higher order language processing. The student may appear to be functioning adequately, but in actuality may need special services. The members of the educational team should work together to make the proper assessment and remediation recommendations. Language-learning deficits should be addressed by the collaborative efforts of the occupational therapist, school psychologist, special educator, teacher, and speech-language clinician.

Appropriate remediation rests upon adequate assessment. Assessment should be conducted in order to determine the individual student's strengths and weaknesses. While patterns of performance have been observed in students with spina bifida, not all students exhibit the same deficits.

While individualized programming is essential, some general implications for intervention can be drawn. Suggestions for the teacher to manage attentional, perceptual, and language deficits in students with spina bifida follow.

Managing Attentional and Perceptual Deficits

Children with spina bifida often exhibit attention deficits which interfere with academic performance (Anderson, 1975). In the classroom they frequently are off task, talk out of turn, don't finish assignments, and need direction. One of the greatest challenges in working with students with spina bifida is to manage these behaviors. However, some of the traditional approaches (e.g., marking incomplete work wrong, having a student stay in during recess, or sending work home) may be counterproductive because they may negatively affect self-image (Todd, 1989). The approaches that are listed below have been suggested specifically for use with the student with spina bifida (Todd, 1989):

1. Frequently give the student positive reinforcement for completing work. Such reinforcers can include acknowledgments for completed assignments, friendly comments when staying on task, earned free time, and awards of stickers, privileges, or small prizes for completed work. The child can be given a selection of rewards to choose from and desirable tasks can be made contingent upon completing less desirable tasks.
2. Provide the child with subtle cues to refocus attention to the task at hand. Such cues can consist of gestures, eye contact, or a secret signal shared by the student and teacher. These are most easily presented when the child is seated close to the teacher. Constantly reminding the child to stay on task may be time-consuming and may draw unwanted attention to the child.
3. Provide the child with preferential seating. Distractions can also be reduced by assisting the child in keeping his or her own desk organized, having only one piece of paper out at a time, and using folders to separate completed from incomplete assignments.
4. Adjust time constraints and the amount of material presented at any

one time. The complexity of input and assignments may need to be modified (Agness, 1983; Fey et al., 1986; Stephens, 1985). Assignments that are too long can be broken into smaller units.

5. Provide as many hands-on learning experiences as possible. Limit the number of paper and pencil tasks and actively involve the child in the learning process.

6. Assist the child in controlling his or her own attentional resources. The student can help in developing goals and charting and recording progress. The student may also be reinforced for finding errors in his or other students' work.

7. Direct the child to important aspects of a task and make sure the child knows why he is engaging in it. Assist the child in identifying what needs to be done before rushing into an assignment. Repeat directions often.

8. Ignore irrelevant comments or limit the number of opportunities for speaking out. A "response cost" system of behavior management can be used in which the child is given a certain number of chances to ask questions or speak out. Each chance may be represented with tokens or check marks and the teacher gives the child a token or mark will be given for each talking-out-of-turn behavior. Privileges are lost when a certain number of tokens or marks has accumulated.

Two final notes of caution may be useful for the teacher. First, the teacher must be aware that success deprivation may interfere with performance. A child who is not successful in performing certain tasks will necessarily want to avoid them. Built-in opportunities for success can increase intrinsic motivation for a particular task or content. Second, the teacher should be relatively certain that the student is capable of doing the work and that he or she understands the task. Asking the child to retell the directions or explain the process may be helpful. It must be remembered that some students can mark responses on worksheets without understanding the principles underlying them.

Managing Language Deficits

In order to make additions to linguistic skills, children with spina bifida need frequent opportunities to relate descriptions of events to actual experiences. If reading a story about planting a garden, some actual experience with the planting process will connect the real event with its verbal description. Additional suggestions for improving language performance in students with spina bifida follow.

1. Comprehension of word knowledge should not be assumed. Because a student can understand a statement in a particular context

does not mean that the student has the ability to comprehend language in other situations or in the absence of visual cues.

2. Comprehension should be evaluated as an ongoing process. A child's comprehension of statements, explanations, and information can be assessed by asking the child to retell the information in his or her own words. Comprehension can also be assessed by asking the child to contrast the information given with known information about the world.

3. The teacher should adjust the level of complexity of input and reduce the complexity of task demands. Complex tasks should be broken up into smaller components.

4. The student should be given opportunities to retell and write about stories and events. Englert and Lichter (1982) provide guidelines for assisting the student's organization of retold events.

5. The teacher should demonstrate and illustrate the relationship between events and their verbal descriptions.

6. The teacher should demonstrate the meanings of words. Lots of exaggerated examples of word meaning should be provided. The teacher should use language the child knows to teach the meaning of new words, and should explain in simple terms the meaning of more complex words.

7. The teacher should gently direct the child's attention to the topic at hand. Reminders to stay on topic can include, "Remember, we're talking about ____," or "We're talking about ____ right now."

8. The teacher should make sure that the complexity of text materials fits the child's comprehension level. It is better to select texts that are below instructional level than above it, particularly when comprehension of connected passages is desired. Comprehension is achieved when the student can identify connections between ideas, state relationships between major topics and supporting details, make inferences between explicitly stated and implied information, and recognize inconsistencies or illogical sequences.

9. Opportunities should be provided for the student to engage in representational play and role-playing.

10. The teacher should specifically model problem-solving skills. The teacher should also present the child with opportunities to problem solve and make predictions about daily events.

11. The teacher should provide frequent references to the main idea of particular texts the child is reading.

12. The teacher should present novel, interesting things to talk about. Attempts can be made to carry out conversations about immediate events or commonly shared experiences.

13. The teacher may need to confine topics to events the child can per-

ceive and has experienced. Conversations can gradually become decontextualized; that is, they can begin to focus on events that are not immediately occurring or that have not been experienced. Additional suggestions for systematically introducing language that is removed from immediate experience can be obtained from the work of Marion Blank and her colleagues (Blank, 1983; Blank & Franklin, 1980; Blank & Marquis, 1987; Blank et al., 1978).

GLOSSARY

Attention span   Length of time an individual can actively focus on certain stimuli or aspects of experiences while inhibiting others.

Attentional deficits   Attention problems characterized by inattention, distractibility, impulsivity, and difficulty ignoring irrelevant background stimuli.

"Cocktail party syndrome"   Pattern of linguistic performance that is characterized by irrelevant expressions, overused statements, and superficial content.

Comprehension deficits   Having problems in the knowledge or understanding of verbal statements and passages.

Figure-ground perception   Ability to abstract or isolate one aspect of an event while ignoring irrelevant aspects of the event.

Inferencing questions   Questions that require one to infer the answer from information that is not explicitly stated; predicting outcomes or drawing conclusions.

Mental age (MA)   Intellectual age as determined by performance on a standardized test; usually expressed in months.

Perceptual abstraction   Separating key incoming sensory information from irrelevant sensory information; ability to single out and attend to one signal in the presence of other signals.

Perceptual deficits   Disturbances involving the interpretation of sensory information.

Performance intelligence score   Score received on subtests of an intelligence test that deal with nonverbal, perceptually based abilities.

Selective attention   Ability of the brain to damp down some information entering a given sensory channel while directing attention to other information entering the same channel.

Speech-language clinician   Professional trained specifically to diagnose and remediate speech and language problems.

Verbal intelligence score   Score received on subtests of an intelligence test that deal with verbal rather than nonverbal abilities.

REFERENCES

Agness, P. (1983). *Learning disabilities and the person with spina bifida*. Chicago: Spina Bifida Association of America.

American Psychiatric Association. (1980). *Diagnostic and statistical manual of mental disorders* (3rd ed.). Washington, DC: Author.

Anderson, E.M. (1975). Cognitive deficits in children with spina bifida and hydrocephalus: A review of the literature. *British Journal of Educational Psychology, 45,* 257–267.

Ayres, J. (1972). *Southern California Integration Tests.* Los Angeles: Western Psychological Services.

Badell-Ribera, A., Shulman, K., & Paddock, N. (1966). The relationship of nonprogressive hydrocephalus to intellectual functioning in students with spina bifida cystica. *Pediatrics, 37,* 787–793.

Baker, H.J., & Leland, B. (1967). *Detroit Tests of Learning Aptitude.* Indianapolis: Bobbs-Merrill.

Baker, L., & Stein, N. (1981). The development of prose comprehension. In C.M. Santa & B.L. Hayes (Eds.), *Children's prose comprehension: Research and practice* (pp. 7–43). Newark, DE: International Reading Association.

Barkley, R.A. (1990). *Attention deficit hyperactivity disorder.* New York: Guilford Press.

Barkley, R.A. (1991). *Attention deficit hyperactivity disorder; A clinical workbook.* New York: Guilford Press.

Beery K.E. (1967). *Developmental Test of Visual-Motor Integration.* Chicago: Follett Educational Corporation.

Blank, M. (1983). *Teaching learning in the preschool: A dialogue approach.* Brookline, Cambridge, MA.

Blank, M., & Franklin, E. (1980). Dialogue with preschoolers: A cognitively-based system of assessment. *Applied Psycholinguistics, 1,* 127–150.

Blank, M., & Marquis, A. (1987). *Teaching discourse.* Tucson: Communication Skill Builders.

Blank, M., Rose, S., & Berlin, L. (1978). *The language of learning: The preschool years.* New York: Grune & Stratton.

Blodgett, E., & Cooper, E. (1987). *Analysis of the language of learning.* Moline, IL: LinguiSystems, Inc.

Burns, M.S., Halper, A.S., & Mogel, S.I. (1985). *Clinical management of right hemisphere dysfunction.* Gaithersburg, MD: Aspen Systems.

Burns, P., & Roe, B. (1989) *Burns/Roe Informal Reading Inventory* (3rd ed.). Boston: Houghton Mifflin.

Colarusso, R., & Hammill, D. (1972). *Motor Free Visual Perception Test.* Novato, CA: Academic Therapy Publications.

Connolly, A.J., Nachtman, W., & Pritchett, E.M. (1976). *Key Math: Diagnostic Arithmetic Test.* Circle Pines, MI: American Guidance Services.

Culatta, B. (1980). Perceptual and linguistic performance of spina bifida hydrocephalic students. *Spina Bifida Therapy, 2,* 235–247.

Culatta, B., & Culatta, R. (1978). Spina bifida children's noncommunicative language: Examples and identification guidelines. *Allied Health and Behavioral Sciences, 1,* 22–30.

Damico, J. (1991). Clinical discourse analysis: A functional approach to language assessment. In C. Simon (Ed.), *Communication skills and classroom success.* Eau Claire, WI: Thinking Publications.

Dennis, M., Fitz, C.R., Netley, C.T., Sugar, J., Derek, C.F., Harwood-Nash, M.B., Henrick, L.B., Hoffman, H.J., & Humphreys, R.P. (1981). The intelligence of hydrocephalic children. *Archives of Neurology, 38,* 607–615.

Dennis, M., Hendrick, E.B., Hoffman, H., & Humphreys, R.P. (1987). Language of hydrocephalic children and adolescents. *Journal of Clinical and Experimental Neuropsychology, 9*, 593–621.

Diller, L., Gordon, W.A., Swinyard, C.A., & Kastner, S. (1969). *Psychological and educational studies in spina bifida students* (Project No. 5-0412). Washington, DC: United States Department of Health, Education, and Welfare (Office of Education).

DuPaul, G.J. (1990a). *The ADHD Rating Scale*. Worcester: University of Massachusetts Medical Center.

DuPaul, G.J. (1990b). *The Home and School Situations Questionnaires—Revised.* Worcester, MA: University of Massachusetts Medical Center.

DuPaul, G.J. (1990c). *Teacher Ratings of Academic Performance: The Development of the Academic Performance Scale*. Worcester: University of Massachusetts Medical Center.

DuPaul, G., Rapport, M., & Perriello, L. (1990). *Teacher ratings of academic performance: The development of the academic performance rating scale.* Unpublished manuscript. University of Massachusetts Medical Center, Worcester.

Edelbrock, C.S. (1989). Child attention profile. In R. Barkley, (Ed.). (1991). *Attention-deficit hyperactivity disorder: A clinical workbook.* New York: Guilford Press.

Englert, C.S., & Lichter, A. (1982). Using statement-pie to teach reading and writing skills. *Teaching Exceptional Children, 14*, 164–170.

Fey, M.E. (1986). *Language intervention with young children*. San Diego: College-Hill Press.

Fey, G., Shurtleff, D., Shurtleff, H., & Wolf, L. (1986). Approaches to facilitate independent self-care and academic success. In D. Shurtleff (Ed.), *Myelodysplasias and exstrophies; Significance, prevention and treatment* (pp. 373–396). New York: Grune & Stratton.

Fleming, C. (1968). The verbal behavior of hydrocephalic children. Studies in hydrocephalus and spina bifida. *Developmental Medicine and Child Neurology, 10*(Suppl. 15), 74–82.

Foster, S. (1985). The development of discourse topic skills by infants and young children. *Topics in Language Disorders, 5*, 31–45.

Frostig, M., Lefever, D.W., & Whittlesey, J.R.B. (1966). *The Marianne Frostig Developmental Test of Visual Perception*. Palo Alto, CA: Consulting Psychologists Press.

Gardner, M.F. (1982). *Test of Visual Perceptual Skills*. Seattle, WA: Special Child Publication.

Gordon, M. (1983). *Gordon Diagnostic System*. Dewitt, NY: Gordon Diagnostic System.

Gruenewald, L., & Pollack, S. (1990). *Language interaction in curriculum and instruction* (2nd ed.). Austin, TX: PRO-ED.

Hagberg, B. (1962). The sequelae of spontaneously arrested hydrocephalus. *Developmental Medicine and Child Neurology, 4*, 583.

Hagberg, B., & Sjorgen, I. (1966). The chronic brain syndrome of infantile hydrocephalus. *American Journal of Diseases of Students, 112*, 189–196.

Halliwell, M.D., Carr, J.G., & Pearson, A.M. (1980). The intellectual and educational functioning of children with neural tube defects. *Zeitschrift fur Kinderchirurgie und Grenzebiete, 31*, 375–381.

Hanner, M., & Richard, G.J. (1985). *Language Processing Test*. Moline, IL: LinguiSystems.

Horn, D., Lorch, E., Lorch, R., & Culatta, B. (1985). Distractibility and vocabulary deficits in children with spina bifida and hydrocephalus. *Developmental Medicine and Child Neurology, 27*, 713–720.

Hunt, G.M. (1981). Spina bifida: Implications for 100 children at school. *Developmental Medicine and Child Neurology, 23*, 160–172.

Hurley, A., Dorman, C., Laatsch, L., Bell, S., & D'Avignon, J. (1990). Cognitive functioning in patients with spina bifida, hydrocephalus, and the "cocktail party" syndrome. *Developmental Neuropsychology, 6*, 151–172.

Hurley, A., Laatsch, L., & Dorman, C. (1983). Comparison of spina bifida, hydrocephalic patients and matched controls on neuropsychological tests. *Zeitschrift fur Kinderchirurgie, 38j*, 116–118.

Ingram, T., & Naughton, J. (1962). Pediatric and psychological aspects of cerebral palsy associated with hydrocephalus. *Developmental Medicine and Child Neurology, 4*, 287–292.

Johns, J. (1981). *Basic Reading Inventory* (2nd ed.). Dubuque, IA: Kendall Hunt.

Jorgenson, C., Barrett, M., Huisingh, R., & Zachman, L. (1981). *The word test: A test of expressive vocabulary and semantics.* Moline, IL: LinguiSystems.

Kagan, J., Rosman, B.L. Albert, J., & Phillips, W. (1964). Information processing in the child: Significance of analytic and reflective attitudes. *Psychological Monographs, 78* (1, Whole No. 578).

Karp, S.A., & Konstand, N. (1971). *Children's Embedded Figures Test.* Palo Alto, CA: Consulting Psychologists Press.

Kirby, E.A., & Grimley, L.K. (1987). *Understanding and treating attention deficit disorder.* Terre Haute: Indiana State University.

Kirk, S.A., McCarthy, J.J., & Kirk, W.D. (1968). *Illinois Test of Psycholinguistic Abilities.* Urbana: University of Illinois Press.

Koppitz, E.M. (1960). The Bender-Gestalt test for children: A normative study. *Journal of Clinical Psychology, 16*, 432.

Kozbelt-Culatta, B. (1975). *The relationship among knowledge of concepts, sensory integration, and relevance of language in spina bifida children.* Unpublished doctoral dissertation, University of Pittsburgh, Pennsylvania.

Laurence, E.R. (1971). Spina bifida children in school—Preliminary report. *Developmental Medicine and Child Neurology, 44*, 71.

Lollar, D.J. (1990). Learning patterns among spina bifida children. *Zeitschrift fur Kinderchirurgie, 45* (Suppl. 1), 39.

Lonton, A.P. (1979). The relationship between intellectual skills and the computerized axial tomograms of students with spina bifida and hydrocephalus. *Zeitschrift fur Kinderchiurgie und Grenzebiete, 28*, 363–374.

Mattson, B. (1982). Learning problems of children with spina bifida. *Clinical Proceedings: Children's Hospital National Medical Center, 8*, 225–230.

Miller, E., & Sethi, L. (1971). The effects of hydrocephalus on perception. *Developmental Medicine and Child Neurology, 13*, 77–81.

Nelson, N.W., (1991). Teacher talk and child listening—fostering a better match. In C. Simon (Ed.), *Communication skills and classroom success* (pp. 78–105). Eau Claire, WI: Thinking Publications.

Owens, R.E. (1991). *Language disorders: A functional approach to assessment and functioning.* New York: Macmillan.

Parsons, J.G. (1968). An investigation into the verbal facility of hydrocephalic children, with special reference to vocabulary, morphology, and fluency. *Developmental Medicine and Child Neurology*, Suppl. 17, 109.

Powers, C.H., & Range, L. (1990). Hydrocephalic, dyseideidetic dyslexic, and low average regular children: Intellectual, visual-perceptual, and spatial reasoning performance. *Children's Health Care, 19*, 106–111.

Richard, G., & Hanner, M.A. (1985). *Language Processing Test.* Moline, IL: LinguiSystems, Inc.

Ross, J.D., & Ross, C.M. (1976). *Ross Test of Higher Cognitive Processes.* Novato, CA: Academic Therapy Publications.

Sands, P.L., Taylor, N., Rawlings, M., & Chitnis, S. (1973). Performance of children with spina bifida manifested on the Frostig Test of Visual Perception. *Perceptual and Motor Skills, 37,* 539–546.

Schwartz, E.R. (1974). Characteristics of speech and language development in the child with myelomeningocele and hydrocephalus. *Journal of Speech and Hearing Disorders, 39,* 465–468.

Shaffer, J., Friedrich, W.N., Shurtleff, D.B., & Wolf, L. (1985). Cognitive and achievement status of students with myelomeningocele. *Journal of Pediatric Psychology, 10,* 325–336.

Shaffer, J., Wolf, Friedrich, W., Shurtleff, H., Shurtleff, D., & Fay, G. (1986). Developmental expectations: Intelligence and fine motor skills. In D. Shurtleff (Ed.), *Myelodysplasias and exstrophies: Significance, prevention, and treatment* (pp. 359–372). New York: Grune & Stratton.

Silvaroli, N. (1986). *Classroom Reading Inventory.* Dubuque, IA: Wm. C. Brown Publications Co.

Simon, C.S. (1991). *Communication skills and classroom success.* Eau Claire, WI: Thinking Publications.

Spache, G.D. (1981). *Diagnostic Reading Scales.* Monterey, CA: CTB/ McGraw-Hill.

Spain, B. (1974). Verbal and performance ability in preschool children with spina bifida. *Developmental Medicine and Child Neurology, 16,* 773–780.

Stephens, S. (1982). Learning difficulties and children born with neural tube defect. *Spina Bifida Therapy, 4*(2), 63–76.

Stephens, S. (1985). *Educating the student with spina bifida.* Austin: Spina Bifida Association of Texas.

Stough, C., Nettlebeck, T., & Ireland, G. (1988). Objectively identifying the cocktail party syndrome among children with spina bifida. *Exceptional Child, 35*(1), 23–30.

Swisher, L., & Pinsker, E. (1971). The language characteristics of hyperverbal, hydropcephalic children. *Developmental Medicine and Child Neurology, 13,* 746–755.

Tew, B. (1988). Spina bifida children in ordinary schools: Handicap, attainment, and behavior. *Zeitschrift fur Kinderchirurgie, 43,* (Suppl. 2), 46–48.

Tew, B. (1979). The "cocktail party syndrome" in children with hydrocephalus and spina bifida. *British Journal of Communication Disorders, 14,* 89–101.

Tew, B.J., & Laurence, K.M. (1972). The ability and attainment of spina bifida patients born in South Wales between 1956–1962. *Developmental Medicine and Child Neurology, 15,* 124.

Tew, B., & Laurence, K.M. (1975). The effects of hydrocephalus on intelligence, visual perception and school attainment. *Developmental Medicine and Student Neurology, 17* (Suppl. 35), 129–134.

Tew, B., & Lawrence, K.M. (1984). The relationship between intelligence and academic achievements in spina bifida adolescents. *Zeitschrift fur Kinderchirurgie,* 39 (Suppl. 2), 122–124.

Thompson, N.M., Fletcher, J.M., Chapieski, L., Landry, S.H., Miner, M.E., & Bicby, J. (1991). Cognitive and motor abilities in preschool hydrocephalics. *Journal of Clinical and Experimental Neuropsychology, 13,* 245–258.

Todd, F. (1989, March). *He's so distractible: Attention deficits in children with spina bifida.* Paper presented at the Spina Bifida Association of Western Pennsylvania Educational Conference, Pittsburgh, PA.

Wallach, G., & Miller, L. (1988). *Language intervention and academic success.* Boston: College-Hill Press.

Wiederholt, J.L., & Bryant, B.R. (1986). *Gray Oral Reading Tests—Revised.* Austin, TX: PRO-ED.

Williamson, G.G. (Ed.). (1987). *Children with spina bifida: Early intervention and preschool programming.* Baltimore: Paul H. Brookes Publishing Co.

Willoughby, R.H., & Hoffman, R.H. (1979). Cognitive and perceptual impairments in children with spina bifida: A look at the evidence. *Spina Bifida Therapy, 2,* 127–134.

Woods, M.L., & Moe, A.J. (1985). *Analytical Reading Inventory.* Columbus, OH: Charles E. Merrill.

Zachman, L., Jorgensen, C., Huisingh, R., & Barrett, M. (1984). *Test of Problem Solving.* Moline, IL: LinguiSystems.

Guidelines for Identifying Language Deficits in Students with Spina Bifida

Certain observational guidelines exist for identifying language deficits in students with spina bifida. If a positive response can be answered to many of the following questions, a language deficit should be suspected.

1. Does the student have difficulty following complex and novel directions, understanding explanations, or obtaining information even though his or her knowledge of language rules (words and grammar) is adequate?
2. Does the student have more difficulty answering inferencing than factual questions?
3. Does the student have difficulty restating explanations?
4. Does the student require demonstrations in order to understand class directions?
5. Does the student frequently change the topic of conversation?
6. Does the student dominate the conversation?
7. Does the student frequently repeat the same idea or frequently relate the same event?
8. Does the student have more difficulty participating in a conversation when the partner introduces the topic?
9. Does the student have difficulty elaborating or expanding on the topic that has been introduced by the conversational partner?
10. Does the student have difficulty relating the various components of a story (setting, characters, initiating event, character's reactions, goals, plans, outcomes)?
11. Does the student have difficulty generating multiple examples of a word's meaning?
12. Does the student have difficulty connecting pronouns with the nouns to which they refer?
13. Does the student infrequently or inappropriately use connective words (*then, so, because, if,* and *therefore*)?
14. Does the student use words in limited or inappropriate contexts?
15. Does the student have difficulty detecting errors or misinformation in other people's speech?

16. Does the student have a limited ability to re-create elaborate themes in play or to take the roles of a variety of characters?

17. Does the student begin to respond before listening to directions or explanations?

18. Does the student require a long time to respond to directions (several seconds between presentation of directions and response)?

19. Does the student have difficulty attending to the speaker throughout presentation of verbal directions or explanations?

20. Does the student's facial expression fail to change with changing content in verbally presented stories, information, and explanations?

21. Does the student have difficulty answering detailed questions about information presented verbally?

22. Can the student respond to language better when the teacher reduces rate of speech, repeats, or breaks up information into smaller units?

23. Does the student have difficulty predicting the outcome of stories read to him or her, identifying story components that are out of sequence, or restating stories in his or her own words?

24. Does the student have difficulty identifying events when provided with a description of the event rather than the label?

25. Does the student have difficulty retelling novel stories told to him or her without the presence of pictures?

26. Does the student have difficulty detecting erroneous information presented in conversations?

27. Does the student have difficulty retelling a novel experience so that a naive listener can understand what happended? Does the student fail to include the details?

28. Does the student talk mostly about very familiar events?

29. Does the student have difficulty using his or her own words to retell directions or explanations during routine classroom activities?

30. Does the student have difficulty describing unusual or novel events?

31. Does the student have more difficulty staying on topic and responding appropriately when content is novel?

Working with Perceptual-Motor Skills

Mary A. Rogosky-Grassi

During the preschool years children compile a tremendous amount of learning. Each becomes aware of his or her body and its associated mobility. Along with gross motor coordination, fine motor coordination develops and most children are able to dress with clothing requiring buttons and snaps, cut with scissors, and copy letters and numbers (Banus, Kent, Norton, Sukiennecki, & Becker, 1979; Clark & Allen, 1985). Also, by the time they reach school age, most children have the ability to sit still, keep their attention on the teacher and follow directions. However, a significant number of students with spina bifida may not have achieved these developmental milestones by the time they are ready for school.

Due to physical limitations, adaptations to the school environment are necessary to accommodate the student with braces and crutches and/or a wheelchair. Early in the school year, school personnel often focus on the accessibility of the school environment. Although accessibility is important, it is equally important to be aware of the learning factors that may affect the child's educational performance.

FACTORS AFFECTING LEARNING IN THE CLASSROOM

Children with spina bifida often exhibit poor upper extremity function, particularly in performance requiring fine motor skills (Anderson, 1976; Sand, Taylor, Hill, Kosky, & Rawlings, 1974; Shurtleff, 1986; Wallace, 1973; Williamson, 1987). Poor visual-motor (eye-hand) coordination interferes with the quality of upper extremity function (Shurtleff, 1986; Soare & Raimondi, 1977; Spain, 1974). Children with spina bifida are also likely to display neurological deficits, in the area of visual perception, that are complex and assume varied forms (Baron & Spiegler, 1982). Finally, many students with spina bifida have difficulty with organizational skills which affects classroom work and learning (Mattson, 1982). Although these deficits may decrease with age and with remediation, most will accompany the individual into adulthood (Wills, Holmbeck, Dillon, & McLone, 1990).

Because of the prevalence of learning deficits, children with spina bifida begin treatment at an early age in infant stimulation and preschool programs. Early identification is important in planning appropriate treatment. Continued assessment and treatment throughout the school years will enable these children to learn and function within the classroom. If these difficulties are not identified and treated, the students' learning problems will increase. They are then at risk for academic failure, frustration, and behavioral problems. Studies have shown that early remediation produces long range improvement in the ability to learn (Gluckman & Barling, 1980).

This chapter discusses the fine motor skills, visual-motor (eye-hand) coordination, visual perception, and organizational skills of students with spina bifida. The description of each area is accompanied by a set of suggested methods of assessment and intervention strategies.

Fine Motor Skills

The Nature of Fine Motor Performance Arm and hand movement allows us to reach, grasp, manipulate, and release objects in a coordinated manner. Therefore, we are able to utilize tools, for example, to pick up and position a pencil, and to perform written communication. The use of the upper extremities and the development of fine motor coordination depend on several factors, which include trunk stability, visual skills, visual perception, sensation, coordination of movement, and muscle strength (Williamson, 1987). The trunk acts as a stable base of movement for the arm as it moves to position the hand for activity. The hand provides information through the sense of touch and by manipulating the object. This manipulation requires coordinated movement of the hand to gather accurate information. Finally, there must be sufficient muscle strength to carry out the movements. Given this complexity, it should be no surprise that fine motor skills of the upper extremities can be affected by pathophysiological deficits such as poor trunk balance, visual deficits, loss of sensation, and muscle weakness (Shurtleff, 1986, chap. 16; Williamson, 1987).

Studies have shown a significant incidence of abnormal upper extremity function in children with spina bifida. Wallace (1973) found that 69% of 225 children participating in her study had abnormal upper limb function. These results were reproduced by Grimm (1976) who found that 82% of children with spina bifida had poor hand function, specifically fine motor skills (Anderson, 1976).

Sand et al. (1974) tested 25 children with spina bifida using the Developmental Hand Function Test (Jebsen, Taylor, & Trieschmann, 1969). The mean total score for this sample was approximately two standard deviations below the mean score of nonimpaired subjects. These results indicate an overt delay in hand function for children with spina bifida. Shurtleff (1986) also tested fine motor skill performance using the Developmental Hand Function Test. Ninety-four children with spina bifida were serially tested over a 10-year period. A high percentage of these subjects scored more than two standard deviations below the mean when compared with normal subjects.

Other factors that affect fine motor skills of the student with spina bifida are hydrocephalus, Arnold-Chiari malformation, and behavioral or environmental factors. Hydrocephalus and Arnold-Chiari malformation are discussed in detail in Chapter 1. These conditions may cause neurological deficits affecting upper extremity function. Development of fine motor skills of children with spina bifida is also delayed due to limited opportunities to practice hand activities (Turner, 1985). Throughout their early years, these children must use their hands for support and mobility, due to decreased lower extremity function, and may rarely have the opportunity to practice manipulation and coordination skills (Turner, 1986). These observations indicate that children with spina bifida are at continued risk for poor hand function.

Implications for the Classroom   In the classroom, poor fine motor skills may interfere with games requiring the use of the fingers and self-help activities such as buttoning. Important educational activities such as printing, cursive writing, and cutting with scissors are also adversely affected. Timed tasks, such as tests and seat work, are often difficult for those with poor fine motor control because they simply cannot write as quickly as the rest of the class (Ziviani, Hayes, & Chant, 1990). Students with spina bifida may not develop evenly spaced handwriting, and therefore their writing samples cannot be fairly compared with their peers.

Assessing Fine Motor Skills   Since the student with spina bifida is likely to have poor fine motor skills, it is important to obtain an accurate assessment of the student's upper extremities. This evaluation can be provided by an occupational therapist.

When assessing the child's skills, the occupational therapist will use standardized tests and observation. The therapist will ask the child to perform many school-related activities such as coloring and writing, cutting with scissors, manipulating pages in a book, and using a pencil sharpener. Standardized testing may include the motor items of the Gesell Developmental Scales (Knoblock & Passaminick, 1980), the Nine-Hole Peg Test (Kellor, Forst, Silberberg, Iversen, & Cummings, 1971), and the Vulpe Assessment Battery (Vulpe, 1979). These and other tests can be found in Table 8.1. The Gesell scales provide a qualitative measure of de-

Table 8.1.   Tests for perceptual-motor evaluation

Fine Motor Skills
Bruininks-Oseretsky Test of Motor Proficiency (Bruininks, 1978)
Gesell Developmental Scales (Knoblock & Passaminick, 1980)
Hawaii Early Learning Profile (Furuno et al., 1984)
Jebsen-Taylor Hand Function Test (Jebsen, Taylor, & Trieschmann, 1969)
Vulpe Assessment Battery (Vulpe, 1979)

Visual-Motor Skills
Beery Test of Visual-Motor Integration (Beery, 1982)
Frostig Developmental Test of Visual Perception (Frostig, Lefever, & Whittlesey, 1966)
Test of Visual-Motor Skills (Gardner, 1986)
Vulpe Assessment Battery (Vulpe, 1979)

Visual Perception
Frostig Developmental Test of Visual Perception (Frostig, Lefever, & Whittlesey, 1966)
Motor-Free Visual Perception Test (Colarusso & Hammill, 1972)
Test of Visual Perception Skills (Gardner, 1982)

velopment by age level. The Nine-Hole Peg Test is a quantitative measure of fine motor dexterity utilizing a timed task. The Vulpe Assessment Battery is used to assess the student's fine motor performance based on expectations for his chronological age.

After compiling test results and clinical observations, the therapist will have an accurate understanding of the student's strengths and weaknesses in fine motor skills. This is essential to help the student utilize his or her strengths and learn to improve or compensate for areas of poor function. The therapist and teacher can work together to develop a program to enable the student to function successfully in the classroom. In some cases, an occupational therapist may not be readily available in the school district to evaluate the student. A therapist can sometimes be obtained on a consultative basis to assess the student and set up a plan with the student's teacher. If, however, an occupational therapist is not available, it is still important to assess the student's skills. This service may be provided by another qualified professional such as a school psychologist.

Intervention Strategies   The following strategies will enable the student with poor fine motor skills to function more successfully in the classroom:

1. The student should always be well positioned during any classroom activity. The desk should be an appropriate height and the chair should be low enough for the child's feet to be positioned flat on the floor. If sitting balance is a problem, a chair with arms will provide more stability for the student. Proper seating, support, and balance free the arms and hands to achieve the best performance of tasks requiring fine motor skills.
2. Activities such as stringing beads, gluing small macaroni on paper,

playing with clay, and cutting with scissors help to improve fine motor coordination. Many of these activities can be performed during art classes. Older students may be interested in sewing, using a computer, playing board games, or assembling models or electronic projects.

3. Writing skills are difficult for the student with poor fine motor coordination. Often a thick grip pencil will give the student more control. The pencil size may be reduced as the student's fine motor skills improve.

4. Students with poor fine motor coordination often need additional time to complete timed tasks. An estimate of the student's speed should be made, and targets for completion time adjusted accordingly.

5. The older student may learn to type or use a word processor for lengthy assignments.

6. Good note-taking is virtually impossible for students with fine motor deficits. It is helpful for the student to obtain notes from the teacher or from a peer.

7. The use of a tape recorder during lectures can be a big asset for these students.

Visual-Motor Skills

Visual-motor skills or eye-hand coordination is the efficient use of the arm and hand for visually directed reach, grasp, and manipulation (Williamson, 1987). We have already discussed the importance of visual skills for adequate fine motor performance. Visual-motor skills guide hand movements by allowing the individual to see the objects before him or her, process the information, and direct the arm and hand to respond in a coordinated manner. This set of skills begins developing soon after birth and continues in a natural sequential pattern as part of the overall developmental process. The use of the hands in visual-motor activities begins when the infant learns to bang two objects together or to stack blocks. This process continues during the preschool years with activities such as coloring, drawing, and ball games. School-age children rely on eye-hand coordination to learn writing skills, both printing and cursive, and to participate in classroom tasks such as copying from the blackboard.

Children with spina bifida often have difficulty with eye-hand coordination. Studies have shown that 80%–90% of students with spina bifida exhibit delayed visual-motor skills (Culatta, 1980; Shurtleff, 1986). Factors that seem to affect visual-motor skills in children with spina bifida are hydrocephalus, Arnold-Chiari malformation (see Chapter 1), and lack of opportunity to practice appropriate eye-hand skills due to limited mobility.

Spain (1974) reports a delay in eye-hand coordination in children with spina bifida and hydrocephalus. In her study of 145 children, a significant percentage scored below average on a test of eye-hand coordination. Soare and Raimondi (1977) found that individuals with spina bifida and hydrocephalus performed poorly on perceptual-motor tests involving visual-motor skills. They suggested that this delay may be due in part to limited experiences as a result of time spent in the hospital and the child's physical limitations. Anderson and Plewis (1977) studied manual skills in 20 children with spina bifida, ages 7–10, and compared them with 20 able-bodied children. The task utilized was dotting between circles while speed and accuracy were measured. Children with spina bifida performed considerably more slowly than their able-bodied peers. Further observation during task performances revealed that children with spina bifida were more immature in pencil control and their movements were uncoordinated rather than smooth. Anderson and Plewis found that all the children in the study improved with practice. These results suggest that, although children with spina bifida exhibit poor manual skills, their abilities may improve with consistent practice.

Shurtleff (1986) evaluated 81 children with spina bifida using the Beery Test of Visual-Motor Integration (Beery & Buktenica, 1967). Of the total number of tests completed, only 42.7% of the scores were within one year of chronological age. These results verify that children with spina bifida frequently exhibit delayed visual-motor skills.

Implications for the Classroom In the classroom, poor visual-motor or eye-hand coordination may interfere with the development of writing skills, both printing and cursive (Ziviani et al., 1990). It can affect the student's ability to copy accurately from the blackboard or from a worksheet and can interfere with successful completion of drawing, tracing, and cutting activities. Poor visual-motor skills may also affect the student's performance on the playground and in physical education activities.

Assessing Visual-Motor Skills Since the student with spina bifida is likely to have poor or delayed visual-motor skills, it is important to obtain an accurate assessment of the student's abilities in this area. This evaluation can be performed by an occupational therapist.

When evaluating a student in the area of visual-motor skills, the occupational therapist will use standardized tests as well as observation during various activities. The therapist will observe the student's performance of many school-related tasks that require appropriate visual-motor skills. These activities may include writing and copying, tracing and cutting tasks, and play activities such as ball games.

The Developmental Test of Visual-Motor Integration (Beery & Buktenica, 1967) measures eye-hand coordination by asking the student to copy increasingly difficult geometric forms (Figure 8.1). These visual-motor skills can also be assessed using the Test of Motor Impairment

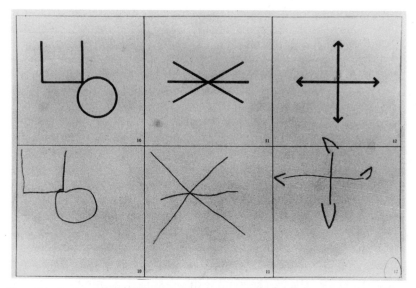

Figure 8.1. Test sample from Beery Developmental Test of Visual-Motor Integration. (From Beery, K.E., & Buktenica, N.A. [1967]. *The Developmental Test of Visual Motor Integration*. Cleveland: Modern Curriculum Press; reprinted by permission of Modern Curriculum Press.)

(Stott, Moyes, & Henderson, 1972) which measures motor impairment compared to able-bodied peers. The Vulpe Assessment Battery (1979) is used to assess the student's visual-motor performance based on expectations for his or her chronological age. These and other tests can be found in the appendix to this chapter. After compiling clinical observations and test results, the therapist will have an accurate understanding of the student's functional abilities in visual-motor skills. This is essential to help the student utilize his or her strengths and learn to improve or compensate for areas of poor function. The therapist and teacher can then work together to develop a program to fit the student's needs. As stated previously, if an occupational therapist is not available to work with the student and teacher, it is important to locate another qualified professional.

Intervention Strategies   The following strategies will enable the student with poor visual-motor skills to function more successfully in the classroom:

1. The student should always be well-positioned for any classroom activity. The desk should be an appropriate height with the chair low enough for the student's feet to be flat on the floor. If sitting balance is a problem, a chair with arms will provide more stability. The student with spina bifida requires a good seating arrangement to achieve the best performance of tasks involving visual-motor skills.

2. The student should be seated in the front of the classroom or close to the blackboard to minimize distractions and to provide a clear view of the teacher and the blackboard.
3. Because copying from the blackboard is a tedious task for students with poor eye-hand coordination, blackboard writing must be clearly written with obvious space between lines to aid the student in copying the material correctly.
4. Workbook material may need to be outlined or highlighted to enable the student to focus on the material and copy it correctly. Outlining and highlighting the material should be continued until the teacher is certain the student understands and can follow through without this aid.
5. Using a ruler to mark the line being copied will help the student copy the material correctly.
6. These students will need additional time to complete written work, especially timed tests and copying from the blackboard or a book.
7. The quantity of written work may need to be decreased for the student so he or she can keep up with classroom learning.

Visual Perception

Visual perception is the ability to recognize and understand what is seen. Visual perception requires the examination of an object, discerning the important features, and integrating and using the information meaningfully (Clark & Allen, 1985). It is the ability to recognize, interpret, and use visual stimuli by relating them to previous experiences (Anderson & Spain, 1977). Visual perceptual skills are needed for activities of daily living such as choosing one's clothing. It is visual perception that enables the student to recognize and use forms and symbols, such as letters and numbers, appropriately.

Visual perception requires visual acuity, ocular-motor control (eye muscle control), and a good attention span (Williamson, 1987). Visual acuity and ocular-motor control are obviously necessary for the eye to provide a good visual image. An appropriate attention span will enable the student to concentrate and focus on tasks. Finally, the visual input must be meaningfully interpreted and appropriately utilized. This complex process of visual perception is required for most classroom activities.

Studies have shown that individuals with spina bifida frequently have deficits in visual perception (Miller & Sethi, 1971; Sand & Taylor, 1973; Tew & Laurence, 1975). Tew and Laurence tested 59 children with spina bifida using the Wechsler Preschool and Primary Scale of Intelligence (Wechsler, 1967), and the Marianne Frostig Developmental Test of Visual Perception (Frostig, Lefever, & Whittlesey, 1966). They compared test results of these children to their normal peers. Children with spina bifida and hydrocephalus scored significantly below their chronological age on the Frostig test. Therefore, Tew and Laurence indicated that these children seem to have greater difficulty with visual-motor organization, which can interfere with learning.

Sand and Taylor (1973) evaluated 37 children with spina bifida using the Frostig test. Fifty-nine percent of this sample scored below average, with the most discrepant scores noted in the areas of eye-hand coordination and figure-ground perception. Sand and Taylor related these perceptual deficits to hydrocephalus as well as to decreased opportunities for learning due to lower extremity motor impairment. They recommended early perceptual assessment to assist with school programming.

Poor memory function has also been documented for children with spina bifida and hydrocephalus. Cull and Wyke (1984) reported impaired memory function in children with spina bifida and hydrocephalus, particularly in learning and recalling unrelated words. This type of deficit in learning verbal material is important since recall is often employed in the educational setting.

There are many different aspects of visual perception: figure-ground, form constancy, spatial relations, visual discrimination, and visual memory. Each of these visual perceptual deficits may reduce school performance. These aspects of visual perception are defined in the next section along with the discussion of their classroom implication.

Implications for the Classroom   *Figure-ground perception* is the ability to focus on relevant visual details. It allows a person to locate a form or object hidden by an extraneous background. It is the ability to identify and concentrate on important items by visually placing them in the foreground while those remaining are placed in the background. Figure-ground perception enables an individual to locate a white shirt lying on a white bedsheet, a specific book on a bookshelf, or a friend in a crowd of people. Students with figure-ground perception deficits may have difficulty focusing on the teacher in the classroom, locating appropriate books in a desk, or identifying an item in a picture with a distracting background (Figure 8.2). (See Hurley, chap. 4., this volume.)

Form constancy is the ability to see, remember, and locate a form in many different locations within the environment, even though it may be smaller, rotated, reversed, or hidden (Gardner, 1982). Students with poor form constancy may have difficulty learning letters and numbers, remembering words, and identifying shapes in different locations (Figure 8.3).

Spatial relations is the ability to perceive one's self in relation to one's surroundings and to identify objects in relation to one another. It is the ability to envision differences between objects. Students with this form of perceptual disturbance often have developed a poor understand-

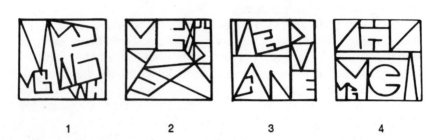

Figure 8.2. Test sample of figure-ground perception from Test of Visual Perceptual Skills (nonmotor). (From Gardner, M. [1982]. *Test of Visual Perceptual Skills [nonmotor] manual*. Seattle: Preston; reprinted by permission of the author.)

ing of the concepts of *in and out, under and over,* and *right and left.* A deficit in spatial relations causes obvious difficulties in classroom learning, particularly in following directions (Figure 8.4).

Visual discrimination is the ability to match similar characteristics of objects and therefore to locate identical items such as two nickels. Visual discrimination is important for developing an understanding of differences and similarities in the environment and the ability to classify objects in categories (Williamson, 1987). Students who have poor visual discrimination skills may be unable to group or classify objects into cate-

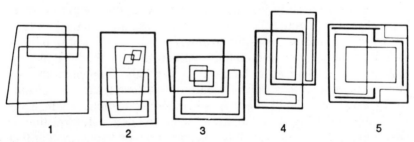

Figure 8.3. Test sample of form constancy from Test of Visual Perceptual Skills (nonmotor). (From Gardner, M. [1982]. *Test of Visual Perceptual Skills [nonmotor] manual*. Seattle: Preston; reprinted by permission of the author.)

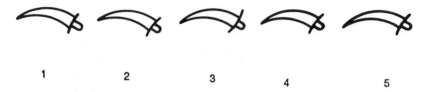

Figure 8.4. Test sample of spatial relations from Test of Visual Perceptual Skills (nonmotor). (From Gardner, M. [1982]. *Test of Visual Perceptual Skills [nonmotor] manual*. Seattle: Preston; reprinted by permission of the author.)

gories. This produces difficulty in distinguishing letters and learning mathematical concepts (Figure 8.5).

Visual memory is the ability to recall a visualized object, including color, shape, and form. Deficits in visual memory will obviously affect many aspects of classroom learning. Poor visual memory skills will impair the student's ability to recall letters and numbers. Comprehension of reading material will also be reduced (Figure 8.6).

Assessing Visual Perception The student susceptible to visual perceptual problems may be evaluated by an occupational therapist or licensed psychologist. The examiner will ask the student to perform school tasks such as reading and writing. Standardized assessments used include the Motor-Free Visual Perception Test (Colarusso & Hammill, 1972), the Test of Visual Perception Skills (nonmotor) (Gardner, 1982), and the Marianne Frostig Developmental Test of Visual Perception (Frostig et al., 1966) (see Table 8.1).

The Motor-Free Visual Perception Test and the Test of Visual Perception Skills (nonmotor) measure visual processing and do not require a motor response from the student. These tests assess only visual percep-

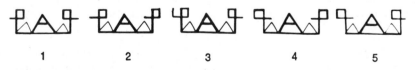

Figure 8.5. Test sample of visual discrimination from Test of Visual Perceptual Skills (nonmotor). (From Gardner, M. [1982]. *Test of Visual Perceptual Skills [nonmotor] manual*. Seattle: Preston; reprinted by permission of the author.)

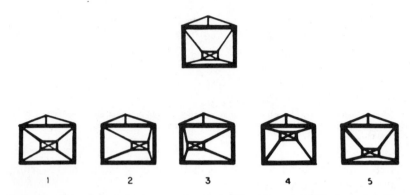

Figure 8.6. Test sample of visual memory from Test of Visual Perceptual Skills (nonmotor). (From Gardner, M. [1982]. *Test of Visual Perceptual Skills [nonmotor] manual*. Seattle: Preston; reprinted by permission of the author.)

tion without the interference of poor fine motor or visual-motor skills. The Test of Visual Perceptual Skills (nonmotor) provides more details about areas of strengths and weaknesses by assessing visual perception in seven areas: visual discrimination, visual memory, visual-spatial relationships, visual form constancy, visual sequential memory, visual figure-ground, and visual closure.

The Frostig Developmental Test of Visual Perception is a paper and pencil test which was developed as a screening tool. This test measures five areas relevant to school performance. These include: eye-hand coordination, figure-ground perception, shape constancy, position in space, and spatial relationships. Since this test relies on the motor skill of writing, students with poor fine motor skills or poor eye-hand coordination may take longer to complete test items. Students who experience difficulty with writing need to be monitored closely when taking this test.

After the assessment, results are compiled and the student's strengths and weaknesses will be noted. The student's program can then be restructured to use his areas of strength for learning, while working to remediate or compensate for problem areas. Thus the evaluator and teacher can work together to design a successful learning experience for the student.

Intervention Strategies The following strategies will enable the student with visual-perceptual deficits to function more successfully in the classroom:

1.   The student's desk should be free of clutter and visual stimuli to allow the student to focus only on work at hand. A portable study carrel is often helpful if the student is very distractible.

2. Sitting in the front of the classroom minimizes distractions.
3. Learning aids for quick reference can be taped to the desk; for example, a copy of the alphabet in upper case and lower case letters, a copy of the multiplication tables.
4. Highlighting or underlining reading material will help the student to focus on relevant details.
5. Tasks should be broken down into small steps to allow the student to tackle one piece at a time.
6. There are visual perception training programs available (e.g., the Frostig Program for Development of Visual Perception, 1964).
7. Often programs must be very individualized on the basis of an accurate assessment of the student's strengths and weaknesses. Areas of strength can be utilized in classroom learning.

Organizational Skills

Many children with spina bifida have difficulty with organizational skills (Hurley, Dorman, Laatsch, Bell, & D'Avignon, 1990; Mattson, 1982). To function adequately in the classroom, the student must be able to follow verbal directions and carry them out in an organized manner. For example, the pupil must follow an organized thought process to complete the following task: "Take out your spelling workbook, turn to page six, and begin work on that page." To complete the task successfully, the student must put away other books on his desk, locate the spelling book, turn to page six, locate a pencil, and then begin to work. The student with spina bifida often has difficulty organizing this type of simple classroom task. He or she may neglect to clear his or her desk, have difficulty finding the correct book, lose his or her pencil, or need to ask the page number again. The teacher will have to offer guidance for organizing the student's belongings and school tasks.

Implications for the Classroom   The student with poor organizational skills will have difficulty functioning in the classroom setting without additional structure. Following verbal or written directions of more than one step will be difficult, as well as changing activities, such as switching from reading to math. Poor organizational skills will also affect the quality and neatness of the student's written work.

Intervention Strategies   The following strategies will enable the student with poor organizational skills to function more successfully in the classroom:

1. The student should have easy access to books and be able to see them clearly. The use of a small bin next to the student's desk may be helpful for book storage and easy access.

2. The student should keep pencils in a specified box or tied to the desk with a string.
3. The teacher should help the student develop methods that enable him or her to organize tasks and activities.
4. The teacher should keep directions simple with as few steps as possible until sure the student understands and can follow through. More complex directions can be introduced gradually by adding steps to the directions that the student has already mastered.
5. The student should be provided with a form (Figure 8.7) or notebook to keep track of homework assignments as they are given throughout the day.
6. A timer often works to aid in completion of seatwork or tests.
7. Assignments can be broken down into steps, giving the student a list to check off as tasks are completed.

A further discussion of organizational skills is included in Chapter 9, pages 223–225.

SUMMARY

Along with the obvious physical manifestations of spina bifida, these students often exhibit perceptual-motor deficits that can affect school performance. Poor fine motor, visual-motor, visual perceptual, and organizational skills will affect the child's ability to function in the classroom. Teachers must be aware that children with spina bifida often exhibit these deficits, so schoolwork can be altered accordingly. Work skills can be improved with carefully structured settings, but most children will need ongoing adaptations to complete tasks and assignments. With appropriate intervention and structured programs, these students can be successful in school and carry this success with them into adulthood.

GLOSSARY

Figure-ground perception Ability to focus on relevant visual details.
Fine motor skills Ability to reach, grasp, and manipulate objects using the hands in a coordinated manner.
Form constancy Ability to see, remember, and locate a form in many different locations within the environment, even though it may be smaller, larger, rotated, or reversed.
Occupational therapist Health care professional with training in the evaluation and treatment of upper extremity function, fine motor and visual-motor skills, perceptual-motor skills, self-care skills, and the use of adaptive equipment.
Spatial relations Ability to perceive one's self in relation to one's surroundings and to identify objects in relation to one another.

Homework

Name _____ **Date** _____

Reading _____

_____

Math _____

_____

Science _____

_____

Language Arts _____

_____

Social Studies _____

_____

Tests _____

_____

_____

Figure 8.7. Homework assignment form to improve organizational skills. (From Spina Bifida Center, Allegheny General Hospital.)

Visual closure Ability to match an incomplete form or picture with a completed form or picture.

Visual discrimination Ability to match similar characteristics of objects.

Visual memory Ability to recall or visualize objects including color, shape, and/or form.

Visual-motor skills (eye-hand coordination) Efficient use of arms and hands for visually directed reach, grasp, and manipulation.

Visual perception Ability to recognize and understand what is seen.
Visual sequential memory Ability to recall a visualized series of forms, letters, or numbers.

REFERENCES

Anderson, E. (1976). Impairment of motor (manual) skills in children with spina bifida myelomeningocele and hydrocephalus. *British Journal of Occupational Therapy, 39*(4), 1–92.

Anderson, E., & Plewis, I. (1977). Impairment of a motor skill in children with spina bifida cystica and hydrocephalus: An exploratory study. *British Journal of Psychology, 68,* 61–70.

Anderson, E., & Spain, B. (1977). *The child with spina bifida.* London: Methuen.

Banus, B., Kent, C., Norton, Y., Sukiennecki, D., & Becker, M. (1979). *The developmental therapist.* Thorofare, NJ: Charles B. Slack.

Baron, I., & Spiegler, B. (1982). Neuropsychological assessment of the child with spina bifida. *Clinical Proceedings: Children's Hospital National Medical Center, 38,* 196–201.

Beery, K.E. (1982). *Administration, scoring and teaching manual for the developmental test of visual-motor integration.* Cleveland, OH: Modern Curriculum Press.

Beery, K.E., & Buktenica, N.A. (1967). *Developmental Test of Visual-Motor Integration.* Cleveland: Modern Curriculum Press.

Bruininks, R.H. (1978). *Bruininks-Oseretsky Test of Motor Proficiency.* Circle Pines, MN: American Guidance Service.

Clark, F., & Allen, P. (1985). *Occupational therapy for children.* St. Louis: C.V. Mosby.

Colarusso, R.P., & Hammill, D.D. (1972). *Motor-Free Visual Perception Test.* Los Angeles: Western Psychological Services.

Cull, C., & Wyke, M. (1984). Memory function of children with spina bifida and shunted hydrocephalus. *Developmental Medicine and Child Neurology, 26,* 177–183.

Cullata, B. (1980). Perceptual and linguistic performance of spina bifida-hydrocephalus children. *Spina Bifida Therapy, 2,* 235–247.

Frostig, M. (1964). *Frostig program for development of visual perception.* Chicago: Follett Publications.

Frostig, M., Lefever, D.W., & Whittlesey, J.R.B. (1966). *The Marianne Frostig Developmental Test of Visual Perception.* Palo Alto, CA: Consulting Psychologists Press.

Furuno, S., Inatsuko, T., O'Reilly, K., Hosaka, C., Zeisloft, B., & Allman, T. (1984). *Hawaii Early Learning Profile.* Palo Alto, CA: Vort Corporation.

Gardner, M. (1982). *Test of Visual Perceptual Skills (non-motor) manual.* Seattle, WA: Preston.

Gardner, M.F. (1986). *Test of Visual-Motor Skills. Manual.* San Francisco: Children's Hospital of San Francisco.

Gesell, A., & Amatruda, C. (1974). *Developmental diagnosis.* New York: Harper & Row.

Gluckman, I., & Barling, J. (1980). Effects of a remedial program on visual-motor perception in spina bifida children. *Journal of Genetic Psychology, 136,* 195–202.

Grimm, R. (1976). Hand function and tactile perception in a sample of children with myelomeningocele. *American Journal of Occupational Therapy, 30,* 234–240.

Hurley, A., Dorman, C., Laatsch, L., Bell, S., & D'Avignon, J. (1990). Cognitive functioning in patients with spina bifida, hydrocephalus, and the "cocktail party" syndrome. *Developmental Psychology, 6*(2), 151–172.

Jebsen, R.H., Taylor, N., & Trieschmann, R.B. (1969). An objective and standardized test for hand function. *Archives of Physical Medicine and Rehabilitation, 50,* 311–319.

Kellor, M., Forst, J., Silberberg, N., Iversen, I., & Cummings, R. (1971). Hand strength and dexterity. *American Journal of Occupational Therapy, 25*(2), 77–83.

Knoblock, H., & Passaminick, B. (1980). *Gesell's manual of developmental diagnosis.* New York: Harper & Row.

Mattson, B. (1982). Learning problems of children with spina bifida. *Clinical Proceedings: Children's Hospital National Medical Center, 38,* 225–230.

Miller, E., & Sethi, L. (1971). The effects of hydrocephalus on perception. *Developmental Medicine and Child Neurology, 13,* Suppl. 25, 77–81.

Sand, P., & Taylor, N. (1973). Performance of children with spina bifida manifesta on the Frostig Developmental Test of Visual Perception. *Perceptual and Motor Skills, 37,* 539–546.

Sand, P., Taylor, N., Hill, M., Kosky, N., & Rawlings, M. (1974). Hand function in children with myelomeningocele. *American Journal of Occupational Therapy, 28*(2), 87–90.

Shurtleff, D. (Ed.). (1986). *Myelodysplasias and exostrophies: significance, prevention and treatment.* New York: Grune & Stratton.

Soare, P.L., & Raimondi, A.J. (1977). Intellectual and perceptual motor characteristics of treated myelomeningocele children. *American Journal of Disabled Child, 131,* 191–204.

Spain, B. (1974). Verbal and performance ability in preschool children with spina bifida. *Developmental Medicine and Child Neurology, 16,* 773–780.

Stott, D.H., Moyes, F.A., & Henderson, S.E. (1972). *Test of Motor Impairment.* Gallph, Ontario: Brook Educational.

Tew, B., & Laurence, K. (1975). The effects of hydrocephalus on intelligence, visual perception and school attainment. *Developmental Medicine and Child Neurology, Suppl. 35,* 129–134.

Turner, A. (1985). Hand function in children with myelomeningocele. *Journal of Bone and Joint Surgery, 67-B*(2), 268–272.

Turner, A. (1986). Upper-limb function of children with myelomeningocele. *Developmental Medicine and Child Neurology, 28,* 790–798.

Vulpe, S. (1979). *Vulpe Assessment Battery.* Toronto, Ontario: National Institute on Mental Retardation.

Wallace, S. (1973). The effect of upper limb function on mobility of children with myelomeningocele. *Developmental Medicine and Child Neurology, 15*(6), Suppl. 29, 84–91.

Wechsler, D. (1967). *Manual for the Wechsler Preschool and Primary Scale of Intelligence.* New York: Psychological Corporation.

Williamson, G. (Ed.). (1987). *Children with spina bifida: Early intervention and preschool programming.* Baltimore: Paul H. Brookes Publishing Co.

Wills, K., Holmbeck, G., Dillon, K., & McLone, D. (1990). Intelligence and achievement in children with myelomeningocele. *Journal of Pediatric Psychology, 15*(2), 161–176.

Ziviani, J., Hayes, A., & Chant, D. (1990). Handwriting: A perceptual-motor disturbance in children with myelomeningocele. *Occupational Therapy Journal of Research, 10*(1), 11–26.

Beyond the Curriculum

Social and Emotional Development

Fern L. Rowley-Kelly

A large body of research has detailed the impact of spina bifida on the social and emotional development of students with spina bifida (Eckart, 1986, 1988; McAndrew, 1979; Rowley, Van Hasselt, & Hersen, 1987; Stein, 1983). This chapter is designed to help educators recognize and deal with classroom behavior that may be encountered when teaching students with spina bifida. It is presented in the belief that the teacher who knows realistically what to expect will be better equipped to promote independent achievement. Each behavior is discussed as it presents itself in the classroom, with a brief description of how it may have been generated from the child's life situation, and with a number of techniques and approaches for dealing effectively with the behavior. These behaviors are of concern because they may limit the student's social and emotional development toward an independent adult life. They may also prevent the student from achieving a maximum degree of academic success.

The discussion focuses on several main topics. The section titled "Learned Helplessness" discusses a student's tendency to act as if disabled in areas where he or she is not disabled. This must be carefully distinguished from those areas where the student is in fact disabled. The section on "Communication" discusses various aspects of verbal communication in young people with spina bifida. "Blocks to Independent Functioning" includes several areas that relate to the student's ability to function competently and responsibly in the current classroom setting and in the future workplace. It focuses on the development of an effective work personality and the development of organizational skills.

"Making Friends" is about socialization, an area of chronic deficiency for adolescents and young adults with spina bifida. "Medical Noncompliance" discusses the reasons why some students do not comply with their medical routines. "Self-Esteem and Body Self-Image" discusses distortions, exaggerations, and exclusions that falsify the student's view of him- or herself. "Positive Traits" considers the need to see past the problems and disabilities to promote the holistic growth of the student.

LEARNED HELPLESSNESS

Learned helplessness or "trained incompetence" (Blum, 1983; Ebner, 1970; Greer & Wethered, 1984; Scheers, Beeker, & Hertogh, 1987) is a form of adult dependency that is present when the students expect someone else to do things for them that they could do for themselves, or could learn to do for themselves. It occurs when the student requires assistance completing tasks that he or she could perform or could *learn* to perform on his or her own initiative. Examples of this form of dependency are when the student does school work only when the teacher is standing beside him or her or when the student waits for someone to push his or her wheelchair. More specifically, academic examples of learned helplessness occur when students let someone else do their thinking for them or proceed from the conviction that they are incapable of learning sophisticated material.

Origin of Learned Helplessness

Learned helplessness develops from many aspects of the life situation of children with spina bifida. Those children require more time and assistance to attain independence in areas such as mobility, toileting, dressing, and bathing. They also have many adults involved in their care, including doctors, occupational therapists, nurses, social workers, physical therapists, and others. Inevitably, these students develop expectations that nondisabled adults will assist them in activities that their peers do for themselves.

Lollar, Reinoehl, Leverette, Martin, and Posid (1989) report that "an insidious dynamic of dependency is often seen among these families. Regardless of socioeconomic status, parental educational level or quality of medical intervention, this dependency undermines appropriate social, emotional, and family functioning as well as actual physical adaptive skills. For parents, it is akin to a 'war'." They note that the quality of care required from parents communicates an unstated message: "The very personal nature of bowel and bladder problems which quickly come to be taken on by the mother or others, communicates to the youngster that even the most basic needs are met by outside forces. This sets the framework for quickly developing an intense dependence in the preschooler with spina bifida" (p. 18).

Feldman and Varni (1982) noted that:

> Parents and significant others may contribute to the lack of independent functioning and the tendency toward "learned helplessness" by responding

in an inappropriate and overprotective manner to the developmental needs of the disabled child, thereby denying the child opportunities for learning age-appropriate skills. (p. 78)

Such parents may lack appropriate models of what degree of independence can and should be expected of their child. They may also have the misconception that overprotecting will shield the child from further unpleasant experiences (Greenspan, 1987).

Learned helplessness may also originate in the frequent failures that many students with spina bifida have experienced. Gardner (1982) discussed the influence of the student's own thinking about himself or herself and about his or her accomplishments. His description of the work of Dweck (Dweck, Davidson, Nelson, & Enna, 1978; Dweck & Goetz, 1978) illustrated the origin of learned helplessness in repeated failure:

> Two experimenters administered problems to children, one posing solvable problems, the other posing unsolvable problems to the same children. After a time the "failure experimenter" began to administer solvable problems, virtually identical to those administered by the other experimenter. Surprisingly, many children failed to solve these problems. Apparently, children can rather quickly acquire the notion that they are incapable of solving a problem, at least under certain circumstances. (p. 92)

In this experiment, the condition of helplessness was generalized from a series of insoluble problems to include all problems posed by the "failure experimenter." Likewise, the student with spina bifida is likely to generalize from genuine helplessness in achieving toilet training, independent mobility, or neat handwriting to an assumed helplessness in the face of any new challenge.

This expectation of failure or presumption of helplessness is confined not only to areas where the student genuinely needs help. Many children and adolescents with spina bifida genuinely believe that they cannot do much for themselves. Although this attitude can be an excuse for not attempting an activity or a ploy to obtain attention, it may also be a reflection of a poor self-concept. There are also secondary gains that accompany the student's status as a helpless person. These include being helped, not having to live up to high expectations, and a sense of being special. Similar gains are of course also available to the student who achieves independence and mastery in a variety of areas. Mastery carries with it a more positive sense of being special, along with other social gains. The student with spina bifida may have decided to settle for the former set of gains, in the belief that the benefits associated with mastery and ability will always be out of reach.

Individuals who are involved in the care of the student with spina bifida may unwittingly promote learned helplessness if they have not dealt with their own feelings and attitudes toward the student and the disability. The adult may feel guilt, anger, inadequacy, misguided sympathy, or a sense of failure toward the student. These unresolved feelings may prompt the adult to do things for the student, rather than allow the student to gain independence. The student may be aware of the adult's desire to take over and feign dependency to please the parent or teacher.

Sometimes it is easier for the student to avoid learning new skills rather than to resist the adult's assistance. An individual who is doing more than 50% of the work for a student is rescuing rather than helping, and is thereby encouraging the student to remain in a helpless position. When the student does reach for new responsibilities, it is crucial that the adult not succumb to the convenience of continuing to do for the student out of habit. It also requires a great deal of patience on the adult's part to refrain from giving assistance as the student haltingly takes over.

Learned Helplessness versus Manipulation

Learned helplessness is distinct from manipulation, but is closely related to it, so that either can be mistaken for the other. Manipulation and learned helplessness lie on opposite ends of a continuum, and the decision about which is present is easy to make at either extreme, but a hard call in the middle. When it is clear to both the student and the teacher that the student is capable of doing what is asked and the student nonetheless seeks to avoid performing, manipulation is present. When the child is genuinely convinced of his or her incompetence, but the teacher knows that he or she can perform or learn to perform, learned helplessness is present. When the child is not sure, either or both may be present.

Left uncorrected, manipulation will lead to short-term coercive successes. In the long term, both peers and teachers will develop the inclination to avoid the manipulative student for the simple reason that they do not like being coerced and feel resentment toward anyone who has attempted to coerce them. If learned helplessness is uncorrected, the student will not grow in skill and competency and will not make effective use of the opportunity for training and education that is provided by the school.

To further complicate matters, the student may genuinely believe that what is being asked is not his or her job and that adults are supposed to perform this service for the student. In this case, the student may suspect that he or she could learn to perform, but is afraid to step out of the dependent role and take on the overwhelming weight of a full measure of adult responsibilities.

When It Is Not Learned Helplessness

A word of caution is in order: Problems with learned helplessness do exist, but often what may look like a problem in personality or motivation is a genuine disability. Students with spina bifida may have neurological or perceptual difficulties that can interfere with independent achievement. These students have difficulty in organizing a mass of data, sorting out the relevant from the irrelevant, and putting things in order. This may show up as a poorly organized desk or locker, or as difficulty in organizing work time. Perceptual problems may also interfere with copying information from a blackboard and taking timed tests. Production of written work may be slowed by deficits in eye-hand coordination. The student may also be distracted or have a short attention span (Knowlton, Peterson, & Putbrese, 1985; Mattson, 1982). (For further discussion of these issues, see Hurley, chap. 4, and Culatta, chap. 7, this volume.)

The teacher needs to be astute to determine whether a given problem is based in learned helplessness or in some pathophysiological problem, perceptual disability, attention deficit, or organizational problem. The teacher can request available documentation of such deficits from the occupational therapist, school psychologist, neuropsychologist, or the student's medical team. In the absence of such documentation, further assessment is appropriate.

There is often a complex interaction between these deficits and learned helplessness. Many teachers are aware of students with attention deficits who become dependent on the teacher for cues to stay on task. In such a case, meeting the student's legitimate needs for support seems to run counter to the need to discourage dependency on the teacher. The same sort of dilemma can be at work in teaching the child with spina bifida and can show up in more than one area of disability. An understanding of both learned helplessness and the specific deficits is equally important in managing the situation.

Enlisting the student's assistance in determining whether learned helplessness is present can be appropriate. The teacher might ask, "Is this something you can't do, something you don't want to do, or something you think you can't do?" The student may be able to answer this sort of question directly. When the situation is not clear to the student, it may be appropriate for the student to answer, "I don't know," at which point the teacher and student can work together in trying things out. A simple and self-defeating attitude of "I can't" can thus be replaced with one of "My teacher and I are going to find a way that I can do this for myself."

Approaches

Fortunately, the intervention strategy is substantially the same whether the student is manipulating, sincerely convinced of his or her incompetence, or reluctant to leave the security of the dependent position. Learned helplessness can be overcome as the student accomplishes new goals and learns new skills. Manipulative behaviors are gradually extinguished as they fail to achieve the desired result and as they are replaced by more acceptable ways of succeeding in interactions with others. All of the approaches outlined below are based on providing continuous positive reinforcement for gradual progress within a context of clear expectations and a warm and supportive relationship. Adaptive teaching approaches will be required to address any genuine learning disabilities identified through professional assessments. Specific approaches should be prescribed by the person who performed the assessments. (See Rogosky-Grassi, chap. 8, this volume.)

1. It is crucial in this and other areas that the teacher establish emotional rapport with the student by inviting, hearing, and acknowledging the student's thoughts and feelings about the matter in question. Recognition and acknowledgment of the student's point of view does not amount to agreement or endorsement of that point of view. It does demonstrate respect and care to the student, and it prepares the student, in turn, to listen to what the teacher has to say. Active or empathic listening will also provide a great deal of information about the problem. Empathic listening is the most effective way to understand the student's perspective and can be an invaluable tool for gaining the student's confidence and cooperation.

2. The teacher should program for growth in small steps in each area of dependency, using reasonable expectations and attainable goals. In working gradually, the student will not have to abandon too many behaviors at one time. The student successively finds reasons to feel competent, and only has to take on one new piece of adult responsibility at a time. This approach allows the student always to have an out, whereas forcing the student into a corner only reinforces dependency, or prompts an escalation of coercive behaviors.

3. The teacher should use lots of encouragement to reduce the fear and lack of self-confidence, and give praise when it is earned. After each task has been achieved, the teacher should encourage the student to feel good about doing this task independently. Just as the student can learn helplessness by generalizing from a series of failures, so can the student learn independence and competence by generalizing from a series of successes.

4. Assistance should be given only as necessary. The teacher should give only as much instruction or prompting as the student needs to complete the task and withdraw from the helping role as soon as possible. The teacher should allow time for the student to get started, to figure out what to do independently, and to complete the task unassisted.

5. The teacher should maintain the expectation that the student will continue to learn to do more things for himself or herself indepen-

dently. The teacher should be explicit about this, with positive anticipation, saying, for example, "You will be amazed at the number of things you'll be doing on your own by the end of the year."

6. Criticism should be avoided, as it only reinforces the conviction of inadequacy and incompetence. The teacher should keep the focus on the new behaviors that he or she wants to see and not on the student's character. This is an example of an effective statement: "I'm really looking forward to the time when you'll be able to keep your desk as organized as we have it now." It would be counterproductive to say, "You really don't seem to be able to get yourself organized," or "How many times do I have to tell you to get this desk organized?"

7. The teacher should communicate the conviction that the student is competent and can fulfill reasonable expectations. The teacher should use the student's achievements as they occur to reinforce and prove the conviction that the student can be both competent and independent.

BLOCKS TO INDEPENDENT FUNCTIONING

Many deficiencies in independent functioning can be diagnosed as a manifestation of learned helplessness, as a manifestation of a perception or coordination problem, or as a combination of both. When present together, the particular disability and the attitude of helplessness are likely to reinforce each other. For example, a particular perceptual disability can be addressed by developing ways to work around the disability, relying on the development of other competencies. A conviction of general incompetence (learned helplessness) would necessarily interfere with this process of remediation to some extent. At the same time, the particular disability seems to "prove" the conviction of general incompetence.

In such cases, effective intervention will require an approach that is designed both to compensate for the identified disability and to treat the general attitude. Specifically, the tendency to overgeneralize from the particular disability needs to be confronted by explicit statements (e.g., "Just because A is hard for you doesn't mean you can't do B") and by the construction of experiences that confirm the child's specific abilities and general competence.

In any of these cases, effective intervention will include the development of adaptive coping mechanisms, including an effective work personality and the ability to organize. An effective work personality will include problem-solving skills, planning skills, and a sense of responsibility. The following discussion focuses on the near- and long-term value of fostering independent functioning in the classroom, suggesting techniques to be used in each of the component areas.

Work Personality

Independent productivity in the school or workplace is a function of a person's work personality. Historically, students with spina bifida have not been put in situations where demands have been placed on them in this area and they may exhibit developmental delays in the work personality (see Grassi, 1986; Hayden, Davenport, & Campbell, 1979; Johnson, 1984; Rowley-Kelly, chap. 12, this volume). The work personality constitutes a person's ability to grasp and deal effectively with an assigned task with a minimum of supervision. It includes problem-solving skills, the ability to plan, and a sense of responsibility. Children develop their work personality to a great extent in school. The student with spina bifida cannot afford to be deficient in this area. In fact, the student with spina bifida needs to develop a good work personality to compensate for any disabilities.

Problem-Solving Skills

Although the student with spina bifida can benefit from learning traditional approaches to solving particular problems, it is also important that he or she learns to develop original approaches to problem-solving. Spina bifida is itself not a traditional problem, and the problems that come along with it are not traditional and usually do not allow for traditional solutions. When the student with spina bifida does encounter a traditional problem, the resources required to apply traditional solutions may not be available. The student will therefore need to develop character traits that are appropriate to original problem-solving, including flexibility, initiative, originality, improvisation, creativity, and effort. This may be very difficult, but is nonetheless necessary.

Approaches

1. The teacher should have the student do the thinking. The student should be encouraged to take the initiative in describing the problem, making certain that it has been clearly defined before proceeding to a solution. Once the student knows what the problem is, he or she can be encouraged to suggest ways to attack it, to analyze unsuccessful attacks, and to redesign further attacks.
2. The normal challenges of everyday life should be used to work on problem-solving skills. Typical challenges include dressing in outdoor clothing, loading a tray in the cafeteria, redesigning tasks to accommodate a wheelchair or braces, and finding the best location for the student's desk in the classroom.
3. The teacher can assign problems that allow many solutions (e.g., "Design a container in which an egg can be safely dropped from a

height of 6 feet," or "How many ways can we find to pick an apple from the top of a 12-foot tree?") The teacher can emphasize the multiplicity of methods that can provide a correct answer in other subject areas, such as mathematics.

4. The teacher should reinforce the student for initiative, effort, and creativity, even when the solutions do not work. The aim is to develop skills and character traits that promote successful problem-solving. Finding the perfect solution to the current problem has only temporary value.

5. The goal of developing a better-than-average set of problem-solving skills should be maintained. Students who have individualized education programs (IEPs) can have goals and objectives in the area of problem-solving incorporated into their program. Goals of students can be incorporated into the teacher's curriculum and lesson plans.

Planning Skills

The ability to plan effectively is an important part of independence. In learning to plan, the student internalizes the supervisory and management functions that adults have been exercising on his or her behalf. Again, because the student's life is harder to manage, more has been managed for him or her. Though necessary, this has probably created expectations that others will continue to manage things for the student. Training in planning can be an important step in turning this management function over to the student (see Rowley-Kelly, chap. 10, this volume). Although the student may be initially reluctant to move away from dependency in this area, the discovery of the capacity to function independently will be a gratifying and pleasant surprise.

Approaches

1. The student should lay out a schedule for the time to be spent doing homework. Which assignment should be done first, and why? How much time does the student think each task will require? When should breaks be scheduled? What materials will be needed before work can begin?

2. In classes where the student is having difficulty completing homework, the student should record each assignment in a notebook. The accuracy of the notebook can be verified by the teacher at the end of each period and the parents can initial each entry as the homework is completed. To further encourage independent responsibility, the student should be expected to approach the teacher or parent with the notebook.

3. After a plan has been developed and executed, the student can critique it and revise it.

4. The teacher should emphasize the experience of planning and re-planning on one's own in a variety of areas. The teacher should give less emphasis to the acquisition of traditional plans that work for most people, and more emphasis to unique or original plans that work for a particular person in a specific set of circumstances. The teacher should not expect plans to be perfect or overly detailed.
5. The student should be taught to identify and consider the following: long-term goals; short-term objectives; performance steps; possible obstacles; time tables; and sources of support, both human (e.g., the librarian) and material (e.g., the library).

Sense of Responsibility

Throughout the educational experience, students with spina bifida have many opportunities to mature in the areas of independence and responsibility. Sooner or later, many of these young people will leave their parents' home. The quality of their lives and the extent of their contribution to society will be largely determined by the level of growth in these two areas that they have achieved in school. In fostering the development of these traits, the teacher has an opportunity to make a real difference in the young adult's adjustment to the world after graduation.

Fostering independence and responsibility can also be of benefit within the school setting. Even if a deficit in attention span is not present, some students function productively only when they are directly supervised by the teacher. Growth in independence and responsibility will ameliorate this frustrating situation, and can be crucial to effective functioning both in school and in the adult world.

Many of the transition problems these children face when they leave high school are due to the suddenness with which large areas of responsibility are thrust upon them (see Rowley-Kelly, chap. 10, this volume). Many have not learned to be responsible in small steps throughout their formative years, both at home and in school. In general, students gain in this area by being given control over areas that they can handle. Resistance to taking control may occur, being based on the expectation that others are supposed to do for the student and on the fear that the student is and will be incompetent. Adults who maintain the belief that students with disabilities cannot do for themselves may communicate this attitude to the student and confirm the student's decision to remain dependent and irresponsible.

Approaches

1. The teacher should give the student control over some appropriate aspect of the work with an explicit statement that this area of responsibility has been given to him or her. The student can later give an

account of his or her stewardship by reporting on how well the task was handled, what was done effectively, and how his or her performance could be improved.

2. The teacher should give the student greater responsibilities in small increments, with feedback, evaluation, and encouragement along the way. The teacher should shape the student's behavior by rewarding successive approximations of the level of responsibility that is being sought.

3. As the child succeeds in handling areas given to him or her, the connection between growth in responsibility and maturation in general should be made clear (e.g., "I see that you're not just getting older; you're also learning to handle more and more things on your own").

Developing Organizational Abilities

Many students with spina bifida have difficulty in organizing what they know and in organizing what they do. In knowing, the student may fail to grasp the organizing principles that unify some body of knowledge. For example, the student may understand what is being said about each individual tree, but may still have difficulty with abstract concepts about the whole forest. Or the student may have receptive knowledge of one or two uses of the phrase "a few," but may not be able to explain the concept involved or use the phrase expressively. (See Culatta, chap. 5, this volume.)

Difficulty with organizing may show up as a disordered locker, desk, or work space, or as an inability to decide where to start working on a task (Mattson, 1982). Again, the student is having trouble finding or using a few organizing principles that will help to order the endeavor. In each of these cases, whether the student is dealing with a cluster of articles, ideas, or tasks, there is an equal inability to impose an order on the whole. This deficiency may have its origin in passivity or helplessness, in physical limits to mobility and exploration, or in deficits in memory, perception, or abstract conceptualization (see Culatta, chap. 5, this volume).

Students with spina bifida may also experience difficulty with the fundamental area of motor control and planning, that is, " . . . the ability of the brain to conceive of, organize, and carry out a sequence of unfamiliar actions" (Mattson, 1982, p. 25). Learning a new physical skill or moving in a new way requires an internal image of the body and its functions and an organized sequence of motions. Deficits in this internal process of imaging and organizing make it much more difficult for a new skill to become automatic or habitual. (See Rogosky-Grassi, chap. 8, this volume.)

Organizing as Active

Organizing is an extremely active process, whether we are organizing our understanding of the motion of the stars and planets or organizing our day's work. We encounter a chaotic reality, explore it thoroughly, identify key features, discover the order that naturally exists, and impose further ordering upon it. Children with spina bifida may have been relatively passive throughout their lives, with things being imposed upon them, rather than their imposing their will on things. The idea of reorganizing reality through their own initiative may be rather foreign to the experience of such students.

Organization and Exploration

Besides requiring energetic activity and a belief in oneself as an active agent instead of a passive individual, organization requires exploration of the environment. The intellectual exploration of an environment is first learned through the physical exploration of environments. Children develop this ability as they crawl and toddle around the home, opening drawers, finding out what is in them, seeing what can be done with the contents, and then advancing to explorations of the backyard and the neighborhood. The child grasps the organized unity of the dining room table, for example, by moving around and under it, seeing it from numerous aspects, and assembling these perspectives into an organized unity of the whole.

This development is problematic for the child with limited mobility. The child in a wheelchair or braces lives in a limited life space. It is difficult to see oneself as having the ability to organize an environment in which one cannot move around. Just as the contents of the upper level of kitchen cabinets are beyond consideration for the typical 4-year-old, so are major portions of the typical person's world beyond consideration for the child with limited mobility.

In reporting a study of goal-directed behavior in children with spina bifida, Landry, Copeland, Lee, and Robinson (1990) discuss the developmental importance of exploratory play:

> The importance of early exploration of the environment has been hypothesized in developmental theories. Exploratory play provides the context for infants and young children to learn and practice their emerging competence, and are most effective in stimulating this developmental process if the experiences are varied and challenging. Harter and Zigler argue that successful mastery attempts must provide an optimal degree of challenge to produce the sense of satisfaction that is reinforcing. An inability to move about could certainly limit the types of mastery experiences available to a child. (p. 310)

Approaches The treatment of deficits in the ability to organize knowledge is discussed elsewhere in the context of deficits in abstract conceptualization (see Culatta, chap. 5, this volume). Suggested approaches to the lack of organization in practical activities are:

1. The teacher should observe the student for evidence of developmental delay in the ability to organize his or her work or surroundings. The teacher should estimate the child's level of development (e.g., is he or she as organized as the average fifth grader? the average first grader?).
2. The teacher should revise expectations according to the child's actual level of development, considering what activities would help him or her move to the next level.
3. The need to organize the work, the work space, or the storage area should be brought to the student's attention. The teacher should ask the student to think about how it might be better organized.
4. The teacher should help the student to develop and apply a written system of organization.
5. The teacher should reinforce the system through periodic monitoring.
6. After the system has had a fair trial, the teacher should obtain feedback from the student. Is it making things easier or more difficult? Can it be improved or made easier to operate?
7. The teacher should look for other opportunities for the child to develop and to apply skills in organizing (e.g., the teacher could help the student to organize the process of gathering belongings at the end of the day).
8. The student should study and report on other systems of organization that are already in use, such as the use of the alphabet to organize the names in the telephone book and the entries in the dictionary, or the use of the Dewey Decimal System to organize the contents of the library.

LEARNED HELPLESSNESS AND COMMUNICATION

Dependency in Communication

The pattern of dependency and inability that tends to manifest itself in other areas is also found in the area of communication (Rowley et al., 1987). In social situations in health care systems, the parents often speak for the child in conferring with doctors, nurses, and other health care professionals. Even when the parents are absent, the child interacts with trained professionals who are generally very good at skills such as active listening, with the unintended result that the child has to carry a relatively small share of the burden of communication. The medical system thus inadvertently conditions the child with the expectation that adults will speak for him or her or will go out of their way to make it easy for him or her to be understood. Because of the depth of involvement in this system, the student with spina bifida may bring into the classroom the expectation that others will speak for him or her. Similarly, the student may have become accustomed to his or her parents anticipating what he or she thinks, feels, needs, or wants. Against this background, it should be no surprise to find that many students with spina bifida have difficulty in expressing their own needs, thoughts, and feelings whether they relate to academics, peer relations, or their own physical situation.

Conversational Deficits

Due to developmental delays in socialization (Rowley et al., 1987) and deficits in perception and abstract conceptualization (see Culatta, chap. 5, this volume), many children with spina bifida are deficient in initiating conversations (Ammerman, Van Hasselt, Hersen, & Moore, 1988) and in responding in such fashion as to keep a conversation going when it has been initiated by someone else. Others display the opposite deficiency, producing numerous statements with good articulation. On further inspection, their conversation may be found to lack depth or relevance. These children generally use conversation as a means of social contact rather than as a means of communication or self-expression (Swisher & Pinsker, 1971). (A more extensive discussion of this and other language processing deficits is provided in Hurley, chap. 4, and Culatta, chap. 7, this volume.) This pattern of verbal behavior may have at least two adverse effects. The first effect is that the casual observer may be led to believe that the child's quantity of conversation indicates a greater degree of intelligence, education, or social maturity than is actually present. The second is that, as the acute observer may notice, this type of hyperverbal conversation lacks organization (Schwartz, 1974; Swisher & Pinsker, 1971; Tew, 1979).

Avoiding Adverse Effects Conversational deficiencies affect the child's progress both socially and academically. In the academic setting of a classroom, desired behaviors include volunteering to answer questions, asking questions when confused, asking for assistance, and other conversational initiatives and responses. The student who has difficulty in initiating, responding appropriately, or maintaining relevance will be at a disadvantage.

In the classroom as a social setting, each student is a unique source of opinions, information, values, and feelings. The individual's sense of independence and worthiness within a social group is based to a large extent on consciousness of this uniqueness, the conviction that he or she has something unique to contribute to the discussion. The student who withholds his or her contribution creates the conviction among himself or herself and others that he or she has no contribution to make, and no independent position from which to make it. Fostering independent communication skills, however, goes a long way toward enhancing social interaction, self-esteem, self-confidence, and independence.

The opportunity to promote development in these areas can be seized with enthusiasm, on the assumption that many children with spina bifida are lacking in one or more of these areas, and all will be well served by an ample supply of self-esteem, self-confidence, and independence, as well as good skills in social interaction.

Gaining Esteem through Communication

Fostering a social and academic situation in which each child is expected to express himself or herself promotes the conviction that everybody is unique and valuable. Although this is good procedure in any classroom, it is of even greater value when the classroom includes a student with spina bifida. That student probably suspects that he or she is not so much unique as simply different and that being different makes him or her less valuable. At the same time, studies indicate that children tend to reject or ignore the different child, even if the difference is as slight as an unusual name or the presence of adaptive equipment (Richardson, Goodman, Hastorf, & Dornbusch, 1961). This rejection is not the active dislike that is felt toward a bully or a student with a conduct disorder. It is rather that peers are not quite sure how to relate to the student who is different, whether the difference is one of language, ethnic group, race, or medical condition.

Using appropriately chosen topics to open communication between the different child and the peer group establishes their common humanity, provides specific information about the extent and nature of the difference, and fosters mutual respect. The different child and his or her peers need to know that this child's information, feelings, and values deserve a hearing, and are as important as anyone else's. Children who are different also need to know that it is their job to express their information, their feelings, and their values.

Approaches

1. Students should be encouraged to speak for themselves. The teacher should not speak for them, or try to guess what they are thinking or feeling. The teacher should tell them they cannot be really understood until they speak for themselves. It should be remembered that learning to speak for oneself is a new skill for most students with spina bifida. The teacher should expect that the student may be very shy, and should provide a lot of encouragement. The teacher should reinforce small steps of progress, and let the student know that there will be future occasions when he or she will be expected to speak for

himself or herself. The teacher should make it clear to the student that this will be worked on at intervals as a long-term project.

2. The student should be taught to stand up for his or her own rights, as this enacts the belief that he or she is just as good as everyone else. The teacher can feel free to role model this behavior by asserting his or her own rights in the relationship with the child.

3. The student should be taught to listen to the thoughts and feelings of others. The teacher should explain that understanding and acknowledging what someone else expresses does not necessarily mean agreeing with it.

4. The student should be encouraged to make wants and needs known, to make requests, and to respond to requests made by others.

5. The student can be encouraged to make "I" statements. In an "I" statement, a person expresses how something is for him or her, without judging the character or intentions of others. To illustrate: When one's toe is stepped on, one can make a "you" statement, judging the other person's character ("You clumsy oaf!") or intentions ("You're trying to hurt me!"); or, one can directly express one's own feelings with an "I" statement ("Ouch, my toe hurts!"). The "I" statement invites the other person to meet the speaker's needs without attempting to compel the other person's compliance.

6. Assertiveness should be taught, as distinct from passivity on the one hand, and aggressiveness on the other. The passive student lets things happen to him or to her. The aggressive student attacks, either verbally or physically. The assertive student sets limits on others by making his or her feelings known clearly. Growth in assertiveness is very helpful in enhancing the student's self-respect, confidence, and independence. Instruction in this area can be formal or it can occur spontaneously on those occasions when it is appropriate to intervene in peer relationships (e.g., stopping an argument or resolving a dispute).

7. The teacher can develop and assign tasks that emphasize expression of thoughts and feelings, such as sharing, show and tell, creative writing tasks, drama activities, and group discussions.

8. The teacher can design a lesson plan or health class that introduces the concept of communication. An understanding of the importance of communicating clearly and of expressing and listening at the level of feelings can be developed.

MAKING FRIENDS

Gaining peer acceptance and developing a normal social life are challenges for the adolescent with spina bifida. An extensive study of elements of psychological and social adjustment of adolescents with spina bifida was recently conducted, using 25 young people with spina bifida from the western Pennsylvania area as a sample population (Ammerman, Van Hasselt, & Hersen, 1986). The study compared a group of adolescents with spina bifida, a group of adolescents with visual impairments, and a group of controls with no impairments. The study found that adolescents with disabilities are more socially isolated and maladjusted than non-disabled controls. These adolescents had serious difficulty with friendship formation and participation in age-appropriate activities. Students with spina bifida had more severe problems in this area than did the study group who had visual impairments. It has been suggested that the difference between the group of adolescents with spina bifida and the group with visual handicaps was caused in part by the limited mobility of the students with spina bifida, especially since those using wheelchairs were more severely isolated than the more mobile individuals with spina bifida.

The second phase of this study included the trial of a variety of treatment methods and found that significant progress can be made in helping adolescents with spina bifida to overcome social isolation (Rowley et al., 1987). This was achieved primarily through training in communication skills and problem-solving, and through the development and execution of a series of social outings.

An extensive discussion of social integration of students with spina bifida into mainstream settings is provided in Chapter 10, this volume. The following section discusses some of the hindrances to normal socialization that exist for students with spina bifida and suggests approaches for helping them to overcome these hindrances in the school setting.

Blocks to Socialization

Spina Bifida—The Difference Without Precedent

The student who is "different" has difficulty in gaining peer acceptance (Ammerman et al., 1986; Richardson et al., 1961). Stein (1983) stated that students who are isolated and not offered the normal range of give and take with peers do not master age-appropriate social skills or mature socially at the same pace as their age-mates. The student with spina bifida presents to the peer group as being different and as being different in a *new* way. This is quite unlike the challenge of gaining acceptance for persons with visual or hearing impairment, which is somewhat mitigated by the many generations of experience that our society has had in dealing with such individuals.

The experience of dealing with children or young adults with spina bifida is novel in our culture because these people are novel: It is only within the last 30 years that medical science has been able to ensure the survival of most of this population into adulthood. Today's typical student may have a parent, uncle, or grandparent who had a friend or acquaintance with visual impairment, and today's student may thereby learn some degree of acceptance of this form of difference. Today's typical student cannot have an older relative who grew up with a student with spina bifida, because such students simply did not grow up in those days. Furthermore, there are few or no fairy tales, nursery rhymes, folk tales, or Bible stories to provide cultural reference about the student with spina bifida.

The nondisabled peer's view of the student with spina bifida can be very important, as socialization is to a great extent a mirror phenomenon. We tend to come to see ourselves as others see us. The self-understanding of the student with spina bifida is thus conditioned in part by the peer group's understanding of him or her. Whether this student sees himself or herself as "different, but acceptable" depends to a great degree on the extent to which he or she has been accepted by the peer group.

Medical Factors

Socialization for the student with spina bifida is also complicated by the continued need for medical care. This student may be out of school frequently for extended periods when major surgeries and long periods of convalescence are indicated. The student will also need time and emotional resources to cope with the stress of hospitalization and surgery, and to return to normal routines.

The medical situation also necessitates a higher degree of involvement between the parent and child for a longer period of time. This often means that the child is relating to his or her mother instead of to peers, or that the time available for unstructured play with peers is more frequently interrupted by routine care. This problem tends to persist in school if the student's care time with the nurse or aide is always scheduled during lunch, recess, or other unstructured times that provide opportunities for social growth. Socialization is also adversely affected by the fact that at any given age the typical student has achieved a greater degree of emotional and practical emancipation from his or her parents than has the student with spina bifida.

The child's development of socialization is further impeded by the social isolation generally experienced by the child's parents.

> What we seem to have failed to do in our institutional arrangements is to recognize the sheer physical hard work and mental strain which is involved and falls largely on the child's mother. Moreover this physical and mental stress is both unremitting in nature and increasingly onerous as both chil-

dren and parents grow older. Caring for handicapped children is in its nature an isolating experience. The lives of parents with a disabled child inevitably diverge from their peers. Isolation is experienced in relation to networks of extended family, friends and neighbours and there is little evidence that informal "community" networks are playing a substantial part in supporting parents. (Bradshaw, 1988, pg. 10)

Mobility

Mobility is clearly a factor in the social isolation of the student with spina bifida (Ammerman et al., 1986), and becomes more of a factor as the student and his or her peers get older. For example, typical 7-year-old children do not cover that much ground on their own for a variety of reasons, including safety, the tendency to get lost, and the need to stay close to adults. Typical 17-year-olds are, however, so mobile as to be hard to locate. The difference in degree of mobility increases dramatically between the student with spina bifida and his or her typical peer as both get older, and correlates to an increasingly dramatic difference in the amount of opportunities that each has for socialization.

This difference is decreased as the parents and other adults permit and encourage the student with spina bifida to probe the limits of the environment. Adults need to accept that this young person needs the opportunity to explore unknown territory, to get lost, and to discover that he or she can still survive. Parents of a student with spina bifida may have a similar need to discover that their son or daughter can survive on his or her own. This kind of letting go in terms of mobility and socialization is necessary if the student is ever to make friends with typical age-peers. Teachers can keep themselves informed of supportive opportunities in the community. Such opportunities might include accessible public transportation, accessible camps, and social organizations with adapted programs.

Heterosocial Issues

Heterosocial isolation becomes more of an issue as adolescence progresses. The same factors that adversely affect socialization with peers of the same sex can come into play as the adolescent pursues relationships with members of the opposite sex. Slower development in learning to relate to peers of the same sex places the child with spina bifida several steps behind when it comes time to begin to relate to the opposite sex. Furthermore, the child with spina bifida may have a great deal of confusion about sexual and reproductive functioning. The degree of physical impairment in these areas varies a great deal between males and females and from case to case, depending primarily on which portion of the spine is affected. Although there are particular exceptions, it is generally true that "adults with meningomyelocele [spina bifida] can perform the sex act, desire sex, satisfy their partners, marry and have children" (Shurtleff & Dunne, 1986, p. 446).

Social Progress, Academic Progress, and the School Setting

Because the school setting is a major area for the development of socialization in our society, it also provides an opportune place for informal remediation of socialization deficits. Furthermore, progress in socialization is of academic relevance. On the one hand, the student who is "making the grade" socially will have a strong sense that he or she is as good as the other children, and will develop the belief that he or she should be as capable of handling independent responsibilities as they are. On the other hand, the student who is not relating well with peers will have less energy and enthusiasm for academic work. Finally, the eventual transition from high school to the workplace requires competence in both academic and nonacademic areas, including peer relations. Since this transition is problematic for many students with spina bifida, it is never too soon to begin to train the student to relate well with today's schoolmates . . . and tomorrow's co-workers.

Approaches

1. The teacher should take advantage of progress in other areas to achieve social gains. Students who learn to communicate effectively, to initiate conversations, and to respond appropriately will make friends more readily and have fewer conflicts. Similarly, students who have overcome learned helplessness and dependency on adults will be perceived by themselves and their peers as worthy associates. (These areas were dealt with at length earlier in this chapter.)

2. The teacher should assist the student in finding ways to contribute. Peer acceptance is conditioned by the value and variety of contributions that the student can make to the group. It is quite likely that the student with spina bifida may never contribute to the peer group in traditional or stereotypical ways, such as driving in the winning run in a baseball game. The teacher should bear in mind that there are literally thousands of characteristics, skills, and talents through which any student can make a positive contribution to group experience. Although academic and athletic pursuits necessarily develop only limited sets of these skills and talents, other programs for youth such as Scouting and YMCAs provide endless opportunities for gains in skill mastery, self-acceptance, and peer acceptance. Some examples that are appropriate to a school setting include dramatics (writing, acting, producing, set design, sound effects), music (singing, playing an instrument, disk jockeying), drawing, cooking, cartooning, creating bulletin boards, and collecting.

The teacher should help the student to find some of the many areas where he or she can shine and contribute to the social life of the group, recalling that the number of avenues that are open to the student with spina bifida is much greater than the number of avenues that are closed. The astute teacher can assist the student in identifying areas of opportunity that the student and his or her peers may not have considered, and can coach the student to pioneer in introducing a new skill, game, or activity to the group.

3. The teacher should use the classroom as a social skills learning laboratory. Whether they do so consciously, students test and evaluate social behaviors by employing them among their peers, and they learn new social behaviors by observing and repeating the behaviors they see their peers and teachers using. Although this process will go on with or without conscious participation by the teacher, it is very useful for him or her to play some role in guiding the experiments. The teacher should observe the social behaviors of the student with spina bifida, noting strengths and deficits. The teacher should reinforce the strengths, and have the student take note of those peers who display the skills that he or she lacks. The teacher can discuss the usefulness of the behaviors that the selected peers display, and encourage the student with spina bifida to try doing the same. For example, the teacher could say, "Fred, have you noticed what Charlie does to get other kids to play checkers with him? He has such a nice way of inviting them. Do you think you could just keep an eye on him and see how he does it?" Then later, after Fred has observed Charlie, the teacher could say, "Well, did you get to check Charlie out? What did he say? Did you notice how he said it? Did you see the smile? Why don't you go and try the same sort of invitation with Larry? It doesn't always work, but it's worth a try." What comes naturally for most students may require some degree of directed learning for others. Although this need is more frequently present in the student with spina bifida, what is said here can be of real benefit to any student at one time or another.

4. The teacher can provide common experiences in which the student with spina bifida can fully participate. Groups of people, and especially adolescents, develop group cohesiveness, or a pack mentality, by going through experiences together. This phenomenon is exploited in boot camp to create esprit de corps in the armed services, and in hazing and initiation rituals to solidify fraternity and sorority membership. The same phenomenon can be employed to promote group bonding that includes the student with spina bifida, simply by arranging matters so that he or she fully shares experiences with his or her classmates.

MEDICAL NONCOMPLIANCE

Causes

Individuals with spina bifida must comply with an extensive set of medical routines, including wearing braces, attending appointments, and emptying the bowel and bladder on a scheduled basis. Although compliance in any of these areas can be an issue, the most significant area of noncompliance that is likely to occur in the school setting relates to bladder management or urinary incontinence. Students with spina bifida may have little or no feeling of pressure in their bladder, and may not feel the wetness when they are incontinent. This area is managed through a program of clean intermittent catheterization. Nondisabled students are often reluctant to stop their activities to go to the bathroom until it is almost too late and are then only driven to the bathroom by the urgent feeling of pressure in the bladder. It should therefore come as no surprise that some students with spina bifida forget or disregard their responsibility to perform self-catheterization, and thus remain wet and smell of urine.

There are a variety of factors that lead to noncompliance in this area. Many students do not identify the areas of the body that they cannot feel or operate as being parts of themselves. Drawings of human figures by students with spina bifida as part of a psychological assessment may include full normal detail of the upper body, but only a vague and distorted outline of the lower extremities. These students lack sensation in their legs and use of them, and appear to be only minimally aware of them. They may have little regard for areas they identify as non-self, and tend not to take care of those areas, or to be careless about them. In other cases, noncompliance with bladder management may be a manifestation of adult dependency, where the expectation remains that some grown person will remind them to catheterize themselves, possibly even doing it for them.

Noncompliance may also be a struggle to maintain a maladaptive identity as a perpetual consumer of medical services (Herskowitz & Marks, 1977). McAnarney (1985) noted that an adolescent with physical disabilities lacks the usual opportunities to experiment that are available to nondisabled peers because of a lack of mobility and a limited network of peers. "Early adolescence may be the most challenging age for a young person with a disability, because identity formation and independence from the family may be so difficult to achieve" (Eckart, 1988, p. 29). Noncompliance with a medical routine may provide an opportunity to test the value of the advice that has been given by adults or to strike out on one's own.

Other students may not have adequately expressed or dealt with their feelings of anger, jealousy, or resentment about their disabilities. Though they may be angry, overt rebellion is atypical for children with spina bifida (Blum, 1983). In these cases, noncompliance is a passive-aggressive behavior: "I don't like having a neurogenic bladder, and I can't really act out, but I don't have to do what is expected of me, either." The message is then communicated through nonverbal behaviors, such as neglect of the catheterization schedule. These students are in need of opportunities to learn assertiveness, and need someone to listen to their more direct expressions of their feelings about their situation.

Additional stress is created through the fact that toileting, which is normally a strictly private and personal matter, tends to become public knowledge. The catheterization procedure can become psychologically invasive if performed by another person. To a lesser degree, control over the schedule and management of the procedure can also be psychologically invasive. Typical peers do not have someone telling them when it is time to go to the bathroom.

In some cases, the neurogenic bladder is the only thing that separates the student with spina bifida from nondisabled peers. It is possible that the student will feel anger toward his or her body and that this anger will be expressed through noncompliance. Continued involvement by the parents in the child's program of bladder control, although it may be necessary, may perpetuate the child's dependency on adults, which is already problematic.

Of course, none of these explanations provide a justification for noncompliance with the bladder management program. The program is necessary to prevent major urological problems, kidney failure, and skin breakdown. It is also the clear responsibility of all human beings to do whatever they can to avoid exposing others to their bodily waste products. The child with spina bifida may already be having difficulty in gaining full acceptance by his or her peers and in finding ways to make a positive contribution to the group. Although peers may understand an occasional unavoidable accident, few behaviors can sabotage peer acceptance as fast as irresponsibility in the area of toileting. Teachers need to understand that toileting behavior is different and more challenging for the child with spina bifida, but they do not need to excuse or expect irresponsibility.

It bears repeating that not all children with spina bifida can achieve perfect continence, even through perfect compliance and the use of medication. This can depend on the severity of the physical handicap, and on the child's level of intelligence. Wetness does not always imply irresponsibility. In cases where perfect continence cannot be achieved, appropriate garments are commercially available.

Approaches

1. The teacher should give clear expectations in a calm and noncritical manner.
2. Compliance should be reinforced when it occurs. For example, the teacher could say, "I notice you have really been following your catheterization schedule on a regular basis lately. You must be proud of yourself, even though it must really be a pain sometimes." Terms should be chosen that are appropriate to the student's age.
3. Occasional, gentle reminders should be given. If more than that is necessary, the teacher should contact other adults, including the parents and the school nurse, to develop a strategy.
4. The teacher should convey respect for all parts of the child's body, especially those parts that he or she cannot feel or use.
5. The teacher should permit or encourage the child to express negative feelings about his or her medical situation in a direct and responsible manner. When this approach is ineffective or insufficient, the student may be referred for counseling in this area.
6. The teacher should consistently convey respect for the privacy of the child's toileting program, and convey the expectation that others should do the same.
7. The teacher can give the child control over the toileting program, maintaining the expectation that this control will be exercised responsibly, especially if it is clear that the child is engaged in a power or control struggle about the catheterization program.

SELF-ESTEEM AND BODY SELF-IMAGE

Self-Esteem

Many, if not all, of the areas mentioned elsewhere in this book relate to issues of self-esteem. Several studies have shown that children with spina bifida have significantly lower self-esteem than their nondisabled peers (Campbell, Hayden, & Davenport, 1977; Hayden et al., 1979; Kazak & Clark, 1986; Lutkemeier, 1979). MacBriar (1983) and Pearson, Carr, and Halliwell (1985), however, found no difference in levels of self-esteem between students with spina bifida and their nondisabled peers. Reviewing these studies, Eckart concluded that:

> Adolescents with spina bifida are likely to experience more difficulties in self-esteem development than do their nondisabled peers. It is also true that some adolescents with spina bifida will suffer from low self-esteem, while others will have a positive self-image. (1988, p. 37)

Since there was a clear risk for deficiencies in self-esteem within the population of young people with spina bifida, Eckart (1988) focused on factors contributing to differences in self-esteem within the population. Eckart (1988) noted that self-esteem improves with age for adolescent girls with spina bifida, and decreases for boys. She concluded that girls with spina bifida were more able to meet gender-related cultural norms of sociability and acceptable behavior. Adolescent boys with spina bifida found themselves at a disadvantage in attempting to meet cultural norms requiring physical competence and achievement.

In general, a student's self-esteem grows as progress is made in gaining peer acceptance, learning to speak for himself or herself, learning to function with a minimum of dependence on adults, achieving academic progress, and learning new skills in a variety of areas. Self-esteem also grows as the student gains competence in handling his or her responsibilities for bladder management and complying effectively with other medical routines. The relationship between these factors is not that of simple cause and effect: Progress in any area promotes self-esteem and, in turn, gains in self-esteem promote progress in every other area.

Body Self-Image

Adolescents are painfully conscious of their appearance and tend to see their flaws in exaggerated proportions. The egocentrism of adolescents is rampant, so that "adolescents are, in general, acutely aware and vehemently insisting that everybody is looking at, and all behavior is meant for, them" (Friedrich & Shaffer, 1986, p. 413). Drovin, Norman, and Issard (1987) detail the social component of the development of body image.

> School children are frequently cruel in their honesty so they make derogatory remarks about a child who is different . . . . It seems that teasing has a lasting effect. According to many studies, people who were teased as children were less satisfied with their bodies as adults. The "ugly" child remembered his misery long into adulthood. Thus, the school experience may either reinforce or weaken the child's feelings about himself as a unique, important person with specific talents or abilities. (p. 100)

The student with spina bifida may view himself or herself primarily in terms of the differences in his or her appearance. Similarly, such a student's self-definition may be stated primarily in terms of disabilities rather than abilities.

Furthermore, as is mentioned in the discussion of bladder management, there is a tendency to ignore or discount those areas of the body that cannot be felt or used. Students with spina bifida may thus see themselves in a far less complimentary light than others see them. It is also likely that their self-image includes significant distortions, including exaggerations of perceived flaws and exclusions of portions of the body. This painful awareness of self-image is not unique to adolescents with disabilities. All students, with or without spina bifida, are self-conscious, and all are likely to be overly aware of their less flattering attributes. This in fact provides an opportunity to share experiences with nondisabled peers, so that a mutual desensitizing can occur.

Approaches

The general strategy of intervention with students with a poor body self-image or low self-esteem is to allow them to experience the positive aspects of themselves repeatedly over a long period of time, while allowing them to desensitize themselves to their flaws by developing an accepting and matter-of-fact attitude. Specific tactics for applying this strategy are:

1. The teacher should establish a no put-down rule.
2. Positive reinforcement should be used whenever possible.
3. The teacher should provide all students with opportunities to identify each other's good points in all areas.
4. The teacher should provide all students with casual opportunities to discuss feelings they may have about their own less flattering features. If necessary, the teacher's own exaggerated adolescent misgivings can be recalled and related.
5. The teacher should target his or her efforts toward revising the students' central beliefs about themselves. Helping a student to see himself or herself as a good learner or as competent and reliable may be difficult, but it will have a significant impact on the life of the child (Canfield & Wells, 1976).

POSITIVE TRAITS

Focusing on the Positive

The reader may at this point be overwhelmed with both the number of social and emotional difficulties that may be encountered and with the amount of effort that could be required to remedy all of them. Should this be the case, it should be noted that this chapter was intended to cover most of the possible difficulties that students with spina bifida may have. They certainly do not all display all of the difficulties mentioned. It would be a mistake to expect to find hidden difficulties in areas where they may not, in fact, exist. It is also important to keep an eye open for the positive traits that all of these children display.

Young people with spina bifida display the same range of delightful attributes that are found in typical students. Some are cheerful, some are resolute, some are humorous, some are imaginative, and so forth. It is possible that the child with spina bifida will be so aware of his or her negative attributes and disabilities as to be only minimally aware of good points, even though they must vastly outnumber the troublesome features. If the teacher also falls into the trap of primarily seeing the problems, the relationship will not be much fun, or of much use, for either the student or the teacher.

Approaches

1. In extreme cases, the positive aspects of the student's personality may be well hidden and may be especially well hidden from the student. The teacher should look for the treasures buried in the student, expose them, and enjoy them in the company of the student and his or her peers. The teacher who applies this process will gradually find a far more enjoyable student to whom to relate, and will greatly assist the student in learning to behold and develop his or her own positive traits and abilities.
2. The teacher should observe quietly, catch the student in the act of doing something well, and call it to his or her attention.
3. The teacher should be sure to relay positive comments that he or she hears other students or teachers make about the student. Nobody needs to hear these things more than the student about whom they were spoken.
4. The disability should be dealt with frankly when it naturally arises in the relationship, but the student should know that he or she is expected to relate to the teachers as a complete person.
5. Those behaviors and attitudes of the student to which the teacher pays attention will grow faster than those that are ignored or played down. The teacher should thus be selective about what he or she attends to, as he or she will probably see more next month of what is looked hard at today.

ASSESSMENT CHECKLIST

The quick-reference checklist in Table 9.1 can be used on a daily basis to target areas for intervention. All of the topics listed were discussed in detail in this chapter.

CONCLUSION

Although many of the problematic characteristics discussed in this chapter are ingrained character traits, they are subject to gradual improvement. It is fortunate that each teacher has several months, and each school system has several years, to chip away at these deficits. When this task is begun early on in the student's education and pursued consistently throughout, the eventual probability that the student will make a successful transition to a happy and productive adult life will be greatly

Table 9.1. Assessment checklist

Obstacles to independent functioning
  Learned helplessness
  Dependency
  Manipulation
  Medical noncompliance
  Socialization
  Conversational deficits
  Incontinence
  Low self-esteem
  Poor self-image

Skills or traits required
  Sense of responsibility
  Problem-solving skills
  Organizing skills
  Planning skills
  Social interaction skills
  Independence
  Communication skills

Remediation strategies
  Identifying learned helplessness
  Overcoming learned helplessness
  Developing the work personality
    Problem-solving skills
    Planning skills
    Organizational skills
  Developing independent communication
  Developing positive peer relationships
  Managing bowel and bladder
  Building self-esteem and self-image

improved. In addition to being of eventual usefulness in the student's future, the approaches suggested here should prove useful in the short term for teachers who encounter passive or unproductive behavior in the student with spina bifida. It is the author's sincere hope that this chapter will prove most useful to the concerned educational professional who finds him- or herself wondering, "Why isn't this student functioning?" or asking, "How can I help this student learn and mature?" Finally, in those cases where students are eligible for specialized services, and the development of an IEP is in order, it is hoped that the ideas and approaches presented here will be useful in developing goals in the areas of communication, socialization, independent functioning, overcoming dependency, and building self-esteem.

GLOSSARY

Active agent In the health care setting, patients are by definition passive, in that they permit or undergo the ministrations of a medical professional. In these terms, the professional is the active agent who does something to and for

the patient. Construing a student with spina bifida as a patient may uncon-
sciously reinforce the student's passivity, making it more difficult to foster the
capacity to act independently in one's own behalf or to become an active agent.

Active listening See *Empathic listening.*

Adaptive coping mechanism Any behavior or set of behaviors that has enabled a person or family to handle a challenging situation effectively.

Body self-image Person's image or conception of his or her own physical
appearance.

Developmental delay Delay in the development of any skill or capacity, as
compared to the normative standard set by nondisabled peers.

Effective work personality Adaptive coping mechanism needed by students
with spina bifida, which includes problem-solving skills, planning skills, and a
sense of responsibility.

Emotional rapport Achievement of a relationship between two or more persons in which communication can comfortably occur on an emotional level.

Empathic listening Ability to enable another person to express his or her feelings by listening attentively and without criticism to the emotional component
of what is expressed.

Genuine disability Inability to perform a desired function because of a pathophysiological condition.

Heterosocial Pertaining to interpersonal relationships with members of the
opposite sex, including dating, courtship, and related activities.

Learned helplessness Acquired conviction that one is capable of very little,
or that one is incapable of performing a given task or function.

Manipulation Any attempt to coerce another person into behaving in a certain
way, or not behaving in a certain way. In the context of the social and emotional
aspects of spina bifida, manipulation is frequently directed toward evading an
expectation.

Pathophysiological Pertaining to any physiological pathology such as a neurogenic bladder or a muscular paralysis.

Performance step In goal planning, any concrete action that is to be taken by a
designated individual within a specified time frame to achieve an objective.

Self-esteem Estimate of the self by the self, or the degree to which a person
values himself or herself.

Self-image Person's image or conception of himself or herself. Self-image includes body self-image, along with other dimensions of the self.

Sense of responsibility Conviction that one can and should perform one or
more tasks effectively and to the satisfaction of other significant persons.

Timetables Previously agreed-upon listing of times and dates.

REFERENCES

Ammerman, R., Van Hasselt, V., & Hersen, M. (1986, November). *Assessment of social functioning in handicapped adolescents and their families.* Paper presented
at the twentieth annual convention of the Association for the Advancement of
Behavior Therapy, Chicago.
Ammerman, R., Van Hasselt, V., Hersen, M., & Moore, L. (1989). Assessment of

social skills in visually impaired adolescents and their parents. *Behavioral Assessment*, *11*, 327–351.

Blum, R.W. (1983). The adolescent with spina bifida. *Clinical Pediatrics*, 22(5).

Bradshaw, J. (1988). The social impact of childhood disablement. *Zeitschrift für Kinderchirurgie*, *43*, Suppl. 11, 5–11.

Campbell, M.M., Hayden, P.W., & Davenport, S.L. (1977). Psychological adjustment of adolescents with myelodysplasia. *Journal of Youth and Adolescence*, 6(4), 397–407.

Canfield, J., & Wells, H.C. (1976). *100 ways to enhance self-concept in the classroom*. Englewood Cliffs, NJ: Prentice Hall.

Drovin, R., Normand, & Issard, B. (1987). I like you just the way you are. *AXON* 8(4), 99–101.

Dweck, C.S., Davidson, W., Nelson, S., & Enna, B. (1978). Sex differences in learned helplessness: II. The contingencies of evaluative feedback in the classroom, III. An experimental analysis. *Developmental Psychology*, *14*, 268–276.

Dweck, C.S., & Goetz, T.E. (1978). Attributions and learned helplessness. In J. Harvey, E. Wickes, & R. Kidd (Eds.), *New directions in attribution research* (Vol. II) (pp. 157–179). Hillsdale, NJ: Lawrence Erlbaum Associates.

Ebner, M. (1970). Accidental training: Unplanned reinforcement. In G.R. Patterson (Ed.), *Families' application of social learning to family life* (pp. 25–36). Champaign, IL: Research Press.

Eckart, M.L. (1986). *Correlates of self esteem in children with myelomeningocele*. Unpublished master's thesis, University of Cincinnati, OH.

Eckart, M.L. (1988). *Correlates of self esteem in adolescents with myelomeningocele*. Unpublished doctoral dissertation, University of Cincinnati, OH.

Feldman, W., & Varni, J. (1982). A parent training program for the child with spina bifida. *Spina Bifida Therapy*, 4(2), 77–89.

Friedrich, W., & Shaffer, J. (1986). Adolescent psychosocial adaptation. In D.B. Shurtleff (Ed.), *Myelodysplasias and exstrophies: Significance, prevention and treatment* (pp. 411–419). New York: Grune & Stratton.

Gardner, H. (1982). Relations with other selves. In H. Gardner (Ed.), *Developmental psychology* (2nd ed., pp. 459–490). Boston: Little, Brown.

Grassi, M.A. (1986). *Attitudes toward independence of mothers and their adolescent children with spina bifida and their relationship to self-care performance*. Unpublished master's thesis, University of Southern California, Los Angeles.

Greer, J.G., & Wethered, C.E. (1984). Learned helplessness: A piece of the burnout puzzle. *Exceptional Children*, *50*, 524–530.

Hayden, P.W., Davenport, S.L., & Campbell, M.M. (1979). Adolescents with myelodysplasia: Impact of physical disability on emotional maturation. *Pediatrics*, 64(1), 53–59.

Herskowitz, J., & Marks, A. (1977). The spina bifida patient as a person. *Developmental Medicine and Child Neurology*, *19*, 413–417.

Johnson, A.F. (1984). Psycho-social achievement in the latency-aged child with spina bifida within the family structure. *Zeitschrifte für Kinderchirurgie*, 39(Suppl. II). 138–140.

Kazak, A., & Clark, M. (1986). Stress in families of children with myelomeningocele. *Developmental Medicine and Child Neurology*, *28*, 220–228.

Knowlton, D., Peterson, K., & Putbrese, A. (1985). Team management of cognitive dysfunction in children with spina bifida. *Rehabilitation Literature*, 46(9–10), pp. 259–263.

Landry, S.H., Copeland, D., Lee, A., & Robinson, S. (1990). Goal directed behavior in children with spina bifida. *Journal of Developmental and Behavioral Pediatrics, 11*(6), 306–311.

Lollar, D.L., Reinoehl, J.K., Leverette, A.T., Martin, J.C., & Posid, V.A. (1989). Facilitating and assessing progress toward independence: Sheperd's program about real experiences (SPARX). *Zeitschrift für Kinderchirurgie. 44* Suppl. 1, 18–20.

Lutkemeier, D. (1979). *Self concept change among adolescents with myelomeningocele in response to a summer camp experience.* Unpublished doctoral dissertation, University of Cincinnati, OH.

MacBriar, B.R. (1983). Self concept of preadolescent and adolescent children with a myelomeningocele. *Issues in Comprehensive Pediatric Nursing, 6*, 1–11.

Mattson, B. (1982). Learning problems of children with spina bifida. *Clinical Proceedings: Children's Hospital National Medical Center, 38*, 225–230.

McAnarney, E.R. (1985). Social maturation: A challenge for handicapped and chronically ill adolescents. *Journal of Adolescent Health Care, 6*, 90–101.

McAndrew, I. (1979). Adolescents and young people with spina bifida. *Developmental Medicine and Child Neurology, 19*, 413–417.

Pearson, A., Carr, J., & Halliwell, M. (1985). The self concept of adolescents with spina bifida. *Zeitschrift für Kinderchirurgie, 40*(Suppl. I). 27–30.

Richardson, S.A., Goodman, N., Hastorf, A.H., & Dornbusch, S.M. (1961). Cultural uniformity in reaction to physical disability. *American Sociological Review, 26*, 241–247.

Rowley, F.L., Van Hasselt, V.B., & Hersen, M. (1987). Behavioral treatment of families with an adolescent with spina bifida: A treatment manual. *Social and Behavioral Science Documents, 16*(2), 9–68.

Scheers, M.M., Beeker, Th.W., & Hertogh, C.M.P.M. (1984). Spina bifida: Feelings, opinions and expectations of parents. *Zeitschrifte für Kinderchirurgie, 39*(Suppl. II), 120–121.

Schwartz, E.R. (1974). Characteristics of speech and language development in the child with myelomeningocele and hydrocephalus. *Journal of Speech and Hearing Disorders, 39*(4), 465–468.

Shurtleff, D., & Dunne, K. (1986). Adults and adolescents with meningomyelocele. In D.B. Shurtleff (Ed.), *Myelodysplasias and exstrophies: Significance, prevention and treatment* (pp. 421–430). New York: Grune & Stratton.

Stein, R. (1983). Growing up with a physical difference. *Child Health Care, 12*(2), 53–61.

Swisher, L.P., & Pinsker, E.J. (1971). The language characteristics of hyperverbal hydrocephalic children. *Developmental Medicine and Child Neurology, 13*, 746–755.

Tew, B. (1979). The "cocktail party" syndrome in children with hydrocephalus and spina bifida. *British Journal of Disorders of Communication, 14*, 89–101.

Social Acceptance and Disability Awareness

Fern L. Rowley-Kelly

Students with spina bifida are often deficient in social skills and social competence, and achieve minimal social acceptance in school, outside of school, and in later life (Ammerman, Van Hasselt, & Hersen, 1986; Anderson, Clarke, & Spain, 1982; McAndrew, 1979). Studies of children with physical disabilities and children with learning disabilities have found them "to be significantly lower in sociometric status than their nonhandicapped peers" (Asher & Taylor, 1982, p. 2). Sociometric status reflects the frequency with which a student is selected as a preferred playmate, workmate, or lunchmate by his or her peers. Simply put, students with disabilities are not often chosen as friends. "Most peer nomination studies of the handicapped have . . . consistently found integrated handicapped children to be both less accepted and more rejected than their nonhandicapped classmates" (Asher & Taylor, 1982, p. 2).

SOCIAL ISOLATION VERSUS SOCIAL ACCEPTANCE

Understanding Social Isolation

Numerous factors have been presented as possible causes of deficiencies in socialization, a variety of which could be at work in any given case. One factor is the "intensification and prolongation of attachment formation between the child and primary caregiver, usually the mother" (Rowley, Van Hasselt, & Hersen, 1986, p. 68). This intense attachment is attributed to the caregiver's increased responsibility for a child with extraordinary medical and developmental needs. Although this cohesiveness has obvious survival value, it can foster overprotectiveness by or social dependence on the caregiving parent. Such children have greater difficulty in transferring their emotional attachment to peers.

Children with disabilities may also have fewer social experiences than nondisabled children (Drabman & Patterson, 1982) and a consequent reduction in opportunities to learn appropriate or welcome behaviors. Borjeson and Lagergren (1990), in studying a group of 26 Swedish adolescents born with spina bifida in the mid-1960s, found that too many individuals did not achieve social acceptance.

> Contact with other pupils in the school classes varied from very extensive, including leisure activities, to being limited to school hours only (the majority of cases). Nine pupils felt no affinity with their schoolmates. Three pupils described their social contact as poor. None of the pupils considered themselves to be socially popular. (p. 700)

Many activities are simply unavailable to the child with physical disabilities. This lack of opportunity to socialize is often exacerbated by the tendency of nondisabled peers to reject or ignore the child with disabilities. Children with physical deformities (Richardson, Goodman, Hastorf, & Dornbusch, 1961) or minor physical anomalies (Halverson & Victor, 1976) tend to be rejected or to be unpopular. Since many students with spina bifida have learning disabilities, it is worth noting the finding that students with learning disabilities are also less popular (Bruininks, 1978).

In addition to the extensive literature on the socialization of children with disabilities in general, a limited number of studies have focused specifically on the socialization deficits of students with spina bifida. Ammerman (1986) found that "adolescents [with spina bifida] have difficulty with friendship formation and age-appropriate activities" (p. 102). Comparing wheelchair users to ambulatory adolescents with spina bifida and to a group of students with visual impairment, Ammerman found "the wheelchair bound spina bifida adolescents were the most severely isolated adolescents" (p. 103). (See Rowley-Kelly, chap. 9, this volume, for further discussion.) In the absence of particular social skill deficits, Ammerman suggested that this social isolation was due to an inability to initiate peer interactions or to a higher degree of rejection by peers.

Blum, Resnick, Nelson, and St. Germaine (1991) found the following in a study of peer relationships of adolescents with spina bifida:

> While most respondents reported both a "best friend" and, in fact, multiple friendships, certain characteristics of these friendships emerge: (1) best friends were often younger than they by as much as 5 years (approximately one-quarter); (2) few individuals (approximately 16%) reported having social contact with their best friends in each other's homes; (3) while many of their peers were starting to date (respondents indicated nearly half of friends were dating), only 14.7% of youths with spina bifida and 28.3% of those with cerebral palsy had had a similar experience, and of those who did, most reported it to be a rare experience. (p. 283)

Hirst (1989) addresses the social isolation discussed here under the term "social handicap" and employs a very useful distinction between impairment, disability, and handicap. "These can be seen as an ordered sequence of disablement experiences, such that disability results from impairment and both can lead to handicap or disadvantage" (p. 1). It is the entire set of impairments associated with spina bifida that puts the individual at risk of disabilities. The interaction of these impairments and disabilities with the social and physical environment then create the social handicap we often see:

> Poor psychological adjustment and extreme social isolation are associated not so much with individual functional limitations as with particular configurations of impairments and disabilities. It seems that social handicap is not a direct consequence of any impairment or disability but arises generally from severe functional loss and is shaped by dependency on others, restricted choices, physical barriers and adverse reaction of others. (Hirst, 1989, p. 1)

The usefulness of this approach lies in the realization that an effective approach must consider all aspects of disablement experiences, and in the opportunity to intervene at any and every stage of disablement. "Intervention at any point in the sequence of disablement experience may modify disease consequences in other dimensions. If so, any intervention which ignores the way impairments, disabilities and handicaps combine is likely to be less effective than if it takes account of the complexity of the disability experience" (Hirst, 1989, p. 10). At the level of the social environment of the classroom, social handicap can, and therefore should, be remediated by opening restricted choices, removing physical barriers, and converting the adverse reaction of others into a welcoming reaction that promotes social acceptance.

Without remediation, such social isolation can have severe negative social, vocational, and academic consequences. "There is increasing evidence that children's friendships serve important, if not essential, functions and that children without friends are at a risk in terms of later peer relationships" (Asher & Taylor, 1982, p. 4). It has also been argued that social learning is an important part of cognitive development and a necessary prerequisite for full academic progress: "Social interactions with peers may be among the best promoters of intellectual advance, even with respect to purely physical concepts" (Gardner, 1982, p. 95).

Mainstreaming and Social Acceptance

Mainstreaming is, in most cases, a critically necessary condition for the remediation of these social deficits. The arguments in favor of mainstreaming clearly outweigh those against this important practice. By itself, mainstreaming is not a sufficient condition for remediation. "All things considered, mainstreaming alone does not result in beneficial outcomes for handicapped children. Mainstreaming, however, can result in beneficial outcomes if it is focused upon teaching handicapped children the social skills necessary for positive interaction and social acceptance" (Gresham, 1982, p. 103).

Citing several other authors, Lord, Varzos, Behrman, Wicks, and Wicks (1990) advocate active intervention to assure that mainstreaming does result in social integration.

> Able-bodied and disabled children do not intermingle spontaneously (Apolloni and Cooke, 1978; Gresham, 1981), and successful social integration of a disabled child in a mainstream classroom requires the active participation of the teacher (Devoney et al., 1974; Cooke et al., 1977; Guralnick, 1978). Thus placing a disabled child in a mainstream classroom without a plan to facilitate integration can actually increase the child's sense of isolation (Gresham, 1981). (p. 21)

Johnson and Johnson (1978) argued that mainstreaming does not provide the least restrictive environment if students with disabilities are only present with their nondisabled peers: They must have genuine access to their peers. "It is when handicapped students are liked, accepted, and chosen as friends that mainstreaming becomes a positive influence on the lives of both handicapped and normal progress students" (Johnson & Johnson, 1978, p. 153).

If the student with spina bifida is to receive a full social, vocational, and academic education, then it is clear that social acceptance must be achieved, and not merely assumed. After the family, the school may be each young person's most important social learning laboratory. "While we tend to think of schools as locales for learning facts and making cognitive strides, they are also the scene of social development, including the child's expanding knowledge of the social world" (Gardner, 1982, p. 96).

In this social learning laboratory, learning may happen only haphazardly, without conscious or conscientious guidance by the teacher. In such classrooms, students with physical handicaps or learning disabilities are liable to discover that they do not belong, will never fit in, and must always remain more "different" than "the same." Without guidance, nondisabled peers may not even be able to accept or reinforce students with disabilities who have received social skills training outside of the classroom:

> In fact, it is possible that regular education peers may directly reduce the generalization of the handicapped child's new skills by ignoring—or even overtly punishing—attempts by the handicapped child to engage in new, not yet perfected, social behavior. (Strain, Odom, & McConnell, 1984, p. 141)

In other classrooms, well-designed programs of guided intervention have succeeded in increasing both the social competence and the social acceptance of children with disabilities (Strain, 1982; Strain et al., 1984). The exercises presented later in this chapter are guided experiments for the social learning laboratory in which all students live together. They are designed to allow all students to discover, to grow, and to belong.

Positive Results of Social Acceptance

Providing the opportunity to achieve social status also serves to enhance self-concept. Coopersmith (1967) found that "for children ages 8–12, competence and status played the largest role in self-concept formation" (Eckart, 1988, p. 12). Self-concept is, in turn, a critical determinant of academic and vocational success. Wattenberg and Clifford (1962) found that self-concept in kindergarten students was a better predictor of reading success in second grade than were scores on IQ tests. Students with spina bifida are at risk of poor self-concept, due to the presence of a number of factors, including limited physical competence and the likelihood of a poor body self-image. Given the crucial role of self-concept in promoting success, all opportunities to enhance self-concept should be seized, and any factors that might diminish self-concept should be limited in their effects (see Rowley-Kelly, chap. 9, this volume).

Social status or acceptance is thus a major determinant of a positive self-concept, which in turn makes a significant contribution to academic success. Both a positive and a negative prognosis for the student's total development can thus be stated, based on the level of peer acceptance achieved. The positive prognosis is that the student who has been accepted as a peer by his or her nondisabled peers will have an important social support network available to overcome other areas of difficulty. Being accepted as a peer is emphasized because being accepted as anything else, such as a mascot, is likely to create more problems than it solves. The negative prognosis is that a student who learns that he or she does not fit in with his or her peers in school will make poor use of the academic skills that are taught, will lack motivation to learn, and will not fit in to the economic and social mainstream as an adult.

Overcoming Social Isolation

There are two approaches to remediation for both students with spina bifida and their nondisabled peers: 1) exercises and programs that develop disability awareness, to promote communication and understanding; and 2) programs that train social skills and social competence, to give the student with spina bifida the capacity to participate in the full social life of the classroom and school. A discussion of disability awareness programming is offered next, followed by a description of age-appropriate programs designed to promote disability awareness in the schools. The issues involved in developing social skills and social competence, and specific approaches for accomplishing those goals, are then presented.

DISABILITY AWARENESS PROGRAMMING

The student with disabilities and his or her nondisabled peers have specific needs that can be met by a disability awareness program.

Needs of Students with Disabilities

The student with disabilities needs to learn that he or she is not the only one who is different. The student with disabilities also needs to learn that he or she has the right to be included. Finally, it is important for the student with disabilities to learn how to take an active role in helping peers achieve understanding and social acceptance:

> Chronically ill teens must learn to live openly with their handicap and to answer graciously questions that their peers may have regarding their condition. This helps to allay fears that their friends may have regarding the relationship between them and so will encourage friendships. (Jelneck, 1977, p. 61)

The students in a classroom may represent the first group of nondisabled peers the student with spina bifida has encountered. There will be many more such groups, and the student will need to achieve social acceptance in each of them. In future situations, the student with spina bifida will have to achieve acceptance without the support provided by a caring teacher. For this reason the student will need to develop attitudes and skills in the classroom that will foster social acceptance in future settings.

Needs of Nondisabled Students

Nondisabled students need the capacity to relate to members of the minority group comprising students with disabilities, just as they need to learn to relate to members of any minority group. Eckart (1986) noted that "persons with disabilities face social pressures and obstacles similar to those experienced by other minority groups" (p. 15). Further, in citing Wright and quoting Rousso (1985), Eckart (1986) stated that "the attitudes of the nondisabled to the disabled are predominantly negative, with the disabled facing many of the same prejudices as other minority groups" (p. 15).

Nondisabled students need to learn how to relate productively to anyone who is noticeably different. During their lifetime, every student will encounter people who differ ethnically, racially, or religiously; who speak a foreign language; who have an unusual name; who were raised in a different culture; who have a different level of education; or whose bodies function differently than their own. They need to learn to deal with people who are different by overcoming their unfamiliarity, by understanding the areas of difference, and by locating the broader areas of commonality. They also need to develop attitudes that will prepare them for the day when they may be the "different" people who need to achieve social acceptance.

Program Goals

To meet these needs, the following goals can be adopted for teachers, nondisabled students, and students with disabilities:

1. Facilitate acceptance of the student with spina bifida by his or her peers. By achieving this goal, the teacher will diminish the student's reliance on the teacher for social interaction. This will allow the student to develop a more appropriate teacher-student relationship and avoid dependency on the teacher.
2. Develop the capacity of all students to understand people who are unlike themselves in certain respects. Students will also learn to identify and enjoy areas of commonality.
3. Nondisabled students will develop the capacity to enjoy a friendship with a person with disabilities.
4. The student with spina bifida will develop the conviction that he or she is a peer among peers, with the same rights, benefits, and responsibilities as his or her classmates.
5. The student with spina bifida will learn to communicate about his or her disabilities to nondisabled students.
6. All participants will learn that people with disabilities have a broad range of possibilities and that they are to be socially accepted among nondisabled persons.

Presenting the Material: Openness and Sensitivity

Before describing specific methods and materials to help achieve these goals, some issues must be addressed about how these types of material should be presented. The first concerns the reluctance that both teachers and students may have to discuss disabilities and people with disabilities openly. Like race, sexuality, death, and other sensitive topics, many people become uncomfortable when the topic of disabilities is brought before a large group. The level of emotional discomfort that is present is in fact a gauge of the importance of the topic. This discomfort is eased and relieved by open discussion. Speaking forthrightly also removes a great deal of the sense of shame and embarrassment that students may have about people with disabilities, or about their feelings and thoughts about people with disabilities. Leaving the topic underground conveys the impression that it is not all right to talk about disabilities. This impression is uncomfortably close to the impression that it is not all right to have disabilities. Both impressions can be resoundingly removed by a teacher's willingness to speak freely about disabilities with the class.

It is also certain that a topic that is not addressed overtly will be discussed covertly. Covert discussion goes on without adult guidance and spreads rumors, half-truths, and misinformation. Covert discussion is also bound to get back to or be overheard by the student with spina bifida. This will of course be more painful and embarrassing than any well-guided, open discussion could be. In a classroom that includes a student with spina bifida, it is inevitable that the other students will talk about disabilities. Since discussion is inevitable, it should be directed in a manner that allows for the correction of misinformation, the quelling of rumors, and the dissipation of embarrassment. The critical gains that the student with spina bifida will make toward acceptance in the social milieu are clearly worth the initial effort to overcome the reluctance to speak freely about disabilities.

Another issue concerns whether the student with spina bifida should be with the class while the material is being presented. Generally, the student with spina bifida should be present to learn what information is being discussed and to supplement it. To minimize discomfort, the teacher should confer with the student ahead of time so the student may anticipate what is to come. When appropriate, the student can make suggestions, or be given an active role or part in the presentation. It is also important to confer with the student's parents.

The student's emotional and social maturity should be a major factor in determining whether he or she should be in class when the material is presented, and in determining his or her level of involvement. The social maturity, attitudes, and behavior of the class should also be considered. Some peers may find it easier to raise questions and make comments in the absence of the student with spina bifida, and may need an opportunity to do so. The teacher is also advised to talk with the student with spina bifida afterward to see if he or she has any concerns about the presentation.

It is also possible to dilute the emotional pressure of the situation through a number of devices. One such device is to provide information about spina bifida in a cluster of material about other disabilities or chronic medical conditions such as cerebral palsy, asthma, epilepsy, or color blindness.

Another such device is to provide dramatic distance, by using plays or stories that are about other people or characters who live far away, who lived long ago, or who exist in a mythical realm. The Hollywood musical "South Pacific" succeeds in addressing racism in America by telling a story about a French planter, a Tonkinese mother and daughter, and several American service people stationed far away. The audience is given a safe opportunity to consider the dimensions of racism by observing the attitudes and decisions of the characters, with relief provided by music and comedy. Many of the currently available materials on disability awareness use similar methods by creating fantastic characters in make-believe situations. Discussion afterward can be used to make the material more immediately relevant to the class.

Finally, it is both useful and important to stress areas of commonality. The student with spina bifida or another disability is like his or her peers in many more ways than he or she is unlike them. Although the similarities may not be as apparent as the differences, it is important to find a way to draw attention to them.

DESCRIPTIONS OF PROGRAMS PROMOTING DISABILITY AWARENESS

The elementary and secondary school years (K–12) represent several levels of cognitive, emotional, and social development. Acknowledging these differences, this section is organized as follows: kindergarten through second grade, third and fourth grades, fifth and sixth grades, seventh and eighth grades, and high school. In addition to specific approaches, a discussion of the developmental issues relevant to each age level is included. Resources for each age group are presented in the appendix at the end of this chapter.

All Ages

The following approach is relevant for students at all age levels.

Approach

Highlighting Competency   The teacher should discover something that the student with spina bifida does well and find a way to highlight it. This may include a coin or stamp collection, crafts, writing skills, board games, or many others. The teacher can then arrange for the student to present this special skill to the class, and have it written up in the school newspaper. The aim of this activity is to present the student's competency and identity to himself or herself and to the student body. Highlighting competency is important and valuable throughout the school years.

Kindergarten through Second Grade

Issues

Students with spina bifida, as well as their nondisabled peers, have a great need for security during kindergarten, first, and second grade. This need for security means that the student requires stable relationships, primarily with the teacher, but also with the peer group. The student is just beginning to handle the complexity of peer relationships outside of the home, and is not well prepared to learn how to deal with new significant others. Students with spina bifida have had extensive dealings with caregiving adults because of their medical and developmental needs, and may have become overly dependent on adults for their social relating. These ongoing relationships with adults may provide the sense of belonging at this age, making it more difficult for the student to launch into peer relationships.

Beginning in kindergarten and developing toward second grade, children will move from playing by themselves or next to their peers to actually playing with small groups. During these years, children learn to wait for their turn, begin to cooperate with peers, become aware of some individuals in their class, develop an interest in competition, and begin to acquire "best friends." They seek approval from their teacher, thriving on praise, and disliking criticism. They develop the capacity to pursue questions, to assert themselves verbally, to nag adults, and to quarrel with peers. They rely on adults to lead groups and to supervise their peer relationships (Lanning & Robbins, 1966). Students with spina bifida may display developmental delays in any of these areas. They may also have some delay in developing the capacity to play with their peers because of limited mobility and the restriction from activity that this entails.

They also may be accustomed to extra attention from adults because of their participation in an infant stimulation program and a special needs preschool. These highly structured programs rely on a one-to-one relationship between trainer and student. This level of intense interaction is critically necessary in allowing children with spina bifida to achieve a maximum degree of cognitive, physical, and social development in the early years. Students who have completed this type of program may have difficulty in learning to compete with other students in the group instructional settings that are typical of kindergarten and first-grade classrooms.

At this early stage, children's social thinking is very concrete and simple. Kindness is understood as giving away a lot of things, preferably things that taste good. Fairness means treating everybody the same, without regard to differences in need or merit, and is based on a conviction that children should have what they desire. Social conventions stand as fixed rules that cannot be changed (Gardner, 1982). Students in these grades may have difficulty accepting that the student with spina bifida is not always treated the same as they.

Students in kindergarten, first, and second grade prefer to participate by cutting, drawing, pasting, and asking questions. Nondisabled peers are prone to frustration at the lack of development in their fine motor skills and the difficulty they may have in coloring within the lines or cutting things out neatly. Students with spina bifida are at greater risk of frustration in this area because of their delayed development of fine motor skills. All students will be less interested in talking about how they feel or maintaining extended discussions. There is also a great deal of natural curiosity among the peers, who want to understand how things work and how they fit. There will probably be a great many questions about the student with spina bifida that peers will need and want to have answered so they can understand how things are for their classmate.

Classmates may also tend to be overly nurturing toward the student with spina bifida, almost as if they were playing with a doll or taking care of a younger sibling. Although this nurturing behavior is kindhearted and well intentioned, it might reinforce the student's tendency to remain dependent. The student with spina bifida may already expect that others are to do things for him or her, and thus may not expect to learn to do things independently. The following exercises are designed to satisfy curiosity, promote understanding, and foster acceptance of the student with spina bifida as a full member of the group.

Approaches

1. *Alike-and-different activities* At this level, alike-and-different activities should focus on concrete comparisons and involve movement. For example: 1) all the students who packed their lunch can go to the front of the room, while all the students who will buy their lunch can move to the back; 2) all the students who came to school on a bus this morning can stand up, while all the students who came some other way can remain seated; 3) all the boys can fold their arms, while all the girls wave theirs; 4) all the students who have ever been in a hospital can tell about what it was like, while all the students who have never been in a hospital can ask questions; or 5) all the students who have been to a baseball, football, basketball, or hockey game can tell about it, while those who have not can ask questions. Similar categories and procedures can be developed at the teacher's initiative.

2. *Situation stories* A situation story is similar to a case study but is written for a younger audience. It allows the reader to better understand the disability being studied. The class reads the story, and the students are asked questions about the person and his or her disability. To avoid singling out the student with spina bifida, the class could begin with one or two of many stories about other disabilities, such as *Tracy* (Mack, 1976), about a girl with cerebral palsy, or *He's My Brother* (Lasker, 1974), about a boy with developmental delays. These and other resources are included in the appendix at the end of this chapter.

3. *Personal talk time* A time could be set aside each week for open discussion on a variety of issues that relate to socialization, feelings, attitudes, and behavior. Students should be encouraged to ask ques-

tions, raise topics, and respond to open-ended questions presented by the teacher. Natural curiosities about braces or wheelchairs could be satisfied as they occur.

The teacher could begin "talk time" in a variety of ways. The teacher could choose one of the senses and ask the class to imagine what it would be like to be without that sense (e.g., "What would be the limitations?" "What could you still do?"). The teacher should make a list of the responses and correct any misconceptions. On another occasion, the teacher could ask the students to imagine not having the use of one hand or some other part of the body.

4. *Adapt a game*   The teacher should ask the students to think of a game that can be played with a person with disabilities. The students could name existing games that would not require modification, change the rules of an existing game, or invent a new game. The activity should be completed by actually playing the new or adapted game.

Third and Fourth Grades

Issues

A sense of belonging continues to be a matter of concern at this age level, because children become more aware of "differences." Third- and fourth-grade students are more interested in achieving competency in areas such as sports and academics, and have begun to choose friends on the basis of what they can achieve. A pecking order based on competence has begun to develop, and there are likely to be one or two peers who are always picked last when choosing up sides for a game.

Developmentally, this is a critical time for establishing peer relationships. Because the student with spina bifida is likely to have different levels of competence than most of the other students, peer acceptance may begin to be a problem. Staring at the student who is different may be an issue, as well as teasing. Third- and fourth-grade students are also more likely to compare themselves to their peers, and to be aware of which students are liked or disliked, and admired or accepted by the other students. These students have begun to adopt the social standards of the peer group as one means of measuring self-esteem and determining their sense of identity.

Children at this stage are less reliant on adult standards of behavior. They are more willing to abide by peer-group decisions, and will insist on the observation of rules in more organized games. Spirits of competition and cooperation are developed as large groups are formed for competitive games (Lanning & Robbins, 1966). The student with spina bifida who is excluded from such large-scale competitive activities in the gym or on the playground is thus denied a critically important opportunity for social development.

Social thinking has gained in complexity. Kindness is now understood as giving by "someone who has" to "someone who does not have," to restore or create equality among group members. What is given may now be expanded beyond the material to the psychological, so that support or advice may be given, instead of candy. Children can now understand the fairness of distributing rewards on the basis of merit, and can differentiate between talent, effort, and other forms of merit. They can evaluate their own performance on a task by comparing it to that of their peers, and can learn from someone else's success or failure (Gardner, 1982). Many students with spina bifida may have learned to defend their self-esteem appropriately by comparing their physical performance to their own physiological capacities, rather than the capacities of their nondisabled peers. Such a student may feel justifiably proud of the ability to walk a long distance with crutches, just as a nondisabled peer feels proud of a victory in a foot race (Eckart, 1986).

While peers are advancing in autonomy, the student with spina bifida may continue to be dependent on adults in important practical respects, including assistance in a bowel and bladder program, mobility, and physical therapy. The student with spina bifida may also have a great deal more with which to cope than the nondisabled peers and may not have the available coping resources needed to advance socially along with the group. In various circumstances, this student's dependence on adults may be due to a practical necessity, a developmental delay, or an instance of unnecessarily immature behavior.

Approaches

1. *Alike-and-different activities*   These activities are designed to show the many ways we can be different from each other, while still remaining alike. One such activity is: Students are matched randomly in pairs and asked to name 10 ways in which they are like their partner, and 10 ways they are different. Students meet with their partner to discuss "likenesses" and "differences" and then report their findings back to the group.

2. *Disabilities unit*   In third and fourth grade, there should be sufficient cognitive development and structure in the educational process to allow for a unit on disabilities in social studies, health class, or in any other suitable area of the curriculum. Students should be given a pretest, a reading assignment, activities, and a posttest. Sample questions for a disability awareness pretest include: 1) Are disabilities contagious? 2) Are disabilities a punishment? Are they someone's fault? 3) Is a disability a sickness that can be cured? 4) Can people with disabilities lead useful and happy lives? 5) Is it all right to stare at someone with disabilities? 6) Is it all right to ask questions of someone with disabilities? 7) Are people with

disabilities sad most of the time? Do they need pity? 8) Are people with disabilities born that way? 9) Will people with disabilities grow out of them?

This test could be readministered as a posttest at the end of the unit (Benham, 1978; Children's Museum of Boston with WGBH Boston, 1978).

3. *Design a room*   The class, or a selected team, could be asked to design a classroom or another room to meet the needs of a student with crutches or wheelchair. The student could be interviewed to determine what he or she can reach, open, move through, or carry. Barriers are identified and alternatives suggested.

4. *Adapt a game*   A team could be appointed to pick one or two active games and adapt them to include the student who uses a wheelchair, crutches, or other assistive device. The project should be successfully completed by actually playing the game.

5. *Name calling and teasing*   The issue of name calling and teasing may be addressed without relying on references to disabilities or spina bifida. The teacher could ask each student to recall a time when they have been teased or called a name, and a time when they have engaged in teasing or name calling. Each student would then be asked to write a short autobiographical or fictionalized account of the situation. An alternative activity would be to have students write a skit or perform a role play. After the stories have been written and read aloud (or after the skits have been performed), the students should discuss their feelings about teasing and being teased (Barnes, Berrigan, & Biklen, 1978).

6. *Wheelchair simulation*   If it is possible to obtain a wheelchair, a nondisabled student could be asked to spend a period of time moving around in a wheelchair. The student could then report on what was different, what was accessible, what was inaccessible, and how it felt.

Fifth and Sixth Grades

Issues

Students in the fifth and sixth grades have begun to develop independence from adult standards. They are reinterpreting their identity in terms of their own perceptions of themselves, and in terms of their peers' perceptions of them. Their body image or sense of what they look like is developing, and this is very important to them.

These developments place the student with spina bifida at risk in many ways. Obviously, for many, this student's body looks different, and the development of a realistic and acceptable body image can be problematic (see Rowley-Kelly, chap. 9, this volume). These are often the years when many students with spina bifida begin to realize how much they are unlike their peers. At the same time, students with spina bifida may remain more dependent on adults than other students of the same age, and the move toward autonomous and peer-oriented self-interpretation may be delayed.

Students in fifth and sixth grades are more aware of and concerned about others' feelings. Peers have become the dominating influence, and their approval is sought. Teamwork is developed, and loyalty is displayed toward the team, club, or troop. There are intense friendships, and a clear sense of the social rank of classmates. There are separate groupings for boys and girls, with some display of hostility between the sexes. Sports and outdoor activities such as camping become valued, and competence and daring become important, especially among boys (Eckart, 1988; Lanning & Robbins, 1966). Development in all of these areas can be problematic for the student with spina bifida.

The growth in sophistication of social thinking continues. Fifth graders are quite likely to understand that social conventions are arbitrary and can be changed at will. They will, accordingly, adopt standards of behavior for their groups, including passwords, initiation rites, and membership requirements (Gardner, 1982). This capacity can be exploited in the activities presented in this section that allow the group to redesign an activity, game, or law to accommodate a person with disabilities.

The needs of fifth and sixth graders for acceptance are similar to those for third and fourth graders, but are acted out at a more sophisticated level. A positive sense of belonging remains important, as does the development of positive self-identity and self-esteem. Nondisabled peers have developed a good deal of social initiative and are now making good use of their independent mobility to visit friends, go to new places, and learn to do new things.

This puts many students with spina bifida at increased risk of isolation. In the activities presented in this section, emphasis should be placed on actively including the student with spina bifida in the activities. The activities themselves, such as "design a city" and "law writing," incorporate the concept of actively including people with spina bifida and other disabilities in the total adult world.

This may also be a good time for the student with spina bifida to be a presenter of information about his or her disabilities. Nothing will make it easier for this student to get included in the social milieu than the ability to be assertive and informative about himself or herself and about his or her needs and strengths. It should be noted, however, that this must be done with a great deal of planning, as all children this age are extremely self-conscious.

Approaches

1. *Alike-and-different activities* The exercise presented to third and fourth graders could be used as is, or adapted as follows. Groups of

four students are randomly selected. Two students serve as subjects, while the third is assigned to "prove" how totally alike they are. The fourth student must "prove" that the first two are totally different. The two debaters may interview the subjects, write their results, and then present their case to the class. Humor should be encouraged as long as it is in good taste and respectful of the students.

2. *Disability unit*   Structured reading assignments with pretests and posttests could be given. The list of pretest and posttest questions in the section for third and fourth graders could be used as is, or adapted. Students could select a disability and do research on it in the library or interview persons with the disabilities as resources. This information could then be presented in writing or in an oral presentation. Emphasis should focus on the experience of having disabilities. Biographies of well-known persons with disabilities (Franklin Delano Roosevelt, Helen Keller, and others) may be included in the resource list. Some students may be interested in examining how persons with disabilities are treated in traditional fairy tales and nursery rhymes (Barnes et al., 1978).

3. *Design a room, school, vehicle, or city*   This activity (as described in the section for third and fourth graders) may be expanded beyond the classroom to include any type of architectural access situation. For example: Can a person in a wheelchair or braces get into the local library, post office, grocery store, movie theater, church, or other public building? What changes would have to be made? (Ross & Freelander, 1977).

4. *Adapt a game*   This activity (as described in the section for third and fourth graders) may be repeated at the fifth- and sixth-grade level, with the expectation that a more sophisticated game or activity would be adapted, and that the student with spina bifida would be more involved in the interaction and planning.

5. *Law writing*   Students could study the laws that currently exist for persons with disabilities. Students could review advocacy material and then suggest other laws that could be passed to assist persons with disabilities (Ross & Freelander, 1977).

Seventh and Eighth Grades

Issues

Cognitive and social sophistication continues to develop. Giving to a friend or a person in need is now likely to be understood by the student in early adolescence as including psychological support. Friendship is now seen as an enduring relationship, with ongoing needs and obligations. Boys and girls begin to take a more active interest in each other, with girls being generally ready to interact socially before boys are ready to reciprocate (Gardner, 1982). Heterosocial issues become difficult areas of adjustment for adolescents, and especially for adolescents with spina bifida. Because social isolation is a major problem for young people with spina bifida after they leave high school, this is an important time to encourage their full participation in the full life of the school.

Identity formation is a key task of adolescence that usually begins in middle school. Cognitively, most students in middle school have arrived at the stage of formal operations. For the student with spina bifida, this means that the magical belief in an eventual recovery can no longer be sustained. The normal challenges of identity formation are thus enormously complicated by the need to integrate the permanence of disability into the developing concept of self. (See the discussion of stages of acceptance in Rowley-Kelly, chap. 12, this volume.)

This stage of development also includes an increasing capacity to criticize the adult world and to differentiate from parents and teachers (Lanning & Robbins, 1966). The traditional way of doing things is subject to review at all levels. This capacity may be directed toward the critical review of the current treatment of persons with disabilities in society. Students in middle school are beginning to develop an awareness of social and political issues such as access and discrimination. They are also capable of dealing with more detailed information. Access to careers for persons with disabilities can be addressed at this age. All students are preparing for an adult level of responsibility and this type of interest can naturally be directed into revisions of the ways that the current adult society advertises, legislates, designs equipment, and so forth. The following activities will channel this interest while developing an awareness of the needs of persons with disabilities.

Approaches

1. *Positive inclusion* These are active years when participation in activities is essential to social growth. The teacher should make a point to include the student with spina bifida in fundraisers, clubs, special projects, and other activities. For example, the teacher should: 1) insist that the student come to the dance—have him or her collect tickets or help with decorating; 2) give the student a useful role to play with the basketball team, such as official timer or public address announcer; or 3) encourage the student's participation in the school choir, band, or orchestra—have the student mail out invitations for open house, hand out programs for concerts and class plays, or serve on the make-up committee. Many dramatic roles can be portrayed by students with spina bifida. There is no need to typecast students with disabilities or to limit them to playing only characters who have disabilities. The teacher may need to

insist on participation and actively facilitate the process. However it is done, the goal is to allow the student with spina bifida to come through on an age-appropriate task that the other students will both benefit from and appreciate.

2. *Ethical situations* The teacher could work with adolescents' growing awareness of moral values by presenting the following situations to the class and asking the accompanying questions:

> A young woman is standing at a busy street corner. She is blind and has a seeing eye dog by her side. The dog is visibly confused and preparing to cross the street even though the light is still red and a car is quickly approaching. What would you do?

> A young man is in a wheelchair in the hallway of a college building. He is about to leave the building to cross the campus for his next class. As he puts his sweater on, a pen accidentally falls from his lap. What do you think you should do? Immediately help him pick it up? Wait to see his response? Is it wrong not to help a person with disabilities? Does this man really need your help?

Similar situations could be constructed to develop an awareness of when it is important to help persons with disabilities and when it is important to allow them to be independent (Barnes et al., 1978).

3. *Accessible building tour* A class trip could be planned to visit a building in the city that is accessible to persons with disabilities. A barriers checklist like the one in Figure 10.1 developed by Barnes et al. (1978) should be taken along to determine whether the building is completely accessible for persons with disabilities. The class may also want to visit a building that is *not* accessible to persons with disabilities and use a barriers checklist to discuss the differences in the two buildings (Barnes et al., 1978). The visit could conclude with a discussion of what it might be like to live in a society where many if not most buildings are not fully accessible.

4. *Investigating public transportation* Students could be given the opportunity to investigate the accessibility of public transportation for persons with disabilities. Students could call or write to different airlines, passenger railroads, bus lines, and ship lines to obtain current information regarding the accessibility of these modes of transportation (Barnes et al., 1978).

5. *I'm the same . . . .* Students could write an essay after reflecting upon one of the following statements: "I'm the same as a person who is blind because . . . ," "I'm the same as a person who is in a wheelchair because . . . ," or "I'm the same as a person who is deaf because . . . " (Barnes et al., 1978, p. 36).

6. *Wheelchair simulation* This activity (described in the section

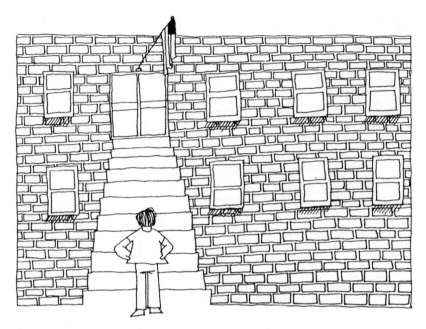

73. BARRIERS CHECKLIST

Materials: Ditto on barriers
Activity: Have the children in small groups assess their school using the following checklist:

Barriers Checklist

A barrier is something that makes it very difficult or impossible for a disabled person to get into or around a building. Is your school barrier free? Use this checklist to find out. And if your school does not do very well on the checklist, don't be too surprised. Most buildings have barriers. And barriers can be changed.

Barrier - Free

If the main entrance to the school has a ramp it is
barrier free. If it has stairs, and no ramp, it has a
barrier.   ☐ Yes ☐ No

Are the door knobs of all main doors 3 feet from the
ground so that people in wheelchairs can reach them?   ☐ Yes ☐ No

Do the hallways have handrails to help people walk?
No handrails is a barrier for some people.   ☐ Yes ☐ No

(continued)

Figure 10.1.   Barriers checklist to measure a building's accessibility. (From Barnes, E., Berrigan, C., & Biklen, D. [1978]. What's the difference? Teaching positive attitudes toward people with disabilities, pp. 81–83. Syracuse, NY: Human Policy Press; reprinted by permission.)

Figure 10.1. (*continued*)

Parking Spaces: Are there parking spaces reserved
for disabled people? Are they near the entrance of the
building? Are they 12 feet wide? Are there at least 2
out of every 100 spaces reserved for people who have
disabilities?   ☐ Yes ☐ No

Are there curb cuts so that people in wheelchairs, or
people with baby carriages or shopping carts can
pass easily?   ☐ Yes ☐ No

Are there tactile markings (can be felt by touch) cut in
the sidewalk to warn people who are blind?   ☐ Yes ☐ No

If your school has more than one floor, does it have an
elevator? (Skip this question if your school is one
floor.)   ☐ Yes ☐ No

Does the elevator have braille markers for the floor
buttons? (Skip this question if your school is one
floor.)   ☐ Yes ☐ No

Does the elevator have light and bell signals to help
people who are blind or deaf to know when the
elevator is ready? (Skip this question if your school is
one floor.)   ☐ Yes ☐ No

Are the doorways to all bathrooms at least 33 inches
wide?   ☐ Yes ☐ No

Are your sinks low enough? Get a chair and see if you
can reach the sink while you're sitting in the chair. If
not, then the sinks will probably be unusable for
people in wheelchairs.   ☐ Yes ☐ No

Are the telephones in the building accessible? Use
the same test as for the sinks. How many inches
should they be lowered?   ☐ Yes ☐ No

Are the fire alarms low enough for people in wheel-
chairs?   ☐ Yes ☐ No

Are there grab bars in the bathroom stalls so that people
can lift themselves from a wheelchair to the toilet and
back again?   ☐ Yes ☐ No

Are the windows 24 inches or 28 inches from the floor
so that short people and people in wheelchairs can see
out?   ☐ Yes ☐ No

Are the aisles in the classroom at least 32 inches wide
so that people in wheelchairs, or on crutches, or with
canes or walkers, can get around easily?   ☐ Yes ☐ No

Are there flashing lights for fire alarms so that deaf
students will know if there's a fire?   ☐ Yes ☐ No

Are there picture signs to show the purpose of each
room so that people who cannot read will know where
to go?   ☐ Yes ☐ No

(*continued*)

Figure 10.1. (*continued*)

Count up the number of Yes answers. Total Yes answers _____

Count up the number of No answers. Total No answers _____

Here is how to figure out whether your school gets a passing grade or not:

$$\frac{\text{Multiply Number of Yes Answers X 100}}{18} = \underline{\hspace{2cm}}\%$$

70% is a passing score.

Now that you have studied your school, you probably know some ways that it can be improved. What are the things that you think should be changed first? Are there some things that you and your friends could fix, like making signs for rooms, or a ramp for a short flight of stairs? Do you know of some buildings that would score better on the checklist? How do these buildings make it easier for disabled people?

Prepare a report of your findings and send a letter or go in person to the Superintendent or the Parent/Teacher Association (PTA) to share your findings and to seek change.

---

for third and fourth graders) is as appropriate for middle school and high school students as it is for younger students. Older students have the capacity to develop an even greater appreciation of what it might be like to see the world from the seat of a wheelchair. No simulation can duplicate the experience of using a wheelchair for a lifetime. An extensive and thorough simulation can significantly improve awareness and sensitivity.

7. *Adapt a game* This activity (described in sections for younger students) may be repeated at the secondary level, with the expectation that a more sophisticated game or activity would be adapted, and that the student with spina bifida would be more involved in the interaction and planning.

Senior High School

Issues

The later stages of adolescence present a number of significant developmental tasks. These include the ongoing development of a sense of identity, a task first taken up in early adolescence (Erikson, 1968). Achievement of autonomy and separation from the family, the development of the ability to form mature attachments, and the development of a career orientation are also critical tasks for this period. As difficult as these issues are for nondisabled adolescents, each has an additional dimension for students with spina bifida.

This struggle for identity includes "the problem of defining oneself as a person with a handicap in a predominantly nondisabled world

(McAnarney quoted in Eckart, 1986, p. 44). Achievement of autonomy from the family is especially problematic in students with spina bifida, who tend to avoid rebellion and assertiveness, and to continue to rely on the comfort and support of a close family relationship (Blum, 1983). There are frequently problems in the formation of mature social relationships with peers (Ammerman et al., 1986; Blum, 1983; McAndrew, 1979). The complications to normal adolescent development for young persons with spina bifida are sufficient to have led Shurtleff and Sousa (1977) to conclude that it would be realistic to expect adolescence to be prolonged for these students.

The achievement of social acceptance is thus made more difficult for students with spina bifida in the high school years. It is also made more important. An effective social adjustment to the high school world will significantly increase the probability that these young persons will move out into the world after graduation rather than moving back into the family. The programs suggested here are designed to promote the conviction that students with spina bifida do fully belong in all aspects of the high school world and will belong in the world of work and higher education after graduation.

Approaches

1. *Positive inclusion*   Participation in activities continues to be essential to social growth and to vocational development. Teachers should continue to involve the student with spina bifida in fundraisers, clubs, proms, class plays, special projects, and other activities. For example, the teacher should: 1) involve the student in athletic activities—if he or she cannot participate directly, the teacher should develop a role as equipment manager or announcer; 2) involve the student as a sports photographer for the school newspaper, or enlist him or her for the editorial staff of the high school yearbook; or 3) encourage the student to join the high school band, orchestra, chorus, or drama club—the student could mail out invitations for open house, hand out programs for concerts and class plays, or serve on the make-up committee. The coach or faculty advisor for each activity will probably need to insist on participation and actively facilitate the process. However it is done, the goal is to allow the student with spina bifida to come through on an age-appropriate task that will allow him or her to work with nondisabled peers while developing initiative, responsibility, and other traits that will be useful in the adult social and vocational world.

2. *Ad analysis*   The teacher should have the students cut out a random selection of magazine and newspaper advertisements, and dis-

cuss the fact that persons with disabilities are not included in advertisements. The teacher could relate this to the exclusion of black people and other minorities from advertising prior to the civil rights movement. The teacher should ask the students: "Is this fair? Are persons with disabilities an invisible part of our society? Should any group of people in our society be made invisible?"

The students could prepare a letter to the editor of a newspaper or magazine and argue that the advertisements should include all types of people. Students could make up their own advertisement and include it as a suggestion. They could ask the editor to respond with his or her opinion and the publication's policy on advertising (Barnes et al., 1978). News coverage can also be monitored to determine how well and how often issues relevant to people with disabilities are presented.

3. *Design a room, school, vehicle, or city* Students could be given the opportunity to design a room, a school, a home, a vehicle, or an entire city that is accessible to persons with disabilities. Current accessibility guidelines and standards should be followed in the students' designs. Depending on the circumstances, students in vocational classes could design or build something to meet an access need in the school (e.g., a wheelchair ramp to provide a way around a stairway). This activity will stimulate a concern and growing appreciation for constructing more accessible buildings for persons with disabilities (Ross & Freelander, 1977).

4. *Law writing* Students could be given the opportunity to study the current legislative decisions established for persons with disabilities in our society. The students could then be asked to write new laws that would improve the quality of life for persons with disabilities (Ross & Freelander, 1977).

5. *Television and persons with disabilities* Students could examine stereotypes observed in television programs regarding persons with disabilities. These stereotypes could be discussed and students could be given the opportunity to rewrite the same television scripts to portray persons with disabilities in a more accurate manner.

Conclusion

Promoting disability awareness should be begun in kindergarten and continued throughout the educational continuum. Fortunately, there are many activities available to assist in this process. Many of them are adaptations of activities that already take place in most schools. All of them will benefit all students and help them to deal with their own issues about being different. Nondisabled students will also have excellent opportunities to learn about persons with disabilities and to learn how to relate to people who are different.

DEVELOPING SOCIAL SKILLS AND SOCIAL COMPETENCY

Learning to achieve social acceptance is a critical area of instruction for students with spina bifida. Educating students with spina bifida toward employment will be much more fruitful if they know how to fit into a group of nondisabled peers, and believe that they belong in the mainstream of life. One cannot safely assume that these students will naturally develop social competency or automatically achieve acceptance.

Specific social competency goals need to be set and incorporated in the IEP at all levels, from kindergarten through 12th grade. Students who do not have IEPs should have social competency goals incorporated in the curriculum. Although this planning can take place when transition planning is done, it is very important that work on social competency and social acceptance begin early and proceed throughout each student's education. (See Rowley-Kelly, chap. 12, this volume.)

Issues

Placement of students with disabilities in mainstream classrooms does not automatically generate increased social interaction between persons with and without disabilities, increased social acceptance of persons with disabilities by the nondisabled persons, or modeling of the behavior of nondisabled peers by students with disabilities (Gresham, 1982). The possession of certain key skills, including cooperation, positive peer interaction, sharing, greeting others, asking for and giving information, and making conversation, has been found to correlate positively with social acceptance (Asher, Oden, & Gottman, 1977; Gresham, 1982). Children with disabilities often lack these key social skills (McHale & Olley, 1982). In particular, students with spina bifida are often deficient in conversational skills. (See Culatta, chap. 7, this volume.)

Although presence in a classroom with nondisabled peers may give the student with spina bifida the opportunity to develop these social skills through modeling, it is not safe to assume that modeling will take place just because the opportunity is present.

> For modeling effects to occur, the observer must attend to relevant modeling stimuli, retain the information or stimuli which were modeled, have the motor-reproduction processes necessary to execute the modeled behavior, and have some incentive or motivation for performing the observed behavior. (Bandura, 1977, quoted in Gresham, 1982, p. 102)

As was noted in the preceding chapters, the student with spina bifida may have difficulty maintaining attention toward the relevant stimuli, and may not have the cognitive or motor capacity to reproduce the modeled behavior. Motivation may or may not be present, as learned helplessness, adult dependency, or low self-esteem may interfere. (See Rowley-Kelly, chap. 9, this volume.)

The full possession of key social skills is indispensable to social acceptance and effective mainstreaming. Yet the possession of these skills by the student with spina bifida is by no means guaranteed and there are likely to be significant obstacles to the development of these skills in an unguided social learning environment. Given this likelihood of deficiency in both social skills and social acceptance, all students with disabilities should be assessed for social skill levels and for social acceptance (Gresham, 1982). Based on this assessment, goals for social acceptance and social skills attainment can be incorporated into each student's IEP. Social skills may be assessed by the Social Behavior Assessment (SBA) (Stephens, 1978). The SBA assesses 136 separate skills and is accompanied by a training manual. Social acceptance can be assessed with conventional sociometric techniques such as peer nomination (Asher & Taylor, 1982). Although not all students with spina bifida are currently eligible for an IEP, the likelihood of deficiency in social skills and social acceptance is so great that all students with spina bifida should be assessed in these areas, and appropriate goals included in their curriculum plan.

The failure of a student with spina bifida to use a particular social skill does not always mean that the skill is absent and needs to be trained. "One must also look to the child's social environment to determine the origins and sustaining events surrounding social isolation" (Strain et al., 1984, p. 139). In many instances, social skills are present but not used because of the social environment provided by the peer group. Social skills training is more likely to produce long-term results if training plans include the student with spina bifida and one or more nondisabled peers. Intervention by adult trainers without the mediation of nondisabled peers may intrude into the student's natural social relationships without actually producing social behaviors that fit into the existing behavior patterns of the peer group. Social skills and social competency training can be designed to take these realities of social reciprocity into account (Strain et al., 1984).

Approaches

There is an extensive body of literature describing techniques of social skills training. Most methods rely on changing the antecedent conditions of the social situation, altering the consequences, or modeling (Gresham, 1982). An additional method relies on peers as intermediaries in training. (Resources for this section are included in the appendix at the end of this chapter.)

Changing the Antecedent Conditions

These approaches are based on providing more occasions in the social environment for positive interchanges between students with disabilities and their nondisabled peers. Numerous specific techniques have proven effective:

1. Nondisabled peers could initiate social interactions by inviting the student with spina bifida to join in a game or work on a project (Strain, Shores, & Timm, 1977).
2. Dramas or sociodramatic activities could be used to create interactions between peers as characters acting out a fairy tale, or as participants in a role play of a social situation. This technique requires group rules to limit confusion and avoid counterproductive behavior. Students may also create their own skits (Necco, Wilson, & Scheidmantel, 1982).
3. The teacher could create play or task activities to increase the frequency of interactions between the student with spina bifida and his or her nondisabled peers.

Altering the Consequences

These procedures are based on the finding of social learning theory that behaviors that are reinforced by a desired stimulus will be learned more rapidly and retained more effectively. The reinforcing stimulus need not be extraordinary to be effective:

> The general procedure in contingent social reinforcement involves having a teacher socially reinforce (praise, hug, etc.) the target child when interacting or cooperating with peers. This same procedure can be used to reinforce nondisabled children whenever they approach and interact positively with mainstreamed disabled children. (Gresham, 1982, p. 105)

The delightful simplicity of this procedure is based on the availability of hugs, smiles, and pats on the shoulder in any classroom. The only difficulty is in remembering to target the desired behaviors and to reinforce them when they occur. There are also a variety of more formal techniques:

1. Tokens could be used to reward a variety of desired interactive behaviors. The student with spina bifida who is socially isolated could be given a token for joining a game on the playground, initiating a greeting, asking for information from another student, complying with a request, sharing materials, or inviting another student to join him or her at the lunch table. A predetermined number of tokens could be exchanged for a privilege or a valued item. Since these behaviors should produce natural social rewards, after they are well established it is important to gradually extinguish the use of the tokens.
2. Group contingencies may also be effective. In this procedure, a reinforcement is provided for the entire class if all students display a predetermined level of desirable social behaviors such as sharing, say-

ing "please" and "thank you," verbal complimenting, or cooperating (Gamble & Strain, 1979). In other circumstances, the reinforcement for the entire group could depend on one or two members achieving certain specific social behavior goals. Care should be exercised to ensure that the target student is actually capable of reaching the selected goals (Gresham, 1982).

Modeling

Peer modeling has been used on several occasions to teach social skills to children with disabilities. Of particular relevance to work with students with spina bifida is the progress that has been made in training students who were socially withdrawn. Film modeling, in which the desired behaviors were demonstrated on a film or videotape, has proven effective, as has the use of live modeling by peers in the classroom (Evers & Schwartz, 1973; Evers-Pasquale & Sherman, 1975; O'Connor, 1972; Peterson, Peterson, & Scriven, 1977). This research has generated several specific suggestions to enhance the training effect of modeling:

1. Film modeling is more effective if a narrator calls attention to the behavior being modeled. Live modeling is similarly enhanced if a teacher or other trainer calls attention to the target behavior.
2. Modeling is more effective if it shows a coping response. For example, the model could first show difficulty or fear about interacting with peers, and could then be seen to gradually overcome this (Thelen, Fry, Fehrenback, & Frautschi, 1979).
3. Students are more likely to imitate a model who is high in social status. They are also more likely to imitate a nondisabled model (Peterson et al., 1977).

Peer-Mediated Training

"The necessity of changing the behavior of both the target child and interactive peers to obtain marked increases in the handicapped child's rate of social interaction" [was demonstrated by Walker, Greenwood, Hops, and Todd (1979)] (quoted in Strain et al., 1984, p. 141). They trained for positive initiations by the child with disabilities toward peers, positive responses to peer initiatives, and continuance of positive interaction patterns. Reinforcing only the behavior of the targeted child with disabilities actually led to a reduction in the level of social interaction, while reinforcing both the child with disabilities and the interacting peers led to a measurable increase in social interaction. On this basis, Strain (1982, Strain et al., 1984) recommended that:

1. Critical skills should be taught to the child with disabilities.
2. The same skills should be taught to the child's peers, if necessary.

3. Reinforcement procedures should be directed toward the interaction of the child with disabilities and the interacting peers, and not just to the child with disabilities (Strain et al., 1984).
4. Specific behaviors that have been connected to positive increases in social status should be trained. These include sharing, showing affection, giving physical assistance, and offering ideas for play (Tremblay, Strain, Hendrickson, & Shores, 1981).
5. The teacher should target and train behaviors that are of specific social value in the current peer group. This may be done by identifying a few well-liked students who are of the same sex, ethnic, and socioeconomic status as the student with spina bifida. The teacher can then observe for those behaviors that contribute to the acceptance of the well-liked peers, and teach them to the student who is not accepted (Strain et al., 1984).
6. Valuable behaviors may also be targeted by asking the rejected child to identify one or two peers with whom he or she would like to become friends. The selected peers may then be asked what behaviors they look for in a friend. The rejected child can then be trained in the desired behaviors the chosen peers have identified (Hoier & Cone, 1980).

SUMMARY

Recognizing that students with spina bifida are at risk of developmental delay in key dimensions of social learning and are at risk of limited acceptance in the mainstream peer group, the classroom can provide excellent guided opportunities for positive social learning and full social acceptance. Levels of social skill development and of peer acceptance can and should be assessed, and a program of activities to overcome these deficiencies can be included in the student's IEP. Recent research provides a wide variety of methods and techniques for assessment and remediation in this area, providing a clear opportunity to ensure optimum social development and acceptance, to promote academic achievement, and to help students with spina bifida prepare to take their full place in the workplace and in the world.

GLOSSARY

Antecedent conditions   Preexisting conditions that form the basis for social learning. Altering the social conditions in the classroom can increase the available opportunities to learn the social skills that lead to acceptance.
Autonomy   Ability to function independently, or to do things for oneself, and under one's own direction and motivation.

Contingent social reinforcement   Procedure in which desired social behaviors are encouraged by applying positive social reinforcement when they occur. The reinforcement is contingent because it depends on the student's behavior and is only provided when the student performs as desired. The reinforcement is social because it rewards positive social behaviors, and because the reward is a social act, such as a smile or a statement of approval from the teacher.

Formal operations   In the work of Piaget, formal operations is a stage of cognitive development following concrete operations. In the stage of formal operations, things are seen as they could be. Formal operations also allows for hypothetical and deductive reasoning. Concrete operations are limited to understanding the relationships between objects. Formal operations can grasp the relationships between other relationships.

Identity formation   Development of the sense of who one is, where one is bound, and what one wants to do with one's life. Identity formation occurs through the integration of all of the roles one has tried out in one's life.

Mainstreaming   Inclusion of students with physical, emotional, or cognitive disabilities among students without such disabilities in a classroom or other learning environment. Full and successful mainstreaming requires that the student with disabilities be accepted as a peer by the other students in the classroom.

Modeling   Behavioral training procedure in which the desired behavior is demonstrated or illustrated by some other person who serves as a model. Behavior can be modeled by an adult or a peer. Modeling is more effective when the model is perceived as having high status by those who are being trained.

Peer-mediated training   Social skills training procedure in which a higher status peer is enlisted as a trainer for another student. The peer-trainer may model the desired behavior, provide reinforcement when the desired behavior occurs, or employ other techniques.

Peer nomination   Sociometric technique in which social status is measured by asking peers to name others with whom they would prefer to work, play, or be associated. Peers who are named more often are thought to have higher social status than those who are named infrequently or not at all.

Posttest   Posttesting serves to assess the extent to which the chosen material has been learned. It also serves to reinforce learning through repetition.

Pretest   Pretesting can provide both student and teacher with an assessment of the extent of the student's knowledge of a subject. This serves to motivate the student to learn the identified material and targets the instruction or training toward areas of deficiency.

Self-concept formation   Development of a concept of the self, including decisions about what one is capable of, the extent to which one is accepted among other people, and what sort of standards one can be expected to meet. Self-concept formation is one aspect of identity formation. Self-concept is derived from the collective view of the self that has been presented to the self by all of the other people with whom the self has related.

Sense of identity   See *Identity formation.*

Social acceptance   Full acceptance of a person with disabilities as a peer by his or her fellow students or fellow workers. Social acceptance can be formally assessed by sociometric techniques, or informally assessed by observing the type and frequency of a student's interactions with peers. Social acceptance is a key determinant of academic and vocational success, and can be enhanced through social skills training and other techniques.

Social competency   Sum of one's social abilities, including specific social skills and the general ability to find a place in the social group. Social competency includes but is not limited to competence in the following areas: assertiveness, asking for help or information, offering help or information, expressing emotions, responding appropriately to expressions of emotion, greeting, providing support, respecting other people's boundaries, extending invitations to play or work together, accepting or declining invitations, conversing for pleasure, and conflict resolution.

Social environment   Set of social conditions surrounding a particular situation. The social environment may encourage or discourage the practice of a given behavior. The social environment is itself subject to alteration through a variety of interventions.

Social isolation   Chronic absence of social experiences, including outings and friendships. Social isolation among children, adolescents, and young adults with disabilities is characterized by the lack of an active social life outside of the home. Social isolation in school is marked by the lack of companions at work or play and limited involvement in the social life of the school, including extracurricular activities.

Social learning laboratory   A social environment in which social learning takes place. Although any social environment provides incidental opportunities for social learning, a social environment is considered a learning laboratory when it provides a major opportunity for social learning, or when one of the stated purposes of the environment is to provide for social learning. A Scout troop intends to provide for social learning, and is therefore a social learning laboratory. A grocery store is a social environment that provides for social learning only incidentally. Because significant social learning occurs in the classroom, it is a learning laboratory and should be consciously used as such for at least part of the time, with guided efforts to provide learning experiences of a positive nature.

Social reciprocity   Give and take between members of a social group, especially as it tends to promote or discourage the practice of particular behaviors.

Social skills   See *Social competency.*

Sociometric status   Person's social status relative to his or her peer group, as measured by a variety of techniques, including peer nomination.

Wheelchair simulation   Structured social learning experience in which one or more people without disabilities use a wheelchair temporarily, experience the practical and social environment from that perspective, and report their experience to their peers.

REFERENCES

Ammerman, R.T. (1986). *Social adjustment in handicapped adolescents and their families.* Unpublished doctoral dissertation, University of Pittsburgh, PA.

Ammerman, R., Van Hasselt, V., & Hersen, M. (1986, November). *Assessment of social functioning in handicapped adolescents and their families.* Paper presented at the 20th annual convention of the Association for the Advancement of Behavior Therapy, Chicago.

Anderson, E.M., Clarke, L., & Spain, B. (1982). *Disability in adolescence.* London: Methuen.

Apolloni, T., Cooke, T. (1978). Integrated programming at the infant, toddler, and preschool levels. In M.J. Guralnick (Ed.), *Early intervention and the integration of handicapped children.* Baltimore: University Park Press.

Asher, S.R., Oden, S.L., & Gottman, J.M. (1977). Children's friendships in school settings. In L.G. Katz (Ed.), *Current topics in early childhood education* (Vol. 1, pp. 33–61). Norwood, NJ: Ablex.

Asher, S.R., & Taylor, A.R. (1982). Social outcomes of mainstreaming: Sociometric assessment and beyond. In P. Strain (Ed.), *Social development of exceptional children* (pp. 1–18). Rockville, MD: Aspen Systems.

Barnes, E., Berrigan, C., & Biklen, D. (1978). *What's the difference? Teaching positive attitudes toward people with disabilities.* Syracuse, NY: Human Policy Press.

Benham, H. (Ed.). (1978). *Scholastic feeling free activities and stories.* New York: Scholastic Book Services. (Copyright by American Institutes for Research and Syracuse University).

Blum, R.W. (1983). The adolescent with spina bifida. *Clinical Pediatrics, 22*(5), 331–335.

Blum, R.W., Resnick, M.D., Nelson R., & St. Germaine, A. (1991). Family and peer issues among adolescents with spina bifida and cerebral palsy. *Pediatrics, 88*(2), 280–285.

Borjeson, M.C., & Lagergren, J. (1990). Life conditions of adolescents with myleomeningocele. *Developmental Medicine and Child Neurology, 32,* 698–706.

Bruininks, V.L. (1978). Actual and perceived peer status of learning disabled students in mainstream programs. *Journal of Special Education, 12,* 51–58.

Children's Museum of Boston, with WGBH Boston. (1978). *What if you couldn't . . . ? An elementary school program about handicaps.* Newton, MA: Selective Educational Equipment.

Cooke, T., Apolloni, T., & Cooke, S. (1977). Normal preschool children as behavioral models for retarded peers. *Exeptional Children, 43,* 531–532.

Coopersmith, S. (1967). *The antecedents of self-esteem.* San Francisco: W.H. Freeman.

Devoney, C., Guralnick, M., & Rubin, H.(1974). Integrating handicapped and nonhandicapped preschool children: Effects on social play. *Childhood Education, 50,* 360–364.

Drabman, R.S., & Patterson, J.N. (1982). Disruptive behavior and the social standing of exceptional children. In P.S. Strain (Ed.), *Social development of exceptional children* (pp. 45–55). Rockville, MD: Aspen Systems.

Eckart, M.L. (1986). *Correlates of self-esteem in children with myelomeningocele.* Unpublished master's thesis, University of Cincinnati, OH.

Eckart, M.L. (1988). *Correlates of self-esteem in adolescents with myelomeningocele.* Unpublished doctoral dissertation, University of Cincinnati, OH.

Erikson, E. (1968). *Identity: Youth and crisis.* New York: Norton.

Evers, W.L., & Schwartz, J.C. (1973). Modifying social withdrawal in preschoolers: The effects of film modeling and teacher praise. *Journal of Abnormal Child Psychology, 1,* 248–256.

Evers-Pasquale, W., & Sherman, M. (1975). The reward value of peers: A variable influencing the efficacy of filmed modeling in modifying social isolation in pre-schoolers. *Journal of Abnormal Child Psychology, 3,* 179–189.

Gamble, A., & Strain, P.S. (1979). The effects of dependent and interdependent group contingencies on socially appropriate responses in classes for emo-tionally handicapped children. *Psychology in the Schools, 16,* 253–260.

Gardner, H. (1982). Relations with other selves. In M. H. Bornstein & M. Lamb (Eds.), *Developmental Psychology* (2nd ed., pp. 72–98). Hillsdale, NJ: Law-rence Erlbaum Associates.

Gresham, F. (1981). Social skills training with handicapped children: A review. *Review of Educational Research, 51,* 139–176.

Gresham, F.M. (1982). Misguided mainstreaming: The case for social skills train-ing with handicapped children. *Exceptional Children, 5,* 99–107.

Guralnick, M. (1978). Integrated preschools as educational and therapeutic en-vironments: Concepts, design, and analysis. In M.J. Guralnick (Ed.), *Early in-tervention and the integration of handicapped and nonhandicapped children.* Baltimore: University Park Press.

Halverson, C.F., & Victor, J.B. (1976). Minor physical anomalies and problem be-havior in elementary school children. *Child Development, 47,* 281–285.

Hirst, M. (1989). Patterns of impairment and disability related to social handicap in young people with cerebral palsy and spina bifida. *Journal of Biosocial Sci-ence, 21*(1), 1–12.

Hoier, T.S., & Cone, J.D. (1980). *Inductive ideographic assessment of social skills in children.* Paper presented at the 14th annual convention of the Association for the Advancement of Behavior Therapy, New York.

Jelneck, L.J. (1977, January/February). The special needs of the adolescent with chronic illness. *Maternal Child Nursing,* 57–61.

Johnson, D.W., & Johnson, R.T. (1978). Mainstreaming: Will handicapped children be liked, rejected, or ignored? *Instructor, 87,* 152–154.

Lanning, F., & Robbins, R. (1966). Chart of development. *Instructor, 76*(1), 130–138.

Lasker, J. (1974). *He's my brother.* Chicago: Albert Whitman & Co.

Lord, J., Varzos, N., Behrman, B., Wicks, J., & Wicks, D. (1990). Implications of mainstream classrooms for adolescents with spina bifida. *Developmental Med-icine and Child Neurology, 32,* 20–29.

Mack, N., (1976). *Tracy.* Milwaukee, WI: Raintree Editions.

McAndrew, I. (1979). Adolescents and young people with spina bifida. *Develop-mental Medicine and Child Neurology, 21,* 619–629.

McHale, S.M., & Olley, J.G. (1982). Using play to facilitate the social development of handicapped children. *Topics in Early Childhood Special Education, 2*(3), 76–86.

Necco, E., Wilson, C., & Scheidmantel, J. (1982, September). Affective learning through drama. *Teaching Exceptional Children,* 22–25.

O'Connor, R.D. (1972). Relative effects of modeling, shaping, and the combined procedures for modification of social withdrawal. *Journal of Abnormal Psychol-ogy, 79,* 327–334.

Peterson, C., Peterson, J., & Scriven, G. (1977). Peer imitation by nonhandicapped and handicapped preschoolers. *Exceptional Children, 43,* 223–224.

Richardson, S.A., Goodman, N., Hastorf, A.H., & Dornbusch, S.M. (1961). Cultural uniformity in reaction to physical disabilities. *American Sociological Review, 26,* 241–247.

Ross, R.E., & Freelander, I.R. (1977). *Handicapped people in society: A curriculum guide.* Burlington: University of Vermont, College of Education, Department of Special Education.

Rousso, H. (1985). The relationship between physical disability and narcissism: A critique of the literature. *Clinical Social Work Journal, 25,* 5–17.

Rowley, F.L., Van Hasselt, V.B., & Hersen, M. (1986). Behavioral treatment of families with an adolescent with spina bifida: A treatment manual. *Social and Behavioral Science Documents: Abstracts and Best Seller List, 16*(2), 68.

Shurtleff, D., & Sousa, J. (1977). The adolescent with myelodysplasia: Development, achievement, sex and deterioration. *Developmental Medicine Journal, 49,* 631–638.

Stephens, T.M. (1978). *Social skills in the classroom.* Columbus, OH: Cedars Press.

Strain, P.S. (1982). Peer-mediated treatment of exceptional children's social withdrawal. In P.S. Strain (Ed.), *Social development of exceptional children* (pp. 93–105). Rockville, MD: Aspen.

Strain, P.S., Odom, S.L., & McConnell, S. (1984). Promoting social reciprocity of exceptional children: Identification, target behavior selection, and intervention. *Remedial and Special Education Journal, 5,* 21–28.

Strain, P.S., Shores, R.E., & Timm, M.A. (1977). Effects of peer social initiations on the behavior of withdrawn preschool children. *Journal of Applied Behavioral Analysis, 10,* 289–298.

Thelen, M.H., Fry, R.A., Fehrenback, P.A., & Frautschi, N.M. (1979). Therapeutic videotape and film modeling: A review. *Psychological Bulletin, 86,* 701–720.

Tremblay, A., Strain, P.S., Hendrickson, J.M., & Shores, R.E. (1981). Social interactions of normal preschool children. *Behavior Modification, 5,* 237–253.

Wattenberg, W., & Clifford, C. (1962). *Relationship of self concept to beginning achievement in reading.* Detroit: Wayne State University.

Additional Reading and Viewing

RESOURCES

The school library is often an excellent source for readings about issues associated with disabilities and the acceptance of persons with disabilities. Children's literature has changed greatly in recent years, and is no longer limited in subject matter to "perfect" families with two parents and no problems. A broad variety of fine books addressing important issues are currently available. Many school librarians will have excellent ideas about which stories will address the particular issues that are current in a given classroom. There are also sources that list and describe books according to the topic or issue that each book addresses and the grade level for which each is written. Two such source books are:

Dreyer, S.S. (1977). *The bookfinder: A guide to children's literature about the needs and problems of youth aged 2–15.* Circle Pines, MN: American Guidance Service.

Dreyer, S.S. (1985). *The bookfinder: When kids need books: Annotations of books published 1979 through 1982.* Circle Pines, MN: American Guidance Service.

The following is a partial list of topics listed in *The Bookfinder* (Dreyer, 1977, 1985) that may be relevant to the needs discussed in this chapter: achievement, appearance, attitude toward belonging, birth defects, body concept, braces on body/limbs, cooperation, courage, determination, differences, disabilities, embarrassment, friendship, handicaps, integration, isolation, learning disabilities, loneliness, making friends, name-calling, ostracism, peer relationships, physical handicaps, prejudice, rejection, self-esteem, self-improvement, and teasing.

FOR STUDENT READING

Grealish, C.A., & von Bruansberg Grealish, M.J. (1975). *The sneely-mouthed snerds and the wonderoctopus.* Syracuse, NY: Human Policy Press. This book addresses being different, teasing, and isolation. It is suitable for ages 5–8.

Kamien, J. (1979). *What if you couldn't . . . ? A book about special needs.*

New York: Charles Scribner's Sons. This book discusses handicaps and human differences, and is suitable for ages 8–12.

Lasker, J. (1974). *He's my brother.* Chicago: Albert Whitman & Co.

Lasker, J. (1980). *Nick joins in.* Chicago: Albert Whitman & Co. This book about mainstreaming, wheelchair dependence, and human differences is suitable for ages 5–8.

Mack, N. (1976). *Tracy.* Milwaukee, WI: Raintree Editions.

Payne, S.N. (1982). *A contest.* Minneapolis: Carolrhoda Books. This book about human differences, wheelchair dependence, and feeling different is suitable for ages 8–10.

Pieper, E. (1979). *A school for Tommy.* Elgin, IL: The Child's World. This book about mainstreaming and wheelchair dependence is suitable for ages 5–8.

Pollock, P. (1982). *Keeping it secret.* New York: G.P. Putnam's Sons. This book is about deafness, self-acceptance, hiding a disability, and making friends, and is suitable for ages 9–12.

Rabe, B. (1981). *The balancing girl.* New York: E.P. Dutton. This story about a student who depends on braces, crutches, and a wheelchair emphasizes a unique ability and is suitable for ages 5–7.

Savitz, H.M. (1979). *Run, don't walk.* New York: Franklin Watts. This book discusses wheelchair dependence, mainstreaming, and self-acceptance, and is suitable for ages 12 and up.

Smith, D.B. (1975). *Kelly's creek.* New York: Thomas Y. Cromwell Co. This book is about a boy with a learning disability and is suitable for ages 8–10.

Wolf, B. (1974). *Don't feel sorry for Paul.* Philadelphia: J.B. Lippincott. This book is about a boy with foot and hand prostheses and is suitable for ages 8–10.

Zelonsky, J. (1980). *I can't always hear you.* Milwaukee, WI: Raintree Editions. This book is about deafness, human differences, and feeling different, and emphasizes the variety of ways in which people can be different. It is suitable for ages 7–10.

SOCIAL SKILLS TRAINING CURRICULUM

Nezer, H.W., Nezer, B.R., & Siperstein, G.N. (1986). *Improving children's social skills: Techniques for teachers.* Boston: University of Massachusetts of Boston, Center for the Study of Social Acceptance.

This curriculum consists of a set of manuals and a videotape. It is structured so that the unique needs of particular elementary school classrooms and individual children can be addressed. Highly adaptable, the curriculum can be used on its own or in conjunction with other classroom activities including academic instruction. It contains: 1) an overview of the successful social skills development process in children; 2) methods for assessing students' problems and for selecting skills to be taught; 3) instructional activities that incorporate techniques such as modeling, coaching, and role playing; 4) discussion of how classroom organization affects students' social functioning; and 5) listings of additional resources, including other curricula and relevant literature.

Mainstream and special education teachers can use this curriculum to identify students in need, target skills for training, and implement specific strategies to improve social functioning. From the curriculum materials, teachers concerned about specific students can acquire the information they need to conduct social skills training in their own classrooms.

An in-service teacher training program dealing with the use of this curriculum is also available. Staff at the Center for the Study of Social Acceptance can answer questions about the program, help to obtain state funds to pay for the training, and provide consultant services to school systems concerned with improving the social functioning of their elementary school children. For further information, contact:

Dr. Pamela Campbell
The Center for the Study of Social Acceptance
University of Massachusetts at Boston
Downtown Center
Boston, Massachusetts 02125-3393
(617) 287-5000

VIDEOTAPE WITH CURRICULUM

"The same inside." [Available from March of Dimes Birth Defects Foundation, 1275 Mamaroneck Ave., White Plains, NY 10605; (914) 428-7100.] This is a 13-minute videotape on disability awareness for elementary school students K–6. It includes lesson plans, activities, and a bibiliography.

Schools and Families Working Together

*William J. Casile
and Fern L. Rowley-Kelly*

Given the challenges and opportunities involved in the task of educating a student with spina bifida, a productive relationship between school and family is of great importance. The following statement reflects both the progress that has been made in developing such relationships, and the challenges that remain. Parents and educators have made dramatic strides:

> in their willingness and ability to work cooperatively, but as the parent of a special education student, you may continue to face some fairly steep barriers as you try to participate fully in decisions concerning your youngster. . . . Forming an effective partnership with the school may take a lot of energy and willingness to communicate on both sides. Educators must recognize and use constructively your knowledge, commitment, and energy, while acknowledging the burden you may bear. You, in turn, must be willing to state assertively your views and concerns while recognizing the constraints affecting educators. (Shore, 1986, pp. 99–100)

The lack of a constructive relationship between parents and schools may create additional stress for the family of a student with spina bifida.

> Parents of congenitally handicapped children . . . are more likely than parents of normal children to be faced with interactions with professionals of various kinds—physicians and other medical personnel, social workers, and education specialists. These encounters, while potentially helpful, are sometimes also stressful as a result of the professionals' immersion in a "clinical perspective" that may blind them to the reality of their clients' everyday needs. (Darling & Darling, 1982, p. 45)

A comfortable and effective relationship between parents and school is thus both desirable and possible, but by no means guaranteed. To promote the development of such a relationship, this chapter provides information in two areas. The opening section describes some typical experiences of many parents of students with spina bifida, detailing the stressors that this situation brings to bear on the family, and the typical adaptations that are be made as the family takes on the task of supporting and rearing a child with a disability. The subsequent sections describe the benefits derived from the mandate for a parent–professional partnership. These sections also include information for parents and educators on how they can work to facilitate the development of a collaborative relationship which, in turn, will work to ensure that each student with spina bifida receives all needed educational services.

Since effective partnerships and relationships rely on effective communication, and since effective two-way communication with parents of students with disabilities presupposes an understanding of typical or common family experiences, this chapter begins with a description of challenges that might confront a family supporting a student with spina bifida.

UNDERSTANDING THE STRESSORS AFFECTING THE FAMILY

One of the best ways to develop a positive parent–teacher relationship is to begin with an appreciation of the experiences the parents of a child with spina bifida have had prior to the child's entry into the school system. Parents are usually willing or anxious to share a great deal of information about their child with the teacher. Sharing of specific information will take place much more efficiently if the teacher has already learned about the possible effects that spina bifida may have on the life of the student's family. Because a broad understanding of the stressors is essential from the beginning of the teacher's relationship with the family, it will be useful to begin by outlining the features of a typical family experience. It should be noted that "there is considerable variation in the observed adaptation of mothers of children with chronic physical disorders and few experience clinical maladjustment" (Wallander et al., 1989, p. 372). Although individual family experiences will be different, this section provides information about the stresses shared by most families who have a child with spina bifida.

Families vary widely in their adaptations to the stress imposed by the child's disability. Although some investigators have described this variance in terms of a pathology model,

> A much more useful theoretical formation for research and clinical intervention with families of congenitally malformed children is a competence or coping-based framework. This is a more appropriate alternative to the previously mentioned pathology model in that it emphasizes the tasks and strategies involved in living with congenitally malformed children. (Friedrich & Schaffer, 1986, p. 400)

Such a competency model avoids the tendency to find something "wrong" with the family and substitutes an appreciation of the difficulty of the tasks that the family system faces. In this framework intervention is not based on treating an identifiable pathology, but on evaluating the effectiveness of the coping strategies that have been adopted, and on providing further strategies that have proven effective.

Typical Stressors

Alexander and Steg (1989) report seven areas of increased stress for the family. These areas include the impact of the birth defect itself, the impact of the initial and subsequent hospital admissions, outpatient visits, genetic counseling and family planning, the stress on the marital relationship, and the added financial burden encountered by the family. Friedrich and Shaffer (1986) reported that:

> Family investigators identify nine hardships or stressors experienced by families with ill children, including strained family relationships, modifications in family activities or goals, increased burden of tasks and time commitments, increased financial burden, need for housing adaptation, social isolation, medical concerns, differences in school achievement, and grieving. (p. 401)

Chronic stressors, including chronic illness, are more potent than acute stressors, and predictable stressors are less potent than unpredictable ones. Many of the stressors that effect families of children with spina bifida are both chronic and unpredictable or unpredicted.

The birth of a child with spina bifida is often unpredicted, and begins a period of chronic stress. The family initially experiences shock, confusion, disappointment, and grief (Herskowitz & Marks, 1977; Klaus & Kennell, 1976). Along with the shock, there is the stress of making very difficult but necessary practical adjustments to the needs of the new family member. Despite advances in prenatal diagnosis, many expectant parents are not forewarned and prepared for a new baby with spina bifida and therefore, "the majority of couples will have immense emotional turmoil and sadness at the birth of their child" (Reigel, 1989). Although such a birth is clearly no one's fault, parents may feel guilty and struggle with the conviction that the condition is punishment for something they have done. In the case of a first-born child, parents often experience self-doubt, fears of inadequacy, and profound guilt (Reigel, 1989).

There are also many uncertainties during this early period and parents may experience "the panic of acknowledged powerlessness because [they] cannot prevent what they fear, because it has already happened" (Featherstone, 1980). Powerlessness may be compounded by meaninglessness:

> Immediately after a diagnosis has been issued, parents are generally in a state of anomie; that is, they feel both meaninglessness and powerlessness in relation to their situation. . . . Most parents feel meaninglessness because they have little knowledge about birth defects in general or their child's defect in particular. (Darling & Darling, 1982, p. 172)

Both the fault finding and the guilt that may be experienced by parents of a newborn with spina bifida can be misguided attempts to overcome this meaninglessness by finding a reason for the disability.

Expectant parents often have an idealized image of their anticipated baby (Klaus & Kennell, 1976) and consequently at the birth of a child with spina bifida, the family mourns the loss of the nondisabled child they had hoped for. Parents may feel alienated by the response of family and friends to the birth of a child with spina bifida because they may also be experiencing loss and sorrow (Williamson, 1987).

Solnit and Stark (1961) suggest that parents must mourn the loss of their anticipated healthy child before they can love their child with a disability. Miller (1968) argues that such mourning is more easily completed in the case of a child who dies than in the case of a living child with a disability. Miller further suggests that the resolution of the mourning process for parents of a child with a disability involves three stages of parent adjustment:

1. Disintegration: At this stage, parents are shocked, disorganized, and completely unable to face reality.
2. Adjustment: This phase involves chronic sorrow and partial acceptance. The defect is recognized, but prognosis may still be denied.
3. Reintegration: Parents maturely acknowledge their child's limitations. (Darling & Darling, 1982, p. 50)

Not all parents complete the final stage of reintegration. Many do not complete it until well into the child's growing years.

There are also many reasons for parents to experience fear about their child's future. There is major surgery to close the opening in the spine within the first 24 hours of the infant's life. Also, a shunt may be inserted at that time, or a second surgery may be necessary within a few days when the need for a shunt becomes evident. During the early years of childhood, other surgeries may be necessary to straighten the spine, reposition a leg, or revise a shunt. Parents may experience deep fear on any of these occasions. There is often a chronic underlying fear that their child may die in spite of the medical care being provided. There may also be chronic sorrow accompanying the realization that their child will never be like other children:

> The sadness, the pain, the anger don't go away. Even the most accepting, best adjusted, most positive people don't "get over" those feelings as they go on to make the best of their lives. The feelings are always there—under the surface—ready to be triggered by new events. Birthdays, holidays, mile-

stones (the year she would have learned to drive . . .), seeing other children his age, all tap into that well of "chronic sorrow." (Simons, 1987, p. 72)

The role assigned to the family by the medical team can also be a source of stress:

> With meningomyelocele (spina bifida), the medically related stress tends to be most intense during the newborn period. The need for constant medical attention and the frequent hospital admissions, along with the communication deficits between health care providers and families, are additional stressors. Parents are called upon to learn about complex medical procedures, assume home treatment responsibilities, deal with incontinence, lift the growing child, prevent and heal skin breakdown, and handle special equipment needed by the child with paralysis. (Friedrich & Shaffer, 1986, 401)

The parents of a child with spina bifida are commissioned by the medical team to provide a broad range of necessary services which are required long after the newborn period. Requiring that the parents keep the child's bladder empty, be aware of the possibility of shunt failure, make medical appointments, and bring their child in for weekly infant stimulation, therapy, or special preschool programs can continue to put stress on the family system. Throughout the preschool years the parents are occupied with many new health care procedures to ensure their child's optimum health, growth, and development. The daily care of a child with spina bifida often depletes the parent's energies, time, and money, resulting in decreased participation in social, recreational, and cultural activities (Breslau, Staruch & Morimer, 1982; Shore, 1986).

A review of 33 research studies involving the impact of spina bifida on the child and family showed a general consensus that "problems, tensions, and anxieties exist within these families" (Nevin, McCubbin, & Birkebak, 1984). Extensive medical, social, psychological, and economic complications account for the increased stress and anxiety common to these families. The mother of a child with spina bifida typically spends twice as much time caring for her child as does the mother of a nondisabled child (Joosten, 1979). These mothers typically "make up" for the extra time by sleeping less rather than abandoning their other responsibilities.

Mothers of children with spina bifida have been found to have higher "stress scores" than mothers of children with other disabilities (Tew & Laurence, 1973). Research also indicates that mothers of children with disabilities also have less reciprocal relationships with their families than do the comparison-group mothers (Kazak & Wilcox, 1984). Although they must rely on members of their extended family to assist them in a variety of ways, their opportunities to return these favors are limited by the obligations they are already carrying.

Along with the difficulties come victories and occasions for joy. Simons (1987) reflects on these experiences:

Luckily, parents learn to handle the assaults. Whether out of practice or necessity, you become resilient, more able to meet the next challenge than you ever thought you would be. My friends say, "How can you handle all the problems you have?" I never thought of myself as a strong person, but I guess I've become one. . . . There are a lot of problems, and many of them are huge. You think, "How can I get through this?" But if you put all the disappointments on a scale and put all the joys on the other side, the joys would weigh a lot more. (p. 15)

Families of children with spina bifida often develop a denser network of family relationships (Kazak & Wilcox, 1984). These families relate to fewer people outside of the family unit and rely on relationships within the family to meet multiple needs that might otherwise be met outside of the family. Although this higher network density may help foster a sense of closeness and cohesiveness, it may also contribute another source of stress to the family unit (Kazak & Wilcox, 1984). Research indicates that dense networks may lack "weak ties" or less intimate types of relationships which can provide access to other resources and provide new input into the family system.

Although broader social support networks appear to be a major predictor of successful coping with the care of a child with a physical disability (Stein, 1983), many families remain isolated. This isolation is a problem for both the parents and the child because it intensifies and prolongs bonding between them, making it more difficult for the child to move out from the family system to form relationships with people outside the extended family. This high level of bonding within the family is one of the many factors that make entry into school a potentially difficult transition for the student with spina bifida and his or her family.

School Entry: A Difficult Milestone

Each of the typical milestones in the life of a child with disabilities will be more difficult. Key transition points in the life cycle of the family include the birth of the infant, the infant's becoming a toddler, entry into school, the beginning of adolescence, and launching into independence. "Families with children who have . . . major malformations . . . are likely to experience difficulty at each of these transition points" (Friedrich & Shaffer, 1986). The birth is traumatic, the baby's first steps come late and require braces, and toilet training is significantly delayed and complicated.

The child's entry into school presents another difficult milestone for the family (Williamson, 1987). A significant emotional task must be accomplished: Parents must achieve separation from the child, surrender a significant degree of control to the school, and maintain confidence that the child will do well. They must establish relationships with a number of education professionals, while maintaining their relationships with the myriad of medical professionals they have come to know since the child's birth. From birth on, the parents may have had a generalized concern about their child's future intellectual development (Reigel, 1989), without being able to predict or anticipate specific areas of difficulty.

Achieving separation is more difficult for many parents of a child with spina bifida because the intensity of parental involvement has been greater. These parents have been very protective of their children, and consequently their children have become more dependent on them. At some level of consciousness, they have also struggled with the fear that their child might die, a realistic fear even though current data reveal that 90%, or more, of newborn children with spina bifida will survive (Reigel, 1989). Given the complexity of the care and the critical medical issues involved, it is difficult for these parents to step back from the caregiving role. They have invested an extensive amount of time, energy, and emotion into their child and are understandably cautious about entrusting other people with the child's care. The normal reluctance that any parent feels at this separation is magnified for the parent of the child with spina bifida, and takes on an added dimension.

As the child enters school, "parents are compelled to see their child as different from his or her peers. The child is beginning to have to negotiate school and peer relations on his or her own" (Friedrich & Shaffer, 1986). Chronic sorrow is likely to recur at this transition point as:

> The parents reexperience the initial sadness they had at the birth of their congenitally malformed child because they are again reminded of the child's limitations. . . . Parents might respond to this reemergence of grief by experiencing their own emotional difficulties or by registering increased concern about their child's progress to the pediatrician or the school. The . . . professional must be sensitive to the cyclical patterns of grief in parents and must respond appropriately. Genuine educational difficulties or learning difficulties . . . must be differentiated from parental grief that is expressed as complaints or concerns about an adequate school and a stable state of health. (Friedrich & Shaffer, 1986, p. 403)

A teacher who is aware of underlying grief and other effects of chronic emotional stress can seize the opportunity to improve the parent-teacher relationship by acknowledging the difficulties inherent in the parents' situation and providing emotional support.

Making a Difficult Job a Little Easier

Parents of children with spina bifida are pioneers. With the medical team they have been breaking new ground in the care and treatment of children with spina bifida. Many parents of children with spina bifida have also been instrumental in establishing organizations to provide support and advocacy (Shore, 1986). Just as their children have become the first generation of long-term survivors with spina bifida, they have become the first generation of parents to deal with the long-term care of children with spina bifida. They have become experts in the process.

Although families of children with spina bifida have more extensive child-rearing responsibilities, these families have done amazingly well. They have faced this chronic medical disability with courage and tenacity. Because of the more extensive child-rearing involved, teachers are likely to have more contact with these families and more opportunities for communication and negotiation.

Operating from a competency-based model that includes good communication, an appreciation of the level of stress present, and a willingness to employ problem-solving and negotiating skills to seek appropriate coping strategies will enhance the development of an effective relationship between home and school. In addition, a commitment to avoid the traps of searching for causes and blaming is equally valuable.

The information in the remainder of this chapter is based on the belief that enhanced levels of interpersonal skills are needed when a high level of stress or conflict is present or possible. The skills and approaches described in the following sections are presented in order to encourage parents and teachers to recognize that desired outcomes for children with spina bifida can best be achieved if an effective parent–professional partnership works in collaboration.

CREATING AN EFFECTIVE PARENT–TEACHER PARTNERSHIP

Creating a strong parent–teacher partnership for a student who has difficulty learning is just as important as designing the right brace for a student who has difficulty walking. Like the brace, the partnership will help the student go a lot further. The relationship between the teacher and parent can be the key to the student's success, a hidden reason for failure, or almost anything between these extremes. Although it may be possible to teach many students effectively without paying a great deal of attention to the parent–teacher relationship, this is not the case with the child who has special needs. In the remainder of this chapter we focus on specific attitudes and skills which tend to foster a productive parent–teacher partnership.

Mandating the Parent–Teacher Partnership

When parents are involved with their children's education, increased learning takes place. Student achievement scores rise, student attendance increases, student motivation and self-esteem improve, discipline problems decrease, the dropout rate declines, and parental perception of the school is enhanced (Henderson, 1987; Kurtz & Barth, 1989; Swap, 1990). A review of empirical studies of academic learning reveals that parents directly or indirectly influence the most significant determinants of learning (Walberg, 1984). In spite of this information, which has been collected over the past two decades, "parental involvement remains more a part of the rhetoric of schools than of their reality" (Steinberg, 1988).

Since the passage of PL 94-142, the Education for All Handicapped Children Act (*Federal Register,* 1977), the invitation for parents of children with disabilities to participate in their child's assessment, educational planning, and placement decisions has not been left to the interest, commitment, and discretion of education professionals. Parental involvement has been mandated. The reason for the prescription of this parent involvement is that virtually everyone agrees that it is important for parents to be involved in their children's education. The outcomes resulting from this partnership benefit the professionals, the parents, and the students. Education professionals gain access to information about the child and the family which enables them to provide more appropriate education. The parents gain by sharing information with the school which enables them to reinforce the goals of the education program and can assist them in developing a healthier attitude toward themselves, their child, and the school (Vaughn, Bos, Harrell, & Lasky, 1988). And finally, since everyone is able to develop a more complete picture of the overall needs of the child, there is greater consistency provided in the child's two most significant environments, the family and the school.

Unfortunately, since the Education for All Handicapped Children Act established parental involvement as one of the basic principles of effective and appropriate special education practice, there has been little research that has focused on the outcomes of parental participation in the education of children with special needs. Much of the extant literature is merely descriptive of the role that parents assume in the decision-making process of the IEP (individualized education program) conference (Goldstein, Strickland, Turnbull, & Curry, 1980; Lynch & Stein, 1982; Smith, 1990). This available research, however, has permitted teachers to examine how they relate to parents and to evaluate if they employ practices that facilitate or interfere with the development of effective parent-teacher relationships. This examination of past and current practices suggests that certain attitudes and skills are essential to the creation of an effective partnership. The following section discusses the keys to this process.

Keys to Effective Parent–Teacher Partnerships

The home–school interactions necessary to plan and implement appropriate educational experiences are never emotionally neutral. They can act to enhance or damage the atmosphere of mutual trust and respect which is essential to the development of a productive relationship between parents and teachers. Mutual trust and respect are essential characteristics of an effective relationship. They are necessary conditions if the home–school partnership is to work to solve problems and resolve conflicts without resorting to the power struggle that too frequently typifies the communication pattern between professionals and parents (Sonnerschein, 1984).

The emergence of the due process procedures afforded by PL 94-142, and the role of the parent as advocate, in both the political arena and in the role as a fully enfranchised member of the multidisciplinary or IEP team, has increased the opportunities for adversarial encounters between parents and schools. As a result, parents and professionals can lose sight of the fact that the parent–teacher partnership can be crucial to the success of the student. To guard against unnecessary ruptures in the relationship, and to promote trust and respect, parents and professionals must be willing to reflect, share, understand, and confront the attitudes and beliefs or values they hold.

Attitudes, Beliefs, and Values Barriers to the development of productive home-school partnerships frequently result from differences in values. Values, or the attitudes and beliefs they generate, are shaped by our experiences and "world view," or the way in which we interpret our perceptions of the reality around us. Because each individual processes reality from a unique perspective, it is likely that parents and professionals will sometimes disagree and come into conflict. However, these differences of perception need not create insurmountable problems that become inevitable wedges driven between the home and the school. Instead, they can be viewed as unique windows of opportunity through which one can reframe the needs of the child, discover creative and innovative program responses to these needs, and promote a more fruitful relationship between parents and teachers.

Although there are many values about which parents and teachers may choose to differ, there are two particular values that all parties must hold. These two values are essential to the development of effective parent–teacher partnerships. First, searching for someone to blame will not solve the problem. Second, parent–professional partnerships are worthwhile. The first will permit you to focus on problem resolution; the second will permit you to focus on the relationship. When there is a problem, it is frequently related to the inadequate educational, medical, and social system responses readily available to construct positive outcomes for students with spina bifida. The probability that these desired outcomes will be achieved is significantly enhanced when parents and professionals work to foster collaborative relationships.

Removing the Obstacle of Blaming The development of an effective parent–professional partnership presupposes that both parties are willing and able to enter into the partnership in an interpersonal environment that is not cluttered with negative and destructive attitudes. If the professional chooses to operate from the conviction that the child's problems are caused by or exacerbated by the parents, or if the parents believe that the teacher is not providing an appropriate educational experience for their child—if people are considered "at fault"—then the energy necessary to foster a relationship will be diverted into nonproductive behavior. The parent or the teacher may become accusatory and defensive. They might generate resentment or even hostility. They may become adversaries, pulling in different directions, or at least pulling independently of each other. When this situation develops, it is inevitable that relationships will deteriorate and desired outcomes will be jeopardized, regardless of any legal mandate or professional responsibility to work collaboratively.

When parents lack confidence in teachers, or if they are suspicious of the teachers' commitment to the child's development, these negative attitudes are communicated to the child. As a result, the child will become confused and lose confidence and trust in the teacher and in the value of the educational experience. If Fran hears Mom tell Dad, "Mr. Pizzicato is not a great violin teacher, but he's all we can afford," then Fran will clearly practice with less vigor and listen with less respect than if Mom says, "Boy, am I glad we found out about Mr. Pizzicato. He knows a lot about music, and a lot about teaching, and he is such a gracious man. I just know you are going to learn to play much better with him."

Dealing with problem areas will also create strains between the teacher and child, and the child will take these complaints to the parents. When this happens, the teacher will not want the parent to respond with, "That is just the way Ms. Skoller is; you'll just have to grin and bear it" or, "I don't know Ms. Skollar, but I guess she knows what she is doing." Criticism of the teacher by the parent, or lukewarm approval, will not be very helpful to the student who is straining to meet Ms. Skollar's expectations. On the other hand, the parent, teacher, and student will all benefit if the student hears the parent say, "Ms. Skollar is asking you to do these things because she knows you can grow that way, and so do I. I know it's hard, but we wouldn't be doing our job if we didn't expect you to learn." This kind of supportive statement by the parent will not just come automatically, and it should not be left to chance. It will be authentic only when it is the fruit of an effective parent–teacher partnership.

Blame is a two-way street. Teachers and other professionals are not immune to this fault-finding behavior. Sonnenschein (1984) discusses several types of professional attitudes and assumptions that usually contribute to difficulties in the parent–professional partnership, and one of the most prevalent is the attribution of the cause of the child's disability to the parents. The assumption that parents are the source of the problem stems from years of research and writings on causation theory. "The impact during this century of causation theories has sent many parents on a tremendous 'guilt trip' and, in turn, has produced barriers to constructive parent–professional relationships—resentment, low self-esteem, lack of trust, and defensiveness" (Turnbull & Turnbull, 1986, p. 4).

Wondering about how students got to be the way they are now is useful only if it provides information that will help in designing interventions. Any other motive for gathering information about a child's history or family should be suspect because it can introduce barriers to the development of an effective parent–professional relationship. The central question to be considered is how best to educate the child. In short, questions about causality are irrelevant except to the extent that they help us answer current questions about what the family and school can do for the child.

Viewing the parents as the cause of the child's problems does not encourage the professional to look to the family as a source of strength or support. This view tends to reinforce the belief that the entire family system is somehow deficient and in need of treatment (Dunst, 1985; Sonnenschein, 1984). However, viewing all families as being capable and having strengths creates an enhanced opportunity for the creation of a partnership rather than a paternalistic approach to the relationship between parent and professional (Dunst, Trivette, & Deal, 1988; Rappaport, 1981).

Regardless of whether "fault" can be correctly or justly attributed, the impact of the fault-finding behavior on the parent–professional relationship can be profound and it can be devastating. Whenever and however the relationship is threatened, the professional must work to establish or reestablish an attitude of collaboration and teamwork between the home and the school. Thus, classroom teachers, because of their extensive contact with families, are clearly responsible for the creation of an atmosphere where blaming and fault-finding can be exposed as nonproductive and eliminated. This is not to say that parents have no responsibility for the relationship or are not capable of fostering a positive and productive climate for the partnership. Certainly parents are capable and responsible for the tenor of their relationships. However, while it is intended that both parties should work to ensure that their assumptions, motives, and goals are clear, explicit, and in service to the child, the professional is legally mandated and ethically required to bring to bear those attitudes and skills that will foster a productive relationship.

Teachers and parents must overtly agree and work towards a relationship which is free from fault-finding and blaming. They must reach an accord based on mutual respect and trust. They must be willing to openly discuss their beliefs and behaviors in terms of the overriding goal or purpose of the relationship—the general welfare and development of the child.

Enlisting Support and Expertise Parents and professionals each have unique information and perspectives on the strengths and needs of exceptional children. They also have unique information and perspectives on their own strengths and needs, and on how these are related to appropriate developmental experiences for a particular child. The only way to ensure that complete information and a more whole perspective is used to plan, implement, and evaluate an individualized education program is to access all available experts, parental and professional. Thus the development and maintenance of a relationship between a child's parents and teachers is essential and worthwhile.

Expertise is gained through the thoughtful reflection of one's experience. Teachers and other school-based professionals are educational experts. They have knowledge of principles and concepts related to teaching and learning. The parents have gained specific knowledge about their child and thus have child-specific expertise. The task of educating any student requires both educational expertise and specific information about the student. This means that the needed expertise is available only from the parent–professional team.

The complexity of the education challenge is increased by students who present disabilities which interfere with efficient learning. This enhanced challenge is precisely one reason that the Education for All Handicapped Children Act (*Federal Register,* 1977) required that educational decisions regarding such students be made by a multidisciplinary team, which of course includes the parents. Given the state-of-the-art in educational assessment and instructional intervention, this team approach is the only way to ensure that appropriate decisions are being made for the individual student. It was clearly Congress's intent to provide parents with a more equal role in the parent–professional partnership. The law contains numerous requirements that grant decision-making rights to parents of students with disabilities and enables them to hold schools accountable and to ensure that their child receives an appropriate education (Turnbull, Turnbull, & Wheat, 1982).

While accountability may have been the driving reason for the team approach to educational decision-making, the task-team environment also provides a fertile physical and psychological environment within which the parent–teacher partnership can be cultivated. Consulting the parents at every stage of the educational process acknowledges their expertise and affirms their worth.

Although this approach can be effective with any parent, it can be especially effective when working with the parent of a child with spina bifida. Such parents have had many opportunities to feel wrong about what they have been doing. They may have worked to overcome the suspicion that the child's condition is their fault. They may feel that they have somehow failed to take perfect care of their child. In short, they have had many opportunities to doubt their effectiveness as parents, in spite of how well they may have actually performed. The teacher who provides a nonjudgmental and empathic environment for such parents will encourage them to share their expertise and feelings. This is not just a ploy to make parents feel good or involved. It is an effective strategy to create an open and productive exchange of relevant information between parent and professional. The parent is in fact an excellent source of valuable information about the child. The teacher is in fact capable of fully accessing and using this vital information. When this is a goal of the parent-teacher relationship, it can be accomplished and everyone wins.

Partnership Development Skills In addition to the development of attitudes which create and foster an open invitation to a long-term working partnership, it is necessary for parents and teachers to develop the skills which effectively demonstrate and communicate a commitment to the values of productive home-school teams. Responsible professionals must develop competence in the communication, negotiation, and problem-solving skills necessary to resolve conflict without jeopardizing their relationships with parents. Specifically, teachers need to be able to listen effectively, respond with empathy, and negotiate collaboratively in order to promote parental involvement in their children's education. Furthermore, as Egan (1990) suggests, effective helping professionals should not keep their skills secret. They should share these effective communication skills with others, including parents, and encourage everyone to employ them to resolve problems and build relationships.

Effective Listening Hearing the words of another is just one component of effective listening. To really listen, one must also be an affective listener. That is, one must be attentive to both the meaning of the words and the emotional or affective content of what is said. To accomplish this, one must develop the ability to accept and care for another as a separate individual, and to accept his or her right to have both positive and negative feelings and experiences (Rogers, 1961). Within the parent–professional relationship, this means accepting and understanding parents' positive and negative expressions of feelings. To accomplish this, the professional must learn to listen for understanding and not just to hear the parent.

The counseling and "helping" literature is replete with references to the skills of affective, active, and nonjudgmental listening (Carkhuff, 1983; Egan, 1990; Gordon, 1970; Ivey, 1971). The bottom line is that listeners must be consciously and purposefully engaged in the act of listening. They must want to hear and understand what the other person has to say without rushing to a premature and perhaps prejudicial conclusion or judgment.

Listening for understanding without judging, evaluating, or labeling the speaker is not a natural or innate human skill. Fortunately it can be learned. To become proficient as a nonjudgmental or active listener, one must genuinely embrace the principles of acceptance, respect, and trust, and then systematically practice, practice, practice.

Gordon (1970) suggests that the thoughtful application of active listening will encourage others to express and accept their ideas and feelings, facilitate cooperative problem-solving, and promote the development of productive and mutually supportive relationships. If teachers are able to listen to parents effectively, they will be less likely to fall into the trap of searching for causes and laying blame. They will be better equipped to focus on the development of a nonjudgmental partnership with parents on behalf of their children.

Listening is the teacher's best tool (Rotter, Robinson, & Fey, 1987). By listening to and acknowledging the parents' feelings and content messages, the teacher can gain three important things. First, the stage is set for the parents to hear the teacher when it is the teacher's turn to express his or her ideas and feelings. Second, as the parents gain confidence in the teacher's ability to tune in to their feelings as well as to hear their words, they develop the important conviction that the teacher cares and will be able to tune in to their child's feelings. Finally, the teacher who listens well to feelings and acknowledges them will be given a great deal of useful information about the emotional or affective aspects of the situation. Knowledge of the student's emotional situation and affective make-up can be very useful when it becomes necessary to increase the child's level of motivation or to address the student's lack of commitment. When the child obviously doesn't feel like working or trying something new, the teacher who is tuned in to the child on a feeling level will not be at a loss for ideas about how to help the student get started again. The teacher who has been listening will also be able to connect with the parents to obtain ideas and assistance when the student's motivation is low. In short, a strong emotional connection will promote a very useful degree of trust and confidence when it comes time to overcome or adjust to any educational challenge.

If teachers and parents listen for understanding, they will be prepared to respond to each other's thoughts and concerns with empathy. Empathic responses require the listener to understand the speaker's perspective; to understand what it is like to view the world through the other person's frame of reference; to understand what it feels like to be in the other person's shoes.

The value of applying effective listening to the parent–teacher partnership becomes apparent when one reviews the available literature on parental involvement. Schultz (1987) suggests that there is a significant discrepancy between the legislative policy of parental participation and the practice of parent involvement. She proposes that "the levels of involvement can be described as active participation, passive participation, and nonparticipation" (p. 104). Although active parental participation is clearly the legislative intent, it is the needs, aspirations, and desires of parents, along with the attitudes and skills of the professional, that ultimately determine their level of involvement.

The professional must consider and respect the complexity and uniqueness of each family system in order to determine the appropriate level and nature of parental involvement (Seligman, 1991). In Turnbull and Turnbull's (1986) words:

> Reassessing current parent involvement policy and practice and recognizing the importance of individualizing for families is indeed an important first step in learning to work cooperatively and successfully with families. However, knowing that families differ in their preferences for participation is not enough. It is important to know the specific ways in which families differ, as well as the specifics relative to the family's needs and preferences. (p. 141)

Beyond the individual assessment of family preferences implied in the preceding quote, and even beyond the specific parent-teacher communication strategies presented here and by others (Schultz, 1987; Seligman, 1991; Shea & Bauer, 1985; Stewart, 1986; Turnbull & Turnbull, 1986), teachers need to develop an approach to negotiating parental involvements that promotes the development of the desired home-school partnerships. It is not enough to assess parental preferences; offer an array of home-school linking mechanisms and cultivate appropriate values and skills. Teachers and parents must learn to negotiate.

Collaborative Negotiating Parents and teachers need to develop a practical method for handling any differences which may arise after they have used effective communication skills to explore each other's positions. Negotiation strategies or conflict-management styles have been frequently characterized into five types: 1) accommodation, 2) avoidance, 3) collaboration, 4) competition, and 5) compromise (Johnson, 1990). These styles are defined in terms of the relative importance of "goal accomplishment," or assertiveness, versus "relationship building," or cooperation. Figure 11.1 conveys a graphic representation of the relationships among these five strategies.

Since relationship building between parents and professionals has been identified as worthwhile, it is obvious that a negotiating strategy from the "high" end of the "Cooperation" axis is preferred. This narrows the options to Accommodation and Collaboration, with Compromise as a possible third choice. Which style should a teacher and parent employ to

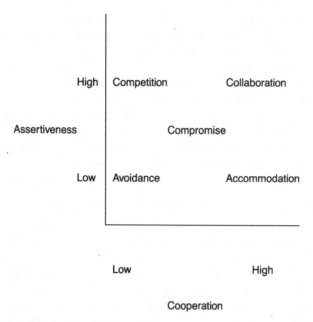

Figure 11.1. Conflict-management styles.

solve problems or resolve conflicts? Is there one style that is always preferable? Probably not. Each style has advantages in different situations.

Accommodation might be a teacher's wisest choice in an initial attempt to encourage nonparticipating parents to become more actively involved, but on their own terms. However, if the parents choose to remain disengaged, the accommodating strategy suggests no way for the teacher to assert his or her needs. The Compromise suggests that each side will move from its original position and meet on some common ground. Ideally, each side will move halfway to reach a fair settlement and both will be satisfied. This sounds logical but, unfortunately, this rarely occurs. More typically, one or both sides feel that there has been an inequitable arrangement made, and they persist in feeling that their interests and needs were not well served. Therefore, even though a compromise may work to solve a presenting problem, it is rare that an arrangement negotiated in such a manner will enhance the relationship.

Collaboration has the advantage of placing an equally high priority on getting the job done and developing the interpersonal relationship between the negotiators. This approach requires that attention be given to ideas and to the feelings of the participants. Collaboration suggests that no one person has the final answer, but that every person has a piece to contribute, and that the "best" solution will emerge when problems or conflicts are brought into the open and faced directly. However, a collaborative strategy presumes that the participants are willing and able to engage in genuine, open, and honest communication.

A negotiation strategy called "Principled Negotiations" developed by the Harvard Negotiation Project (Fisher & Ury, 1991) is based on the principle of collaboration. This approach emphasizes that the participants are not adversaries, nor need they be friends. They are problem-solvers—people who are committed to work together to create the best solutions possible. Participants are not interested in a victory or a compromise; the outcome desired is a wise decision achieved without damaging the relationship between the participants.

The four steps to this approach can be summarized as follows:

1. "Separate the people from the problems" (p. 17). Separate the substantive issues which define the problem from the personalities who comprise the relationship. By dealing with each of these two dimensions separately, you can be "hard on problems, yet soft on people." If you successfully make this separation, you can attack the problem without attacking the person. You do not have to be concerned that the relationship is dependent on what you want and how you respond to the other person's demands.

Ideally, parents and professionals will not be strangers; they will have taken the opportunity to get to know each other personally. They will have already worked together to develop their relationship before a problem or difference emerges. That is why it is so important for teachers to initiate positive communications with parents. This is best done through frequent communications that emphasize the students' successes and accomplishments. This is especially important when dealing with students whose disabilities may have already contributed to a failure mindset. If communication between home and school is characterized by more good news than bad, there is a better chance to build a working relationship that will be able to withstand the stress of negotiations when honest differences of opinion are present.

Separating the people from the problem is not something that can be done once and then forgotten. It must be addressed continuously as part of the process for maintaining the relationship. The key is to treat people with respect and to deal with the problem on its merits. Fisher and Ury (1991) suggest that the next three steps help to address the latter.

2. "Focus on interests, not positions" (p. 401). Use available resources to explore each participant's interests and needs. By attempting to determine what each person needs, and by avoiding having a bottom-line position, the negotiators can focus on creative problem-solving rather than defending their positions. Entering negotiations with a bottom-line, "take it or leave it" demand will interfere with the creative process.

The basic problem in negotiations is not that there is a difference in positions, but that there is a conflict of needs, interests, and concerns. A parent might say, "I know my daughter's speech is significantly delayed, and I want her to have three sessions with the speech therapist each week." This represents the parent's position, but there might be a more basic interest which drives the request. For example, the parent's concern might be that his child is socially immature and does not relate well to peers. One barrier to her social development is her delayed speech, thus the basis for the parent's position. However, if the discussion with the school professionals focuses only on the minutes of speech therapy that the child will receive, only two outcomes are possible. The parents and school will agree or an impasse will be reached. Neither result assures that the underlying concern for social development is addressed unless this concern is openly discussed. If it is discussed, an alternative to formal speech therapy sessions might be discovered.

3. "Invent options for mutual gain" (p. 56). Successful negotiators generate mutually beneficial alternatives which address the expressed needs or interests of the participants. This is best accomplished if you separate the creative process of inventing solutions from the systematic decision or selection process. Create now—decide later; do not let the left-brain evaluation and selection process interfere with the predominantly right-brain creative process. If you are focused on the solution you want, if you have already made a judgment on the best course of action to take, you will not be as open to search for or respond to a solution that was not originally apparent. Collaboration requires that each negotiator become familiar with the needs of all others, and that together they search for individualized solutions which may lie outside of the obvious, historical, or habitual.

In the example above, if the parents and professionals are focused on negotiating between one and three speech therapy sessions per week, neither side may spend time thinking of satisfactory alternatives to achieve their goals. They become position-bound and are not prepared to recognize the spark of inspiration which might lead to a productive solution.

4. "Insist on objective criteria" (p. 81). Once a course of action or decision has been negotiated, do not stop until objective criteria or a fair standard or procedure is identified for use in the evaluation of your strategy. Agree upon some criteria that will tell you if your strategy has been successful. Objective criteria or fair standards are independent of either party in the negotiation. They establish the yardstick by which anyone can measure success or achievement.

Again, in the example above, there might be research available which suggests an optimum level at which individual speech therapy influences social development. Better yet, the parents and professional might negotiate a more individualized objective criterion related to their socialization goal. Perhaps the number of student-initiated conversations during a 30-minute cooperative learning session each week would be more appropriate. If no standard or criterion can be negotiated, then a fair procedure to evaluate progress might be established. The Education of the Handicapped Act (1975) already guaranteed one form of fair procedure when it established the due process procedure to protect the educational rights of students with disabilities. During due process, the participants are encouraged to present their interests and positions to an independent third party for review at a "fair hearing."

Whenever possible, parents and professionals should strive to negotiate fair standards or fair procedures to monitor the effectiveness of their agreements. These individualized, local criteria are usually more relevant to the specific educational challenge at hand. In addition, they will promote an objective and principled evaluation process rather than an adversarial power struggle.

These four steps summarize principled negotiation, one approach to a collaborative style of conflict resolution. From this example, it is clear that it is not an approach that emphasizes winning and losing. It is a practical method to deal with differences between people who also have a vested interest in maintaining and fostering a productive relationship.

CONCLUSION

The values and skills discussed in this chapter are considered essential to the development of effective parent-professional partnerships. The development of these fruitful and productive relationships is dependent on the participants' desire to make it happen and their willingness to work collaboratively. We have emphasized that this process also takes effort. Parents and professionals must work to understand each other's perspective, needs, and feelings. They must work to create an environment of trust and respect. They must work to develop effective communication and problem-resolution skills. If parents and professionals are willing and able to engage each other in a constructive relationship, the benefits to the child, the family, and the professional will justify the effort.

If parents and professionals want to join together in the interest of children, the time has never been better. At this juncture in history, the evolution of educational research and the revolution of the disability advocacy movement have met, and all vectors point toward the worth and correctness of a cooperative approach. It is a time when the quality education of students with special needs demands that parent-professional collaboration be a "best practice."

GLOSSARY

Competency model Distinct from pathology model, a competency model seeks to identify the skills or abilities that an individual or family possesses and that can be applied in coping with a given situation or set of stressors. Treatment consists of identifying and mobilizing existing competencies as coping mechanisms and of developing additional competencies through training.

Due process An established course of judicial or administrative activities designed to safeguard the legal rights of the individual. In special education, these activities include: Written notification to parents of an intent to evaluate, place, or change the placement of a student who is disabled; the parental right to review the student's school records and offer outside evaluations of the student; the opportunity to request a due process hearing whenever the parents and school cannot agree on an appropriate course of action.

Education for All Handicapped Children Act Originally passed as PL 94-142 in 1975, amended in 1986 by PL 99-457, and amended and reauthorized by PL 101-476 under the name of the Individuals with Disabilities Education Act (IDEA), this landmark federal legislation ensures a free appropriate public education (FAPE) in the least restrictive environment (LRE) for all students with disabilities.

Empathy The communication skill which requires the listener to understand the world-view of the speaker and to communicate this understanding back to the speaker for confirmation or clarification.

Individualized education program (IEP) A written plan for instruction required for every student receiving special education services. The plan, written by the student's multidisciplinary or IEP team, includes a statement of the student's strengths, weaknesses, and current levels of performance; annual goals and short-term objectives; all special services required; and a description of the least restrictive alternative for the student.

Infant stimulation A program of development and therapeutic activities from birth through preschool for children with developmental disabilities and their parents. Sensory stimulation, language development, and adaptive skills are usually stressed.

Milestones Those life-cycle events referred to when measuring an individual's growth and progress, or lack thereof. For example, sleeping through the night, cutting a first tooth, walking, beginning to date, graduating, voting, and getting one's first full-time job are typical events that parents or professionals might use as points of comparison between or among individuals.

Multidisciplinary team A school-based team composed of a student's parents and professionals representing various disciplines involved in and responsible for the evaluation, planning, and decision-making regarding that student's educational program.

Pathology model An approach to the treatment of human discomfort and dysfunction that identifies an illness or pathology that can be treated and often cured, thus relieving or limiting the discomfort or dysfunction. A pathology model is used with good effect in medicine and sometimes in psychotherapy and other treatment regimens. The model is misapplied when attempts are made to "find what's wrong and fix it" even when no pathology is present.

Principled negotiations   A collaborative approach to conflict management developed by the Harvard Negotiations Project.

Stressors   Events, experiences, or situations that create or can create stress. Stress can itself be harmful to the person experiencing it, and is then termed *distress*. Stress that is beneficial to the person is termed *eustress*. The same stressor can create distress for one person and eustress for another. Similarly, a stressor can be eustressful for a person is some circumstances and distressful for the same person in other circumstances.

REFERENCES

Alexander, M.A., & Steg, N.L., (1989). Myelomeningocele: Comprehensive treatment. *Physical Medicine and Rehabilitation, 70,* 637–641.

Breslau, N., Staruch, K., & Morimer, E.A. (1982). Psychological distress in mothers of disabled children. *American Journal of Disabled Child, 136,* 682–686.

Carkhuff, R.R. (1983). *The art of helping.* Amherst, MA: Human Resources Development Press.

Darling, R., & Darling, J. (1982). *Children who are different: Meeting the challenges of birth defects in society.* St. Louis: C.V. Mosby.

Dunst, C.J. (1985). Rethinking early intervention. *Analysis and Intervention in Developmental Disabilities, 5,* 165–201.

Dunst, C.J., Trivette, C.M., & Deal, A.G. (1988). *Enabling and empowering families: Principles and guidelines for practice.* Cambridge, MA: Brookline Books.

Egan, G. (1990). *The skilled helper: Systematic approach to effective helping.* Pacific Grove, CA: Brooks/Cole Publishing Company.

Featherstone, H. (1980). *A difference in the family.* New York: Basic Books.

Federal Register. (1977, August 23). Education for All Handicapped Children Act of 1975. Volume 42, page 163. Washington, DC: U.S. Government Printing Office.

Fisher, R., & Ury, W., with Patton, B. (1991). *Getting to yes: Negotiating agreement without giving in* (2nd ed.). Boston: Penguin Books.

Friedrich, W., & Shaffer, J. (1986). Adolescent psychosocial adaptation. In D.B. Shurtleff (Ed.) 411–419, *Myelodysplasias and exstrophies: Significance, prevention and treatment.* Orlando, FL: Grune & Stratton.

Goldstein, S., Strickland, B., Turnbull, A.P., & Curry, L. (1980). An observational analysis of the IEP conference. *Exceptional Children, 48,* 278–286.

Gordon, T. (1970). *Parent effectiveness training.* New York: Wyden.

Henderson, A. (1987). *The evidence continues to grow: Parent involvement improves student achievement.* Columbia, MD: National Committee for Citizens in Education.

Herskowitz, J., & Marks, A.N. (1977). The spina bifida patient as a person. *Developmental Medicine and Child Neurology, 19,* 413–417.

Ivey, A. (1971). *Microcounseling: Innovations in interviewing training.* Springfield, IL: Charles C Thomas.

Johnson, A.F. (1980). *Developmental achievement in the child with spina bifida.* Oak Brook, IL: Eterna Press.

Joosten, J. (1979). Accounting for changes in family life of families with spina bifida children. *Zeitscrifte fur Kinderchirurgie, 28*(4), 412–417.

Kazak, A.E., & Wilcox, B.L. (1984). The structure and function of social support networks in families with handicapped children. *American Journal of Community Psychology, 12,* 645–661.

Klaus, M.H., & Kennell, J.M. (1976). *Maternal–infant bonding: The impact of early separation or loss on family development.* St. Louis: C.V. Mosby.

Kurtz, P., & Barth, R. (1989). Parent involvement: Cornerstone of school social work practice. *Social Work, 34,* 407–413.

Lynch, E.W., & Stein, R. (1982). Perspectives on parent participation in special education. *Exceptional Education Quarterly, 3,* 55–63.

Miller, L.G. (1968). Toward a greater understanding of parents of the mentally retarded child. *Journal of Pediatrics, 72,* 699–705.

Nevin, R., McCubbin, H., & Birkebak, R. (1984). *Stress and coping with spina bifida: A family perspective.* Oak Brook, IL: Eterna Press.

Rappaport, J. (1981). In praise of paradox: A social policy of empowerment over prevention. *American Journal of Community Psychology, 9,* 1–25.

Reigel, D.H. (1989). *Spina bifida; Pediatric neurosurgery: Surgery of the developing nervous system* (2nd ed.). Philadelphia: W.B. Saunders.

Rogers, C.R. (1961). *On becoming a person.* Boston: Houghton Mifflin.

Rotter, J.C., Robinson, E.H., & Fey, M.A. (1987). *Parent-teacher conferencing.* Washington, DC: National Education Association.

Schultz, J.B. (1987). *Parents and professionals in special education.* Boston: Allyn & Bacon.

Seligman, M. (1991). *The family with a handicapped child.* Boston: Allyn & Bacon.

Shea, T.M., & Bauer, A.M. (1985). *Parents and teachers of exceptional students: A handbook for involvement.* Boston: Allyn & Bacon.

Shore, K. (1986). *The special education handbook: A comprehensive guide for parents and teachers.* New York: Teachers College Press.

Simons, R. (1987). *After the tears: Parents talk about raising a child with a disability.* Orlando, FL: Harcourt, Brace, Jovanovich.

Smith, S. (1990). Individualized Education Programs (IEPs) in special education—From intent to acquiescence. *Exceptional Children, 57,* 6–14.

Solnit, A.J., & Stark, M.H. (1961). Mourning and the birth of a defective child. *Psychoanalytic Study of the Child, 16,* 523–537.

Sonnerschein, P. (1984). Parents and professionals: An uneasy relationship. In M.L. Henniger & E.M. Nesselroad (Eds.), *Working with parents of handicapped children: A book of readings for school personnel* (pp. 129–139). Lanham, MD: University Press of America.

Stein, R. (1983). Growing up with a physical difference. *Child Health Care, 12,* 53–61.

Steinberg, A. (Ed.). (1988). Parents and schools. *Harvard Education Letter, 4,* 1–4.

Stewart, J.C. (1986). *Counseling parents of exceptional children* (2nd ed.). Columbus, OH: Charles E. Merrill.

Swap, S. (1990). Comparing three philosophies of home-school collaboration. *Equity and Choice, 6,* 9–19.

Tew, B., & Laurence, K.M. (1973). Mothers, brothers, and sisters of patients with spina bifida. *Developmental Medicine and Child Neurology, 15*(Suppl. 29), 69–76.

Turnbull, A.P., & Turnbull, H.R. (1986). *Families, professionals, and exceptionality: A special partnership.* Columbus, OH: Charles E. Merrill.

Turnbull, A.P., Turnbull, H.R., & Wheat, M. (1982). Assumptions about parental participation: A legislative history. *Exceptional Education Quarterly, 3,* 1–8.

Vaughn, S., Bos, C.S., Harrell, J.E., & Lasky, B.A. (1988). Parent participation in the initial placement/IEP conference: Ten years after mandated involvement. *Journal of Learning Disabilities, 21,* 82–90.

Walberg, H.J. (1984). Families as partners in educational productivity. *Phi Delta Kappan, 21,* 17–20.

Williamson, G.G. (Ed.). (1987). *Children with spina bifida: Early intervention and preschool programming.* Baltimore: Paul H. Brookes Publishing Co.

Transition Planning to Adulthood

Fern L. Rowley-Kelly

For the most part, the medical problems posed by spina bifida are treatable. (See Reigel, chap. 1, this volume.) Young people with spina bifida are doing fine as "patients," but many are having a difficult time flourishing as *people*—socially, vocationally, or economically. Although they may succeed in mainstream educational settings, a significant number do not make an effective transition to meaningful work or continuing education after graduation (Castree & Walker, 1981; Smith, 1983). The following statement by the President's Committee on Employment of the Handicapped describes the problem of employment for high school graduates with disabilities. The level of opportunities for graduates with spina bifida is equally disappointing.

> Each year, approximately 650,000 handicapped young people either graduate from high school or become too old to qualify for public education. Only twenty-one percent will become fully employed. Forty percent will be underemployed and at the poverty level, and twenty-six percent will be on welfare. The statistics have potential for disastrous economic and social problems. (Pennsylvania Departments of Education and Labor and Industry, 1986, p. 3)

Vandergoot, Gottlieb, and Martin (1988) cited similarly disturbing statistics from a Harris poll and from the United States Bureau of the Census:

> A recent survey of persons with disabilities by Louis Harris and Associates (1986) found the prevalence of disability to be 15% of Americans between the ages of 16 and 65. A stunning 62% of persons with disabilities are unemployed. Only one person in 4 was found to work full-time and 50% of people with disabilities earn less than the amount necessary to surpass the poverty level. (p. 1)
> According to the Current Population Survey of the Bureau of the Census of 1985, 18% of the people between the ages of 15 and 64 were thought to have a functional limitation, and "77% of people without disabilities were in the

labor force compared to only 53% of those with limitations." The Census Bureau also found that "Only 8.3% of people without disabilities earned less than $600 per month, as compared to 18.8% of people with disabilities. Conversely, over 34% of people without disabilities earned over $3000 per month while only 19% of people with disabilities did so." (p. 7, 8)

This picture of unemployment and income discrepancy fits into a broader pattern of delayed maturation typical of many youth with spina bifida. These young people are often delayed in the acquisition of work skills and other key life skills. (See Rowley-Kelly, chap. 9, this volume.) For many, active participation in life sharply declines following their high school graduation. Most remain in their parents' home. Many do not work and many lack a meaningful daily routine. When many attempt vocational training, higher education, independent living, or employment, they often fail.

At the same time, a study by the National Council on the Handicapped (1987) cited a recent Harris Poll on employment indicating that jobs are available. The study also cited the lack of qualified applicants as the single most important barrier to employment for persons with disabilities. It is not primarily a lack of specific vocational skills that disqualifies the applicant for a particular job:

> Research and experience show that most employment-related failures or difficulties have been attributed to inappropriate worker traits rather than a lack of vocational skills. Usually, these negative work habits have been evident during school years, and often have contributed to failure in vocational education or school in general. (Maryland State Department of Education, Division of Vocational-Technical Education, 1984, p. 57)

A similar conclusion was presented by both the Vice President's Task Force on Youth Employment in 1980 and the Pennsylvania Departments of Education and Labor and Industry in 1986:

> Specific vocational skill training is not viewed as being critical to the long-term employability of youths as are positive work habits and sound basic interpersonal work skills. Problem solving skills and adaptability to the work environment are significant employer needs. (p. 3)

The findings of Vandergoot et al. (1988) reinforced this point:

> Recent surveys of employers regarding their expectations of youthful entrants into the labor market indicated their preferences for those that have a good, general orientation to work. Employers also prefer to hire on the basis of what they perceive as socialization skills, perhaps in preference to occupational skills. (p. 45)

Acquisition of basic "academic skills in reading, writing, and computation" are, of course, also important to employers of youth (National Commission for Employment Policy, 1979, p. 3).

The work habits and interpersonal skills employers require are the very skills that are difficult for students with spina bifida to develop. The traits that predispose these youth to vocational failure are likely to be present in the school setting, where identification and treatment are possible. Students with spina bifida have a definite need for training during their school years that will help them achieve positive work habits, interpersonal skills, and work skills. Suggestions for providing this training are presented in a subsequent section of this chapter, entitled "Preparing the Student for a Successful Transition." Research has shown that 90% of children with disabilities who are capable of entering the mainstream of jobs and family life will confront significant social and physical barriers to that process (Kramer, 1985). Enhancing their ability to overcome these barriers will promote adolescent adjustment and serve society's future need for productive and independent citizens.

TRANSITION PLANNING AND THE NEEDS OF EARLY ADOLESCENCE

Transition from the school environment to the work environment involves a critical period of adjustment for the family and student with spina bifida.

> For any family, the transition of children from adolescence to adulthood is the most stressful time of all (Carter & McGoldrick, 1980; Olson et al., 1984). . . . as stressful as the transition to adulthood is for most families, it becomes even more stressful when the son or daughter is disabled. (Wikler, 1981, p. 19)

The most significant factor causing many mothers stress during the launching of transition was whether or not a family was " 'off schedule'— that is, whether the child's leaving was delayed later than peer and societal expectations dictate for the achievement of independence" (Harkins, 1978, cited in Brotherson, Backus, Summers, & Turnbull, 1986, p. 19). "Many parents of sons and daughters who are disabled have reported that the uncertainty of their child's future has caused the family deep concern" (Brotherson et al., 1986, p. 21). Parents worry about the welfare of their child as he or she becomes an adult, particularly when he or she approaches adulthood. Careful planning for the child's future can reduce some of the stress associated with this transition.

Neurologic and developmental factors may make it difficult for adolescents with spina bifida to pursue the complex goal-directed behavior required to transform themselves from public school students to workers or vocational trainees. Studying much simpler forms of goal-directed behavior among children with spina bifida in play situations, Landry, Copeland, Anjanette, and Robinson (1990) reported "these results suggest that children with spina bifida may have specific problems with sustaining goal-directed behavior, and need assistance in formulating and implementing a sequence of actions in order to achieve concrete, short-term goals" (p. 306). It is prudent to assume that the adolescent with spina bifida may require significant assistance in setting and achieving the abstract and long-term goals involved in the transition to work.

This transition planning process comes at a very difficult stage in the development of the adolescent with spina bifida. Fortunately, the process of transition planning can help the young person to achieve the developmental tasks of this stage. Friedrich and Shaffer (1986) compared the developmental tasks of the adolescent with spina bifida to the normative crisis of all adolescents. Citing Offer (1969), they noted that all "adolescents must develop an independent personality, increase their self-confidence, establish comfort and strength in their abilities, make important decisions about their futures, and free themselves from earlier attachments to their parents" (p. 411).

Although the vast majority of adolescents pass through this crisis fairly well, "adolescence for the congenitally impaired is typically a very difficult time and psychologically more problematic than Offer's normative crisis" (Friedrich & Shaffer, 1986, p. 412). Anderson and Clarke (1982) found that 51% of adolescents with physical disabilities had problems with independence, responsibility, social life, heterosexual relations, or psychological adjustment. Most adolescents have arrived at the stage of cognitive development known as "formal operations." They are now capable of seeing things as they could be, and not just things as they are ("concrete operations"). They can perform hypothetical reasoning and deductive reasoning. At this stage of cognitive development, illusions about the temporary nature of their malformations can no longer be maintained.

> Adolescents use formal operations and, thus, realize that their impairments are going to be with them for the rest of their lives. As an example, adolescents with myelomeningocele must realize that they will chronically and consistently have to deal with all of the concomitant issues that comprise their clinical pictures, such as decubiti, obesity, toileting accidents, urinary tract infections, shunting complications, scoliosis, arthritis, limited mobility, subtle impairment of intellectual function, etc. (Friedrich & Shaffer, 1986, p. 415)

In a study of the correlates of self-esteem for adolescents with spina bifida, Eckart (1988) investigated differences in self-esteem between adolescents of different ages, and differences in internal and external perceptions of control. Generally, high self-esteem is correlated with taking credit for one's successes and denying responsibility for failure. The denial of responsibility for failure is especially adaptive in circumstances that are essentially beyond the control of the individual, as may be the case for a member of a minority group or for an adolescent with disabilities. Specifically, Eckart found that:

> For early adolescents with spina bifida, ages 12–14, taking credit for successes and not for failures is associated with high self-esteem. The value of the "self-serving bias" in preserving self-esteem is supported for this age group. . . . Older adolescents seem to both feel and display less self-esteem in regards to being able to affect outcomes. . . . One could speculate that as adolescents with spina bifida grow older, the types of outcomes which they are trying to affect may change. . . . As the developmental tasks facing them change—from being well-liked in school and doing well academically, to finding a job and relating to the opposite sex—there may be a period in which the reinforcements for control and lack of control are not so clear-cut. (pp. 114–115)

Older adolescents with spina bifida thus tend to lose the capacity to preserve self-esteem by refusing to accept responsibility for failures. This type of loss of self-esteem differs from what has been found with nondisabled populations:

> Studies of nondisabled populations have generally shown that perceptions of internal control increase with age (Knoop, 1981, Sherman, 1984). Rosenberg (1979) states that as children reach adolescence, they begin to shift from external to internal attributions for many outcomes. However, in the present study, perception of internal control over positive outcomes was *negatively* correlated with age for adolescents with spina bifida. . . . The older adolescents in the study perceived significantly less internal control than did the younger ones. (Eckart, 1988, p. 118)

As did Friedrich and Shaffer (1986), Eckart (1988) suggested that the tasks of adolescence involve a great deal more for adolescents with spina bifida than for adolescents without disabilities. The change in perception of control can be attributed to the difficulty these young people have in mastering key tasks:

> This finding may reflect a real developmental change which occurs as adolescents with spina bifida grow older. . . . Harter (1979) states that success experiences are necessary for the development of a sense of internal control. Lefcourt (1981) states that changes in the sense of personal control depend on mastery of the key tasks of life. It may be that as the tasks of adolescence change with age, they become increasingly difficult for the adolescent with spina bifida to master. (Eckart, 1988, p. 119)

The tasks of adolescence are not only more difficult for the young person with spina bifida; there are also more tasks, including coming to terms with the permanence of the disabilities and taking over responsibility for managing a broad program of medical care. Given the greater stressors of adolescence for the young person with spina bifida, a period of hopelessness and depression is a realistic outcome for some students at this stage. Thorough, effective assessment and transition planning can go a long way toward rebuilding hope on a realistic basis.

> At the stage of formal operations, an awareness of an individual's pattern of cognitive strengths and weaknesses would be particularly helpful along with creative problem solving from people working with the individual. This is evident and essential in the school setting. (Friedrich & Shaffer, 1986, p. 415)

Creative problem-solving should include finding ways to compensate for areas of deficiency that have not yet responded to efforts at remediation. Finding new ways to achieve, survive, and succeed can provide a brighter outlook in a potentially difficult situation.

> There are multiple ways to learn the contents of a worthwhile book, to learn how to live and earn a living, and to communicate the understanding of concepts. For both the impaired adolescent and the parent, active problem solving as well as learning a vocation, compensation, and an avocation are recommended as a potential antidote for a sense of hopelessness and associated depression resulting from school and social failure. (Friedrich & Shaffer, 1986, p. 416)

Effective transition planning can thus serve as a key intervention at this important stage in the life of the young person with spina bifida, as well as providing a planning tool for the family, school, and vocational service agency. The planning process will serve both purposes much more effectively if the student, family, and school can arrive at this stage with a great deal of progress already in hand in the key areas of work habits, work skills, and interpersonal skills.

TRANSITION PLANNING AND TRANSITION PREPARATION

With an understanding of the significance of the key traits and skills described above, an important distinction can be drawn between transition planning and transition preparation. *Transition planning* is a process mandated by law (section 204 of the Carl D. Perkins Act) that must begin at age 14, and preferably well before that. *Transition preparation* is a process that could and should occur throughout the student's educational experience. Early personal development must occur in several critical areas if the child is eventually to make a successful transition to the work force.

> Preparing all students to be independent in their living skills and employable in the marketplace are major goals. However, it takes careful planning and preparation for post-school placement. Key to the success of these goals is the role of parental concern and involvement. To ensure effective parent/guardian involvement in the transition process, schools should encourage parents to participate in planning for their child's post-secondary life as early as elementary school. . . . Parents can be encouraged to work

with their children at home to promote appropriate behavior, good groom-
ing, completion of chores, wise handling of money, as much independence
as possible, and as many opportunities as possible to explore and enjoy the
community. (Council of Chief State School Officers, Resource Center on Educational Equity, 1988, p. 5)

The prognosis for a successful transition at the end of high school will be
greatly enhanced if the parents and the school system start as early as
possible and work together in developing the necessary skills and traits.

To meet individual needs and to overcome current barriers to smooth transitions, all cooperative programs among agencies should encourage the following generic components: 1. A continuum of educational services which
begin in the early grades increasingly exposing all children with disabilities
to the post-school world and its responsibilities. Knowledge and skills
should be those identified as essential to all individuals in their personal,
family, home, community, and work responsibilities. . . . (Council of Chief
State School Officers, 1988, p. 6)

There is thus a documented need for programming in the areas of transition planning and transition preparation. (A subsequent discussion presents recommended approaches for both areas.) It is also important that
the recommended approaches be adapted with due consideration to
what has already been stated about the developmental needs of adolescents with spina bifida. It is especially important to tailor the approaches
to each student's current stage of acceptance of his or her disabilities.

In the least mature stage, the student has not fully grasped the permanence of the disabilities, and continues to believe that they will dis-
appear magically with maturation, or that parents and other adults will
always be willing and able to provide care and to compensate for the disabilities. Younger students, as well as older students who remain at this
stage of acceptance, will rely more heavily on parents, teachers, and
other adult caregiving figures. They can be expected to take individual
experiences of failure less seriously, as they have not yet fully confronted
the need to function independently and competently. A student who remains at this stage during the time when the individualized transition
plan (ITP) is being developed may respond to the planning process with
passivity, allowing parents and professionals to lead the way while
providing little in the way of genuine input or participation. Such a response would of course indicate that a great deal of further transition
preparation is needed. Even in the presence of such passivity, it remains
important to encourage and prompt participation by the young person. In
a comparable context, Borjerson and Lagergren (1990) stress the need to
outgrow the pattern of professional-to-parent communication that had
been appropriate in managing sophisticated pediatric care: "Often too
much communication with adolescents had been through their parents,

but this attitude must change to communicating with the adolescents themselves and to discussion with them in person. They have the right to participate directly" (p. 704).

In the second stage, the student has begun to grasp the reality of the permanence of his or her disabilities. As noted earlier, such a student tends to suffer from depression or discouragement, to have low self-esteem, and to have a limited belief in his or her capacity to control or influence a situation. Some will tend to retreat into hopelessness or help-lessness. The student in this stage is well served by inclusion into the process of planning his or her individualized education program (IEP). The connection between current programming and the student's future life situation should be made very clear to the student. The student should also be given ample opportunity to appreciate his or her pattern of abilities and history of successes, while realistic plans are formulated to overcome or compensate for specific disabilities. In the event that the student is occupying this stage during the transition planning process, full involvement in the process may help the student to conclude the developmental tasks of this stage and move toward the most mature level of acceptance.

A student in the most mature stage of acceptance has stopped asking, "What do you expect of a person with disabilities?" and has proceeded to the task of getting on with his or her life and finding ways to meet realistic self-determined expectations. A student in this stage would be likely to take an active or leading role in the transition planning process and would be taking some independent initiatives in the area of transition preparation. The student who is functioning effectively in this stage can be expected to display a gradual increase in self-esteem and an increasing confidence in his or her ability to control the outcome of situations that are important to life goals.

Planning in the area of meeting medical needs can be helpful at any stage. Extending opportunities to take responsibility for managing routines and scheduling appointments will allow more mature students to move forward, and will prompt less mature students to begin to think about managing their disabilities without the perpetual assistance of their mothers and fathers. Students who are beginning to confront the permanence of their disabilities will find an occasion to be competent rather than helpless as they face their many physical needs. They will also be in a better position to find answers to their own questions about their capabilities and impairments as they initiate contacts with the medical profession. Exercises to promote medical self-management can be introduced as a part of transition preparation at any age level. In transition planning, medical needs must of course be provided for and taken into consideration.

To summarize, transition planning has been presented as a formal process, mandated by law, beginning at age 14. It has also been seen as an opportunity to assist the young person with spina bifida in working through key developmental tasks that are specific to adolescents with spina bifida. Transition preparation is a process that can and should continue throughout the educational career of the student with spina bifida, providing the opportunity to develop those key personality traits and skills that can make possible a successful transition to a position of adult responsibility. Both processes are best undertaken with an understanding of the developmental needs of adolescents with spina bifida and can be tailored to correspond to each student's stage of acceptance of his or her disabilities. The following discussion provides recommended approaches to the area of transition preparation, with an emphasis on the identification and development of key traits and skills.

PREPARING THE STUDENT FOR A SUCCESSFUL TRANSITION

There are specific positive traits that employers require, but that develop slowly for students with spina bifida. For example, how a student talks to the person working nearest him or her is important in second grade, and equally important at work 20 years later. These positive employment traits can be grouped into personality traits, work habits, work skills, and interpersonal communication skills.

Personality Traits

Personality traits crucial for a successful adaptation to the adult world of work and advanced training include independence, adaptability, and a sense of responsibility. Children with spina bifida often remain psychologically dependent on their parents much longer than their nondisabled peers, and many do not assume increasing responsibility as they grow older (see Rowley-Kelly, chap. 9, this volume). Many young adults with spina bifida also remain dependent on established routines. Although some areas of dependency are based on realistic medical considerations, dependency in other areas may provide security and structure that the young person is reluctant to abandon. In the area of medical needs, where a structured routine is necessary, the youth may not accept responsibility for administering the routine and may depend on parents to tell him or her what to do and when to do it (see Rowley-Kelly, chap. 9, this volume). In the following discussion about growth in responsibility, what is said about the role of the parents can be applied, with appropriate modifications, to the role of the teacher:

> [Parents] provide training and guidance so that the children can gradually begin to assume those responsibilities for themselves. In most families, this

process is a reciprocal one in that parents relegate responsibility as they receive cues about their children's increasing abilities, or as their children demand or take more freedom. However, in families with a disabled child, parents may not receive those cues. They may not expect a growing sense of responsibility, nor may it occur to the disabled child to make demands. Thus, parents with developmentally disabled children must consciously plan the transfer of responsibility rather than simply rely on the natural process of change. (Brotherson et al., 1986, p. 22)

Blum, Resnick, Nelson, and St. Germaine (1991) reinforce this point in discussing household chores as a means of gaining social worth within the family:

The process of transferring responsibility from parent to the individual cannot begin in the middle of adolescence with the expectation that the young adult will be able to manage his or her own needs. Rather, transition is a process best started in childhood in a progressive manner with the child, and subsequently the adolescent, assuming responsibilities commensurate with his or her developmental capacitation. In addition, parents need ongoing support as they facilitate their child's assuming additional responsibilities. (p. 284)

Parents of nondisabled students operate from the presupposition that the student will be able to do more and more independently as he or she "gets bigger." The parents of a student with spina bifida may be locked into the presupposition that the student will continue to be helpless and dependent for life. The fact that the student with spina bifida must remain dependent in some areas does not imply dependency in other areas. Teachers and parents need to plan transfers of responsibility to the student consistently and consciously, even in the face of the student's frequently erroneous conviction that "I can't."

Approaches

1. Assigning chores in the classroom and assuring the worth of these activities can help in creating a greater awareness and appreciation of work, and a conviction that the student can make a contribution to the well-being of the class. In elementary school, such chores might include passing out papers, feeding the fish, changing the date on the blackboard, or organizing the bookshelf. In secondary education, the student with spina bifida could be a library aide, work on the student newspaper, or operate the public address system.

2. Adapting these tasks by putting tools or equipment within reach can encourage the student's willingness to adapt work spaces, especially if the student is asked to think about how the adaptation can be made. The student should be encouraged and expected to take control of the process of identifying those situations that require adaptation, of adapting the situations to fit his or her needs and abilities, and of adjusting himself or herself to the situation.

3. The teacher should expect the student with spina bifida and his or her peers to be equally responsible for homework. Do not be afraid to have high expectations. Papers and homework should be in on time and spelling should be correct. Each pupil should be allowed to develop responsibility for his or her own work and to accept the consequences of poor work. The teacher should be aware of specific disabilities that may require adjusting the expectations. (A thorough discussion of this topic is presented in Rowley-Kelly, chap. 9, this volume, under the heading "Learned Helplessness.")

4. The teacher should provide opportunities for the student to be creative and to use his or her strengths and abilities.

Work Habits

Although medical problems may occasionally create extended absenteeism, attendance is not usually a problem for students or employees with spina bifida. They may, however, lack initiative, have difficulty remaining on a task, and be dependent on adult figures (parents, teachers, supervisors) for direction. (See Rowley-Kelly, chap. 9, this volume.) Deficits in these areas can show up in many elements of the student's school performance, and should be addressed as they occur.

Approaches

1. The student should be expected to learn to get himself or herself started and to keep on the job.

2. The student should be encouraged to talk to the teacher when direction is needed, but the initiative should be given back to the student by encouraging him or her to think about what should be done next.

3. The teacher should ask the student to evaluate his or her own work, naming areas of which he or she is proud and areas that can be improved.

4. The teacher should encourage initiative by providing creative opportunities where the student may choose, design, and execute a task independently.

5. The student should be given special consideration only when necessary. The teacher should provide modifications when needed (e.g., if eye-hand coordination problems have been documented, the student may require extra time to complete written work) (see Culatta, chaps. 5, 6 and 7, and Rogosky-Grassi, chap. 8, this volume). A little creativity can turn an inaccessible setting into a workable environment where real learning can take place.

6. The teacher should express appreciation for the good attendance and punctuality and other positive work habits that the student displays. The teacher should let the student know that a future employer will also appreciate these traits.

The student or worker with spina bifida may have difficulty organizing work, time, and work space (see Baker and Rogosky-Grassi, Rogosky-Grassi, and Rowley-Kelly, chaps. 2, 8, and 9, this volume). Problem-solving may be difficult because of the inability to recognize a scheme of organization hidden within the problem and the inability to develop a systematic approach to solving the problem.

Approaches

1. The teacher should observe the student in order to identify areas of difficulty with organization.
2. Organizing skills should be taught whenever opportunities arise (e.g., scheduling independent work time, straightening out the storage area in the desk, or assisting in the inventory of band equipment).
3. The teacher should ask the child to study other people's systems of organization: "How does the librarian keep track of all the books?" "How do your parents organize the pots and pans?" "Why is a dashboard laid out that way?"
4. Commonly used methods of organization, such as alphabetical order, should be taught.
5. The student should be encouraged to develop and employ his or her own systems of organization, and to adapt other people's systems to personal use.
6. The teacher should encourage work in problem-solving in all areas, such as word problems in the math book, brain teasers, and detective stories.

Interpersonal Communication Skills

Students with spina bifida often lack social skills, depend on adults for socialization and interaction, and are generally passive in the social realm. (See Rowley-Kelly, chap. 10, this volume.) Some students do not initiate conversations, while others may be quite talkative (see Culatta and Rowley-Kelly, chaps. 7 and 9, this volume). Some students with spina bifida may lack assertiveness and may be reluctant or deficient in expressing their feelings, stating their points of view, describing their experiences, defending their rights, or contributing their ideas (Rowley, Van Hasselt, & Hersen, 1986). Such students are likely to be deficient in their ability to develop cooperative work relationships with peers and supervisors.

Approaches

1. Relevant discussion should be encouraged. The teacher should reinforce appropriate responses to conversational initiatives, and expect the student to maintain relevance in his or her verbal interactions.
2. Opportunities to discuss feelings should be provided. The teacher should welcome spontaneous verbal expressions of feeling by paying

attention to and responding to the pupil. Although the student may be more comfortable in initially learning and practicing this behavior with the teacher, it is important to encourage the transfer of this skill to the student's interactions with classmates.

3. The teacher should expect contributions to general discussions. Students should be asked to summarize each other's remarks.

4. The teacher should encourage expression in a variety of media: writing stories, drawing cartoons, putting on puppet shows, or talking into a tape recorder or videocamera. Again, it is most important that these opportunities are structured to emphasize the student's communicating to peers and interacting with them, rather than with the teacher.

5. The teacher should assign joint projects that require two-way communication.

6. Communication games should be played. For example, one student in a blindfold could play pilot as another student directs him or her to "land the airplane" by moving safely between two rows of chairs.

7. The teacher should observe peer interactions, teaching the student with spina bifida to assert his or her needs in a responsible fashion. The student should be taught how to set limits on the amount of help given by peers. For example, the student should learn to say, "No, thank you. I'd rather do that myself" or, "It was nice of you to offer, but I can do this on my own."

8. The student should be taught how to ask for help when it is genuinely needed. For example, the student should learn to say, "Would you please get me that book from the top shelf?"

9. The teacher should encourage participation in extracurricular activities and school social functions.

DEVELOPING THE INDIVIDUALIZED TRANSITION PLAN

"The transition plan is the bridge between the security and structure offered by the school and the opportunities and risks of adult life." (Will, 1984, p. 1) Starting at age 14, each student with disabilities should have an ITP in place. This plan is created by the school, adult rehabilitation agencies, the spina bifida treatment center, the family, and the student. The state vocational rehabilitation agency should play a strategic role in this process. The planning process focuses on the final development of the nonacademic work traits mentioned earlier, while maintaining an emphasis on traditional academic and vocational training. This process must also be continually guided by realistic assessments of the student's physical ability and intellectual potential. Resources for these assessments should include the spina bifida treatment program and the school psychologist.

During the formal transition planning process, the vocational rehabilitation counselor will take the role of case manager, maintaining a view of the whole project and coordinating services. A similar role should be assigned during the transition preparation process, so that the full benefits of a team approach can be realized.

To aid in the transition planning, the checklist in Table 12.1 was developed to monitor the student's development in critical areas, and to assist in the development of the ITP. This checklist emphasizes known areas of difficulty for students with spina bifida. Not all students with spina bifida will have difficulties in the areas mentioned. The appendix to this chapter provides many useful suggestions about the key areas of work experience for teenagers with spina bifida.

SUMMARY AND CONCLUSIONS

The lists of approaches presented in this chapter are of course not complete. Many readers will be able to develop additions or modifications as they encounter the unique needs of each student with spina bifida. Similarly, all possible developmental needs have not been mentioned. It is hoped, though, that a theme has emerged: We may not safely assume that a child with spina bifida has achieved any particular developmental milestone that his or her nondisabled peers have surmounted. The teacher should be alert for particular deficiencies, and be aware that what has not yet been learned can probably be learned in school, and usually without major modifications to normal programming. Teachers

Table 12.1. Checklist of strengths and needs

1. Does the student work independently?
2. Does the student have adequate organizational ability?
3. Does the student have a perceptual deficit? poor eye-hand coordination? fine motor difficulties?
4. Does the student have learning disabilities?
5. Does the student avoid responsibility, accept responsibility, or seek responsibility?
6. To what extent has the student overcome dependency on adults?
7. To whom does the student relate more effectively: peers? adults? peers and adults equally? neither effectively?
8. Does the student socialize effectively with peers? Does the student have a friend or friends? Does the student join activities? Is the student shunned by peers, tolerated, or welcomed?
9. Can the student communicate information effectively when sharing a task?
10. Does the student show initiative?
11. How well does the student remain on task?
12. Does the student complete assignments in a timely and conscientious manner?
13. Does the student display good study habits?

are of course encouraged to consult and confer with the parents, as progress in developing work habits happens much faster when all significant adults share the same expectations. Finally, the teacher must look to the development of the traits and skills that may not be in the curriculum, but will be in demand in the workplace.

Of course, each student has his or her own set of positive traits. While working on overcoming developmental delays, it is important to identify, recognize, and reinforce the positive qualities of each student. It is also often possible to "build from the strengths" by making use of positive traits in developing strategies for compensating for areas of weakness.

The checklist in Table 12.1, as well as the other information provided in this chapter, is designed to call attention to those areas where the student with spina bifida may not be receiving adequate preparation during his or her public education. The author's recommendation that these areas be considered in transition planning does not rule out training in these areas throughout the student's educational experience.

The process of transition preparation described in this chapter should begin long before the age of 14, as early as possible in the formal education process. Students who have IEPs should have goals and programs in place to help them prepare for the eventual transition. Students who do not qualify for individualized educational planning will still require early preparation. In fact, as in many other areas, early intervention is likely to be both easier to execute and more effective. In the best cases, by the age of 14, assessment will indicate that the school district has already made considerable progress in preparing the young person with spina bifida for a successful transition to a full and meaningful adult life, and that the task of preparation was well begun in the first year of enrollment.

GLOSSARY

Adaptability Generally, the capacity to fit oneself into the needs of a work situation. Specifically, the ability to adapt a work environment, work space, or task to fit one's own pattern of abilities or disabilities, and one's own ability to move and handle things.

Individualized transition plan (ITP) Legally mandated plan of services to be provided to a student with a disability, beginning at age 14 and covering the student's transition from public education to employment, vocational training, or further education. The school, state office of vocational rehabilitation, family, and student are participants in the planning process, along with representatives from the local spina bifida treatment team.

Interpersonal work skills Interpersonal skills required for success in the workplace, training center, or further education, including: the ability to receive, transmit, and request information; the capacity to be a pleasant companion; the ability to request or provide assistance; the capacity to be assertive without being aggressive; and the ability to cooperate effectively with supervisors, clients, co-workers, and subordinates.

Normative crisis   For the nondisabled, that phase of adolescence in which decisions about one's future adult role are confronted, including career, marriage, and childbearing. For the adolescent with spina bifida, this crisis is intensified by confrontation with the permanence of the disability, taking over responsibility for medical care and decisions, and other challenges.

Perception of control   Perception that one is or is not responsible for outcomes and events in one's life. High self-esteem correlates positively with the perception that one is responsible for favorable outcomes, and not responsible for unfavorable outcomes. Being able to understand that unfavorable outcomes are largely due to factors beyond the individual's control allows the individual to retain a sense of mastery.

Positive work habits   See *Work habits.*

Transition   Specifically, the process involved in leaving high school and going on to employment, training, or further education. Generally, the developmental process that prepares a young person to achieve eventual emancipation from dependence on adult supervision and adult support, including the development of necessary traits and skills.

Transition preparation   All of the structured and unstructured experiences that promote the development of skills and character traits important to a successful transition. These experiences can and should occur in school, at home, and in other programs of socialization and development. Goals related to transition preparation should be a part of each student's individualized education program (IEP).

Work habits   Routines and behaviors that are useful in any work setting, including timeliness, punctuality, courtesy, cleanliness, thoroughness, task completion, and good work quality.

Work skills   Needed work skills include the ability to get oneself started and to stay on task; problem-solving; and the ability to organize work, time, and workspace. Related traits include a sense of responsibility and pride in workmanship.

REFERENCES

Anderson, E.M., & Clarke, L. (1982). *Disability in adolescence.* London: Methuen.

Blum, R.W., Resnick, M.D., Nelson, R., & St. Germaine, A. (1991). Family and peer issues among adolescents with spina bifida and cerebral palsy. *Pediatrics, 88*(2), 280–285.

Borjerson, M.C., & Lagergren, J., (1990). Life conditions of adolescents with myelomeningocele. *Developmental Medicine and Child Neurology, 32*, 698–706.

Brotherson, M.J., Backus, L.H., Summers, J.A., & Turnbull, A.P. (1986). Transition to adulthood. In J.A., Summers (Ed.), *The right to grow up: An introduction to adults with developmental disabilities* (pp. 17–44). Baltimore: Paul H. Brookes Publishing Co.

Carl D. Perkins Act, section 204. (Public Law 98-524), 20 U.S.C. §§2301 et seq. (1984).

Castree, B.J., & Walker, J.H. (1981). The young adult with spina bifida. *British Medical Journal, 283*, 1040–1042.

Council of Chief State School Officers, Resource Center on Educational Equity. (1988). *The disabled student in transition*. Washington, DC: Author.

Eckart, M.L. (1988). *Correlates of self-esteem in adolescents with myelomeningocele*. Unpublished doctoral dissertation, University of Cincinnati.

Friedrich, W., & Shaffer, J. (1986). Adolescent psychosocial adjustment. In D.B. Shurtleff (Ed.), *Myelodysplasias and exstrophies: Significance, prevention and treatment* (pp. 411–419). New York: Grune & Stratton.

Harkins, E. (1978). Effects of empty nest transition on self-report of psychological and physical well-being. *Journal of Marriage and the Family, 40*(3), 549–556.

Harris poll on employment: Disabled employees rated excellent (Spring 1987). *Focus* (newsletter of National Council on the Handicapped), p. 3.

Kramer, R.A. (1985). Long-term outlook for handicapped children. *Pediatrics in Review, 6*(10), 305–309.

Landry, S.H., Copeland, D., Anjanette, L., & Robinson, S. (1990). Goal-directed behavior in children with spina bifida. *Journal of Developmental and Behavioral Pediatrics, 11*(6), 306–311.

Maryland State Department of Education, Division of Vocational-Technical Education. (1984). *Handbook for vocational support service teams in Maryland*. Annapolis: Author.

McLone, D.G. (1986). Treatment of myelomeningocele and arguments against selection. *Clinical Neurosurgery, 33*, 359–370.

Offer, D. (1969). *The psychological world of the teenager.* New York: Basic Books.

Pennsylvania Departments of Education—Labor and Industry. (1986). *Pennsylvania transition from school to work*. Harrisburg: Author.

Rowley, F.L., Van Hasselt, V.B., & Hersen, M. (1986). Behavioral treatment of families with an adolescent with spina bifida: A treatment manual. *Social and Behavioral Science Documents, 16*(2), 68.

Smith, A.D. (1983). Adult spina bifida survey in Scotland, educational attainment and employment. *Zeitschrifts fur Kinderchirurgie, 38* (Supp. 2), 107–109.

Vandergoot, D., Gottlieb, A., & Martin, E.W. (1988). *The transition to adulthood of youth with disabilities*. Paper prepared for Youth and America's Future by The William T. Grant Foundation Commission on Work, Family and Citizenship of the Human Resources Center at the National Center on Employment and Disability, Research and Training Institute, National Center for Disability Services, Albertson, NY 11507.

Wikler, L. (1981). Chronic stresses of families of mentally retarded children. *Family Relations, 30*(2), 281–288.

Will, M. (1984). *The disabled student in transition—Developing cooperative state models to meet the transition needs of disabled youth: An interagency approach.* Washington, DC: Council of Chief State School Officers Resource Center for Education Equity.

Further
Recommendations

The following recommendations have been selected from *The Transition to Adulthood of Youth with Disabilities* (Vandergoot et al., 1988) as having special relevance for teachers and other educational professionals. The majority of recommendations included in this appendix share the focus of the chapter and its emphasis on transition preparation and ongoing developmental needs. Some recommendations that are of specific relevance to persons involved in the more vocational aspects of transition planning have also been included.

- "Establish direct training and recruiting programs involving schools, vocational rehabilitation agencies and employers so that employers can meet more qualified young job applicants who have disabilities; also, employers should become involved earlier in the transition process so that when training is needed, youth and employer-based training sites are prepared more adequately" (p. 1).
- "Support more programs that teach job-seeking skills (JSS) for youth with disabilities" (p. 22).
- "Make occupational information available to youth with disabilities and their families so that adequate transition planning can occur; typical information should be supplemented with suggestions about availability of aids and devices, transportation and enhanced opportunities through rehabilitation engineering; technological applications will be crucial to ongoing career development of these youth" (p. 22).
- "Continue work experience programs that are built on close cooperation between school and local employers" (p. 44).
- "Make the development of social, as well as vocational, skills equally important goals for work experience programs" (p. 44).
- "Make a range of work experience opportunities available to youth with disabilities who, depending on the disability, may need different levels and types of support and supervision to help them become independent workers" (p. 44).
- "Emphasize a balance between academic studies, social pursuits and work experience during the transition years" (p. 44).
- "Emphasize the development of general socialization skills that can be applied across employers and employment settings" (p. 46).

- "Conduct work-skills preparation and training programs in integrated settings where youth with and without disabilities interact and cooperate" (p. 47).
- "Provide a balance between academic preparation and vocational training for each student with special needs which meets his/her individual needs and aspirations" (p. 47).
- "Actively involve employers in the transition process for youth with disabilities through their input in the planning and development of education and rehabilitation programs that meet their needs" (p. 50).
- "Develop activities which include contacts between youth with disabilities and employer representatives with the intention of developing employer networks for locating work opportunities for these youths" (p. 51).
- "Equip school personnel with access to rehabilitation engineering and information about aids and devices." Rehabilitation engineering involves the use of "aids or devices from one branch of technology or another . . . to enable a person with a disability to perform a task or function previously not possible" (p. 53).
- "Provide rehabilitation engineering applications for youth with disabilities in academic and vocational education settings" (p. 53).
- "Continue to emphasize job-seeking skills in transition planning for youth with special needs" (p. 56).
- "Place a vocational rehabilitation representative in the schools to provide direct services to students such as evaluation, counseling, adjustment training and skills training. Use vocational rehabilitation services to provide more in depth vocational assessments while students are in school" (p. 68).
- "Develop work experience programs using school personnel to provide on-site supervisors" (p. 68).
- "Use the summer break for developing extensive work experience, using school personnel as job coaches" (p. 69).
- "Provide consultation to vocational education personnel regarding curriculum modification as needed, including consultation for work experience site modification" (p. 69).

Rights and Recourses

*Nancy A. Hubley, Ellen Mancuso,
and Pamela Meyer Kunkle*

P arents and professionals involved in the education of a student with spina bifida need to be fully informed about existing laws guaranteeing educational rights, about the practical situations in which these legal rights apply, and about how they can be secured. The first section of this chapter is written from the perspective of education law and describes the rights guaranteed by the two most influential federal laws, PL 101-476, the Individuals with Disabilities Education Act (IDEA), and Section 504 of the 1973 Rehabilitation Act (PL 93-112). The second section presents the existing array of systems for providing education (e.g., special, compensatory, and regular or general education) and describes the various programs available at different ages from infancy to 21. Within each age range and type of system, detailed information about obtaining the services needed for the age and setting is provided. The emphasis in this section is on becoming aware of what services are needed, how they can be arranged, and who should be contacted. There is additional information about expected changes in the types of educational systems that may come about because of current educational reform initiatives. This information will allow parents and professionals to continue to ensure appropriate education as established service delivery models are replaced by new models. Finally, the appendix at the end of this chapter provides a step-by-step review of the process of obtaining an appropriate individualized education program (IEP).

LEGAL RIGHTS

This section provides a general introduction to the legal rights of children with disabilities to special education and related services pursuant to two federal statutes, the Individuals with Disabilities Education Act (IDEA) and Section 504 of the Rehabilitation Act of 1973.

Although this section looks exclusively at these two significant federal statutes, it is important to keep in mind that these are not the only sources of educational rights and protections for children with disabilities. The federal and state constitutions and other federal laws also provide general legal protections for children in the area of education. The Carl D. Perkins Act (vocational education) and the Family Education Rights and Privacy Act of 1974 (34 C.F.R. Part 99) (educational records) are two examples. There are also federal and state judicial decisions affecting the rights of children with disabilities to educational services.

Each state also has its own statutes and regulations governing education for children with disabilities. Thus, this information must be read in conjunction with each individual state's laws and regulations. State laws may provide students with disabilities rights and protections in addition to those set forth in the IDEA and Section 504. However, state laws may not contradict, violate, or limit the mandates of these, or any other, federal laws. For example, in Pennsylvania, children who are mentally gifted and need special instruction are also entitled to special education services under Pennsylvania law.

The right to special education services for children with disabilities continues to evolve. It is important that teachers, parents, advocates, and others involved in the education system are aware of the constant need to update research and to stay informed of the current status of these rights at the state and federal level.

THE INDIVIDUALS WITH DISABILITIES EDUCATION ACT (IDEA)[1]

Background

The most significant federal law in the area of special education is the Education of the Handicapped Act (EHA). This law was enacted in 1975 as PL 94-142, the Education For All Handicapped Children Act. It has been amended several times in the past few years and now encompasses several pieces of legislation and is referred to as the Individuals with Disabilities Education Act (IDEA).

The IDEA is further explained and implemented by the federal regulations promulgated by the United States Department of Education. These regulations are published in Title 34 of the Code of Federal Regulations (C.F.R.). The Office of Special Education Programs (OSEP), a division of the United States Department of Education, is the federal agency charged with administering and enforcing the IDEA.

---

[1]The sections of this chapter on the IDEA and Section 504 were authored by Nancy A. Hubley, Esq.and Ellen Mancuso. These sections have been revised and expanded from an earlier publication of the Education Law Center: *The Right to Special Education in Pennsylvania: A Guide for Parents.* (Mancuso, Rieser, & Stotland, 1991). Reprinted by permission.

Each state's Department of Education is also responsible for ensuring that local school districts (as well as other public and certain private agencies in the state that provide educational services) comply with the IDEA. At the individual level, the IDEA is enforced through the use of administrative and judicial actions brought by parents and advocates who allege violations of the rights guaranteed by the IDEA.

States that elect to receive federal funds under Part B of the IDEA must make available a "free appropriate public education" (FAPE) and a system of procedural safeguards to all eligible children with disabilities from age 3 through 21 years of age. These rights were extended to children ages 3 through 5 at the beginning of the 1991–1992 school year.

The IDEA and its regulations set out an extremely detailed scheme by which children are to be evaluated and appropriate programs of special education and related services developed for them. Extensive parental involvement is mandated by this law in the evaluation and program planning process. Services to be provided to each child must be set out in a written individualized education program (IEP).

The Act and its regulations also set forth extensive procedural and substantive rights that must be provided to children with disabilities and their families under the IDEA. These rights are enforceable through multilevel administrative and judicial procedures.

Children Who Are Protected by the IDEA   Generally, children with spina bifida are protected by the IDEA. However, a child who has a medical diagnosis of spina bifida is not automatically entitled to the substantive and procedural protections of the IDEA. The IDEA protects only those students who are found to be "children with disabilities" within the meaning of the IDEA.

The IDEA defines "children with disabilities" as:

> Children with mental retardation, hearing impairments, including deafness, speech or language impairments, visual impairments, including blindness, serious emotional disturbance, orthopedic impairments, autism, traumatic brain injury, other health impairments or specific learning disabilities and *who, by reason thereof need special education and related services.* (20 U.S.C. §1401(a)(1)(A) [emphasis added]).

The regulations implementing the IDEA further define each of these disabilities. (See Appendix A, Reg. 300.5, Handicapped Children.) Spina bifida is not specifically listed as a disability in either the IDEA or its regulations. However, a student with spina bifida may fall within any one or a number of the expressed categories of disabilities. For example, a child with spina bifida may also have mental retardation, a specific learning disability, be physically impaired, or meet the definition of the other listed physical, mental, or emotional impairments. If the child meets any of these definitions and, because of his or her disability, requires specialized instruction, the child is entitled to all of the substantive and procedural protections of the IDEA.

Children with spina bifida who do not fall within any of the categories of disabilities or who do not require specialized instruction may still be entitled to some special education and support services under Section 504 of the Rehabilitation Act discussed later in this chapter.

The IDEA covers all children with disabilities who require special education, regardless of the severity of the student's disability. States and local school systems may not refuse to provide services on the basis that the child is too severely disabled to benefit from education. (See *Timothy W. v. Rochester School District*, 875 F2d 954 (1st Cir. 1989) cert denied, 110 S.Ct. 519.) In this case, the Supreme Court let stand a decision of a New Hampshire court that held that Timothy W., a child with multiple disabilities and severe mental retardation, was eligible for services under the IDEA. The Court found that there was nothing in the IDEA that required that a child demonstrate that he could benefit from special education in order to be eligible for education services under the IDEA.

Age Range   The IDEA mandates that each state provide all children with disabilities between the ages of 3 and 21 (or up to high school graduation, whichever occurs first) with a free appropriate public education. New federal laws now also require states to provide services to certain infants and toddlers from birth through age 3. These services are referred to as early intervention services and are to be provided in compliance with Part H of IDEA, PL 99-457 and its regulations, 34 C.F.R. Part 303.

Program Responsibility   The responsibility for providing each eligible child age 3 through 21 with a free appropriate public education and all of the procedural protections rests first with the child's local education agency (LEA) (20 U.S.C. §1412(6), 34 C.F.R. 300.220–240, 300.600). In many states, the responsible local educational agency is the school district in which the child's parents reside. Children who reside in foster care, group homes, or residential placements are also entitled to receive appropriate educational programs from the district in which the foster home or residential placement is located. The state education agency is responsible for assuring that the requirements of the IDEA are met within the particular state (20 U.S.C. §1412(6)).

The Right to a Free Appropriate Public Education: The Special Services the Law Provides

What Is "Appropriate"?   The law mandates that states that receive federal educational funds under the IDEA provide each eligible child with a "free appropriate public education" consisting of special education and related services (20 U.S.C. §1401(a)(18)). The IDEA mandates that such special education and related services meet state and federal standards, be provided at public expense, at no cost to the child or family, be provided under public supervision, and be in conformity with the child's IEP.

It is important to note that the IDEA does not provide an explicit definition of "appropriate." However, the U.S. Supreme Court offered some guidance about what constitutes an "appropriate" program under the IDEA in its landmark decision, *Board of Education of the Hendrick Hudson Central School District v. Rowley* 458 U.S. 176, 102 S.Ct. 3034 (1982). In this case, the Court ruled that special education and related services provided to a child with disabilities must meet a two-part test in order to be "appropriate" under the IDEA. The child's IEP must:

1. Be developed in accordance with the procedures set forth in the IDEA, including those governing resolution of disputes between the parties and the school systems, and
2. Be "reasonably calculated to enable the child to receive educational benefits." (458 U.S. at 206–7 102 S.Ct. at 305)

There is no requirement in the IDEA that a school system maximize the potential of a child with disabilities. However, an appropriate educational program is a planned program of education and special services that takes account of the child's individual needs and allows the child to make meaningful progress.

In addition, as stated previously, state law can set a higher standard for the quality of education than that set by the IDEA. Many states do require that the educational program maximize a child's skills. Thus, it is important that state law be reviewed carefully when determining whether a child's education program is appropriate.

What Does "Free" Mean? The IDEA requires that special education and related services provided to a child with disabilities must be provided at no cost or financial liability to the child and family (20 U.S.C. §§1401(a)(16) and (18): 34 C.F.R. §300.4, 300.14). The local education agency is not required to provide the particular service itself, but must arrange for it and ensure that all services are provided at no cost to the child or family. This includes all evaluations, special education instruction, and related services.

What Is "Special Education"? Special education is a planned program of specialized instruction and related services that is based on and responsive to the child's individual needs as identified through the evaluation process. A child with disabilities is entitled, under the IDEA, to a program of "specialized instruction" and those "related services" necessary for the child to benefit from the education program. The IDEA re-

quires that each child's program must be individualized and must provide specially designed instruction to meet the child's unique learning
needs.

Specialized instruction does not mean the child with disabilities
must be placed in a special education classroom, school building, or
other environment where only children with disabilities are educated. In
fact, many children with disabilities are able to receive specialized instruction in the same classrooms and school buildings they would attend
if they were without disabilities.

For example, children with spina bifida may need specialized instruction in physical education to address their unique physical needs,
but may be able to receive the needed specialized instruction within the
regular physical education class. Some children may need the assistance
of an aide or other support services, such as occupational or physical
therapy.

Specially designed instruction includes instruction in the same subject provided to regular education students, with the teaching methods
modified to take account of the child's individual needs. A teacher may
need to modify the method of presenting material to a child with spina
bifida or make other accommodations for the child's disability.

Specially designed instruction can also include instruction in self-
help skills, mobility training, or other skills necessary to participate in
the community. Often children with spina bifida receive educational services in areas not traditionally taught to nondisabled students, such as
dressing skills, brace management, mobility training, or other self-help
skills.

The IDEA explicitly defines "special education" to include instruction conducted in the classroom, in the home, in hospitals and institu-
tions, and in other settings and instruction in physical education and in
vocational education (20 U.S.C. §1401(a)(16)(A) and (B)).

What Are "Related Services"?   Children with disabilities are entitled to necessary and appropriate related services. Related services
consist of "transportation, and such developmental, corrective and other
supportive services . . . as may be required to assist a child with disabilities to benefit from special education" (20 U.S.C. §1401(a)(17). (See also
Appendix B, Reg. 300.13, Related Services.) The federal regulations expressly include physical and occupational therapy, speech therapy, and
psychological counseling as related services.

For children with spina bifida and certain other disabilities, having a
full- or part-time aide or using assistive technology, such as a computer,
calculator, or tape recorder, may constitute a required related service. It
is important to keep in mind that the federal regulations do not provide

an exhaustive list of related services. A service that a child with disabilities needs in order to benefit from education that is developmental, supportive, or corrective may also be a related service, even if it is not expressly listed in the IDEA.

It should be noted that the standard for determining eligibility for related services differs from the standard for "specialized instruction." To receive a related service, a child with disabilities must show not only that it is needed, but that it is *needed in order to benefit from the educational program.* For example, a child with spina bifida may, indeed, benefit in a general way from three sessions of physical therapy per week, but fewer sessions per week may be all that is required to assist the child to benefit from education.

Medical Services Children with disabilities are also entitled to certain "medical services" as related services. Only those "medical services" that are for diagnostic or evaluation purposes are related services. The federal regulations define medical services as those "provided by a licensed physician to determine a child's medically related handicapping condition which results in the child's need for special education and related services." (34 C.F.R. §300.13(b)(4) Other medical services such as the prescribing of medication are not related services.

School Health Services Children with spina bifida, like many other children with disabilities, often require certain health-related assistance during the school day in order to benefit from their educational program. Federal regulations explicitly include "school health services" among the list of related services. School health services are those services that can be provided by a qualified school nurse or other qualified person (34 C.F.R. §300.13(b)(10)).

For example, a child may need assistance with clean intermittent catheterization or the care of a tracheostomy, in order to attend school. If the necessary health-related service can be provided by a school nurse, trained layperson, or other nonphysician, the child is usually entitled to the service as a related service.

The issue of what constitutes a related service was specifically addressed by the U.S. Supreme Court in the case of *Irving Independent School District v. Tatro,* 468 U.S. 883, 104 S.Ct. 3371 (1984). In this case, the Court held that a child with spina bifida was entitled to clean intermittent catheterization as a related service because she needed it during the school day and it could be provided by a nonphysician. The Court referred to such assistance as a "supportive service" necessary to assist the child to benefit from her educational program. This case has set the standard for determining when a support service is, in fact, a related service.

THE RIGHT TO EVALUATIONS AND RE-EVALUATIONS

The Duty To Evaluate

The IDEA imposes on state and local education agencies an affirmative duty to identify, locate, and evaluate all children within the state or educational system who have disabilities or are suspected of having disabilities and are in need of special education and related services (20 U.S.C. §1412(2)(C) and 1441(a)(a)(A); 34 C.F.R. §300.128, 220).

Children who are suspected of having disabilities are most often referred for evaluations by parents, teachers, or other school professionals. Although the IDEA mandates that states identify and evaluate children with disabilities and those suspected of having disabilities, it is the law of each state that determines the specific manner in which this will be done. State law, for example, determines when a referral must be made and by whom.

The IDEA further requires that all children with disabilities be re-evaluated at least once every 3 years and more often if needed or requested by either the parent or an IEP team member. When a child's educational program is not working or does not appear to be appropriate, it is often very helpful to have the child re-evaluated to determine what, if anything, needs to be changed.

What Is the Purpose of an Evaluation?

In order to know what type of specialized instruction a student needs, it is important to understand the child's learning strengths and weaknesses. Therefore, an in-depth evaluation must be done before a child can be recommended for special education. No child may be identified as a child with disabilities, have his or her classification changed (e.g., from "other health impaired" to "learning disabled"), be put in a special education class, or be moved from one type of class into another until a full and free evaluation has been done and recommendations made about such changes.

An evaluation should determine whether a child meets the federal and state criteria for a "child with disabilities" and describe the child's learning style and the types of instruction that will be successful or not successful with the child. An evaluation should provide a basis for developing educational goals and objectives and for deciding which educational placement would be appropriate for the child. Evaluations should also be used to determine what, if any, related services are needed. The IDEA requires that an evaluation be done before a child can be recommended for special education services for the first time.

Legal Protections in the Evaluation Process

Nondiscriminatory   The IDEA and its regulations prohibit racially or culturally discriminatory testing and establish extensive protections to ensure accurate testing. School systems are required, among other things, to administer tests and other evaluation materials in the child's native language or other primary way in which the child communicates. School systems may not use a single test or procedure as the basis for deciding that a child should be placed in a special education program or as the basis for designing a child's special education program (34 C.F.R. 300.532).

Evaluations Must Be Reviewed by a Multidisciplinary Team The IDEA requires that all evaluations be reviewed by a multidisciplinary team or group of persons, including at least one teacher or specialist knowledgeable about the child's suspected area of disability (34 C.F.R. 300.532(e)). The purpose of the "team" approach is to ensure that the student is given a full and complete evaluation and that decisions are not made on the basis of any one test, such as an IQ test.

School systems are further required to assess a child in all areas related to the child's suspected disability, including health, vision, hearing, social and emotional status, general intelligence, academic performance, communication abilities, and motor skills where appropriate. There are additional requirements for children who are suspected of having learning disabilities (34 C.F.R. §300.540–543). As with other special education services, evaluations must be provided at no cost to the child or the child's parent.

Required Notice and Consent of Parent If a school system wishes to conduct an evaluation of a child, it must give the parent prior written notice that it proposes to conduct an evaluation. If a parent requests an evaluation and the school system refuses to evaluate, it must give the parent written notice of its refusal. Such written notice applies to all initial evaluations as well as any re-evaluations.

The IDEA sets forth very specific requirements for the content of notices to parents (34 C.F.R. 300.505). The notice must include, among other things, a full explanation of all of the procedural safeguards available to the parents under the law; a description of the action proposed or refused by the school system with an explanation of why the action is being proposed or refused; and a description of any options the school system considered and why those were rejected. The IDEA further requires that the notice be written in language understandable to the general public and provided in the native language or other mode of communication of the parent.

A school system must obtain a parent's written consent before conducting an initial evaluation and prior to initial special education placement. There are some circumstances where a school system can override a parent's refusal to permit evaluation based on the applicable law of certain states. However, absent a state law governing this situation, a school system would be required to seek a due process hearing. See discussion of due process hearings later in this chapter.

Parent's Right to an Independent Evaluation A parent has the right to obtain evaluation reports from professionals outside the school system and to submit them to school officials. These reports are called "independent evaluations." School officials must consider the results of any independent evaluation submitted by a parent.

At Public Expense A parent can request that the school system pay for an independent evaluation if the parent believes that the school's evaluation was not appropriate. School officials may deny the request for payment. However, if payment is denied, the school system must offer the parent a due process hearing at which time an impartial hearing officer will decide who should pay for the evaluation.

At Parents' Expense Parents can always obtain an independent evaluation of their child at their own expense. However, it is important that the independent evaluator be qualified to conduct the particular evaluation and understand the eligibility rules for special education and related services. With such an understanding, the independent evaluator will be better able to discuss why the child is a "child with disabilities" and what types of services the child needs. It is not unusual for an independent evaluator to observe the child's classroom or a proposed classroom to evaluate its appropriateness for the child and to make recommendations about the child's program.

Parents' Rights Regarding Child's Records Parents or guardians have the right to inspect and review their child's educational records (34 C.F.R. 300.560 et. seq.). Educational records include most information concerning the student except personal notes kept by an individual school employee for his or her private use only. Once a school official shares personal notes with any other school official, the notes become part of the student's educational records subject to review by the parent or guardian.

Parents have the right to request that school records be amended to correct any inaccurate or misleading information. If school officials refuse to make amendments or changes to a child's record, a parent can request a due process hearing. After the hearing, the school officials must either amend the records or allow the parent to put a statement in the records explaining their objections.

School records must be kept private and cannot be released to persons outside the school system without the consent of the parent. However, consent is not needed before sending a student's records to another school system where the student has enrolled or has asked to be enrolled.

THE RIGHT TO AN INDIVIDUALIZED EDUCATION PROGRAM

Every exceptional student is entitled to an individualized education program (IEP). The IEP is a written plan that tells what special education programs and services the child will receive. The IEP is written at a conference by a team which includes the child's parent and the child's current teacher or the teacher of the class being proposed for the child. An IEP must be reviewed each year and, when needed, revised by the IEP team. An IEP must include all the programs and services necessary to meet a child's individual needs as identified during the evaluation or reevaluation process.

The IEP Conference

The law requires that the IEP be developed at a conference with the child's parents, and prohibits school officials from presenting a completed IEP to the parent at the IEP conference. Parents must be invited to attend even if their child lives away from home in a residential setting. The conference must be scheduled at a time and place convenient for the parents and the school officials.

The law also requires school officials to make every effort to ensure that parents attend IEP conferences. Parents must be notified in writing of the purpose, time, and location of the conference and of the other people who are invited to attend. Parents must also be notified of all of their rights. The notice must be in the language the parent uses and must be sent to them early enough so that they have an opportunity to make arrangements to attend the conference.

At the end of the IEP conference, the parent will either be given or mailed a copy of the IEP. The parent also should get a written notice of the proposed placement for the child and notice of their legal rights. If the IEP is the first one for a child, the parent must approve the IEP, in writing, before it can be put in effect. For later IEPs, if the parents disagree with the IEP, they must indicate their disagreement in writing or the school system can assume that the parent approves the IEP.

The IEP Team

At the IEP conference, the IEP team is responsible for reviewing the evaluation report and deciding whether a child needs special education. If the team decides that the child does need special education, it then decides the kind of program and services needed. If the team decides that the child is not eligible for special education, it must give or send the parent written notice of the decision which explains the right to disagree and to request a special education due process hearing.

The IEP team must include:

- The child's parent(s), guardian, or surrogate parent
- One or more of the child's current teachers; or if the student is entering school, a regular education teacher who teaches students of the same age
- Someone qualified to provide or supervise the provision of special education programs
- The student, if over 18 or if the parent would like the child to attend
- Any other people the parent or school officials want to attend the conference

The Content of an IEP

Each IEP must contain information in the following areas:

- A statement of the child's present levels of educational performance
- A statement of annual goals, including short-term instructional objectives
- A statement of the specific special education and related services to be provided to the child (e.g., the type, amount, and frequency of the related services needed by the student)
- The date services and programs will begin and the anticipated duration of such services
- Appropriate objective criteria and evaluation procedures and schedules for determining, on at least an annual basis, whether the student is achieving the short-term instructional objectives
- The amount of time the child will spend in programs and activities with regular education students
- If the student will be in a regular education class, what modifications, if any, are needed for the child to succeed in that class

In addition, needed services in the following areas should also be included in the IEP where appropriate for the child:

- *Assistive Technology*—for students who have physical impairments or other disabilities and require special equipment to help them participate in school.
- *Vocational Education*—for students for whom vocational training is appropriate. As with other services, the need for vocational education depends on the individual child's needs, and not on an arbitrary age requirement, achievement level, or other rule set by the school system.

- *Graduation Planning*—for all students beginning at least 3 years prior to expected graduation. The IEP must contain a plan for the student's graduation from high school.
- *Behavior Programs*—for students classified as "seriously emotionally disturbed" and for students with other disabilities who have behavior problems that interfere with their learning. The IEP should contain a program designed to teach the student appropriate behavior and social skills. All behavior programs should use positive—not negative—approaches.
- *Transition Services*—for all students with disabilities, beginning no later than age 16. Transition services are activities designed to provide the student with the skills needed for post-school life, including vocational training, employment, and independent living.
- *Extended School Year (ESY) Programs*—for students who are eligible, the type and length of the ESY program must appear on the IEP (see below).

Extended School Year (ESY) Programs

Extended School Year programs are special education programs for children with disabilities who regress in basic skills during breaks in the school year and then take a long time to regain those skills once the program begins again. Programs can be provided during the summer months or on weekends.

Children who have autism, severe mental retardation, severe multiple disabilities, or severe emotional disturbances are most likely to require ESY programs. Other children who are likely to regress and have difficulty catching up may also qualify. If a parent or teacher believes a child qualifies for ESY services, he or she can request that the youngster be considered for such services. For children who are found to be eligible, the type and length of ESY program must appear on the child's IEP.

Related Services

The IEP must contain the "related services" needed to help the child benefit from or gain access to the education program, such as transportation or physical or occupational therapy. It is important the IEP state the type, amount, and frequency of the related services to be provided. For example, instead of just stating "physical therapy," the IEP should state "individual physical therapy, 30-minute session, three times per week." In this way, the parent, teacher, and therapist all know exactly what the child should receive.

It is important to remember that a student is entitled only to the type, frequency, and amount of related services needed to assist the youngster to benefit from or gain access to the program.

Transportation Transportation to and from school is probably the most frequently needed related service. Transportation must be appropriate for the child. For example, if the child uses a wheelchair, transportation should be provided with a lift bus or other vehicle able to handle the wheelchair in a safe manner. Additionally, transportation within a school building must also be provided when needed by a child with a mobility impairment. Transportation, like all other related services, must be provided for the child without cost to the parent or family. The length of the transportation provided must also be appropriate in view of the child's age and special needs.

Tips on Developing IEPs

The child's teacher should review the evaluation report prior to the IEP conference. He or she should focus on areas identified by the evaluators as posing difficulty for the child. Any other problem areas that the teacher has seen, or expects to see, in the child must be considered as well. The educator must be prepared to answer questions about the child's current levels of functioning and what may be appropriate short-term objectives and possible annual goals. In addition, he or she must be prepared to discuss what teaching methods may work best with this child.

It might also be helpful for the teacher to be prepared to answer some of the following questions:

- In what subject and skill areas does this child need special help? Which are priorities for children with this disability at this age?
- What kinds of help does the child need in these areas? For example, what teaching methods work best with the child? What types have been tried and have not worked? Does the child learn best by repetition? Does the child need to have material presented visually as well as orally? What needs to be *special* about the way this child is taught?
- What activities especially interest or motivate this child? Are enough of these included in the child's school day? Is there a need to give the child more opportunities for success in school?
- Are there parts of the school day that the child is finding particularly frustrating? How can they be improved? Are there areas that shouldn't be included in the child's program at all?
- Should the child be spending more (or less) of the day in regular education classes? Which ones? Should the child be spending more time with nonexceptional students in activities such as gym, music, art, or lunch?

It is often helpful to make a list of the specific ideas of what might be appropriate to include in the child's IEP. Take the list to the IEP conference and feel free to raise those issues that may be appropriate to ensure that the child be educated appropriately.

IEP Time Lines

The IEP must be completed within 30 calendar days after the determination that the child needs special education and related services. IEP conferences must be held for each child with disabilities at least once per year. Additional conferences must be held if a member of the IEP team, including teachers and parents, requests an IEP conference.

THE RIGHT TO AN APPROPRIATE SCHOOL PLACEMENT

The law requires that an IEP be developed for a child before it is decided where the program should be provided. This is because, to be appropriate, the placement must be able to implement the program and services described in the IEP. Unfortunately, many school officials try to decide the child's placement first—based on what is available—and want to discuss the program issues later. Teachers often want to "get to know" a student before developing his or her IEP. However, the law requires that the education program and placement be fitted to the child, not the child to a prepackaged program and placement. Teachers can always request that an IEP conference be reconvened to revise a child's IEP once the child is actually placed if goals or objectives need to be modified.

Placement decisions may not be made on the basis of administrative convenience, lack of staff, lack of available space, lack of established program, or solely on the classification of the child.

Once an IEP is developed, school officials must give or send parents notice of the placement that is being recommended for the child. This notice must also include information about a parent's rights to due process procedures.

A parent should disapprove the recommended placement and begin the due process procedures if he or she believes that the placement being recommended is not appropriate for the child. Even when a parent agrees with the IEP, he or she may still disagree about the proposed placement for several reasons. For example, the placement may be located at a school too far from the child's home, the other children in the classroom may not be within the child's age range, the placement may not offer the child the amount of integration with children without disabilities which the child may need, or the placement may not be the school the child would attend if not disabled. If these disagreements cannot be resolved by the IEP team, due process procedures may be initiated to determine the appropriate placement for the child.

The Appropriate Classroom

The appropriate class for the child depends on the amount and type of special instruction or related services the child needs. The law mandates that a child with disabilities, consistent with his or her individual needs, be included with nondisabled peers to the maximum amount that is appropriate for the child with the disabilities (20 U.S.C. 1412(5)(B) and 1414(a)(1)(c)(iv); 34 C.F.R. §§300.550–556).

A child with disabilities must be educated in the class and school building he or she would attend if not disabled except where the child's needs dictate otherwise. This is often referred to as mainstreaming or integration and sometimes as *inclusion*.

Generally, a child with disabilities, including a child with spina bifida, can be educated in the same classrooms and school building he or she would attend if not disabled. Some children with spina bifida can be educated in regular classrooms with support and consultative services of other professionals such as special education teachers, school nurses, and physical and occupational therapists. Other children require a more specialized setting.

If the child will receive only some special education support services, the child can probably remain in the regular education classroom. Even if the child needs some courses in special education, it should be possible for the child to be in a regular education class for most of the day. As discussed earlier in this chapter, special education services can be provided to children in their regular education classrooms or the child can receive them in a separate classroom.

However, for some children, placement in a special education class for most or all of the day is necessary. Even in those situations, however, the law requires that, if appropriate, the student spend time with regular education students in academic, nonacademic, or after-school activities.

Procedural Safeguards and Dispute Resolution

The IDEA establishes an elaborate scheme of procedural safeguards designed to ensure that parents are involved in decisions regarding their child's education and that when disputes arise, there is a process for challenging these decisions. (See 20 U.S.C. §1415, where the procedural protections are set forth in the IDEA.)

In the Supreme Court case of *Board of Education of the Hendrick Hudson Central School District v. Rowley*, 458 U.S. 176, 205–06, 102 S.Ct. 3034, 3050–51(1982), the Court emphasized that these procedural protections are not meant to be technicalities, but rather, are the primary mechanism through which the IDEA attempts to guarantee that an "appropriate" education is actually provided to each child with disabilities.

In drafting the IDEA, Congress recognized that, even under the best of circumstances, there may still be disagreements between school officials and parents about special education services. Disagreements can occur at any stage of the special education process—whether to do an evaluation or reevaluation of a child or what tests to use; whether the child has a disability and if so, what program and related services are needed and in what amounts; whether the child's program is or isn't working well; or what class and school is needed to help the child learn. Thus, the IDEA provides elaborate procedures for resolving these disputes.

The Right to an Administrative Hearing

The IDEA entitles parents and students to an impartial administrative hearing on any matter related to the provision of a free appropriate public education, including, but not limited to, identification, evaluation, and placement issues (20 U.S.C. §1415(b)(1)(E) and (b)(2)). There are also provisions that permit school officials to request administrative hearings.

The IDEA gives states the option of implementing a one- or two-tiered hearing and review system. In states that choose a single-tier system, the state education agency conducts administrative hearings. In these states, the hearing officer's decision must be final and binding, subject only to an aggrieved party bringing an action in court. It cannot be subject to any further administrative review.

In states that choose a two-tiered system, administrative hearings are conducted at a local level and any aggrieved party has the right to appeal the decision to the state education agency. The state education agency must then conduct an impartial review of the hearing and make an independent decision about the issues presented in the case. The impartial official conducting the review must examine the entire record of the hearing; ensure that proper procedures were followed; give the parties an opportunity to give written and/or oral arguments; seek additional evidence if necessary; and must issue written findings and conclusions to be distributed to the parties. Under the two-tiered system, the impartial reviewing official's decision is final and binding unless appealed to a court.

In both systems, the official conducting the hearing cannot be an employee of an education agency or unit involved in the education or care of the child. Nor can the person have a personal or professional interest that would undermine his or her objectivity in deciding the case. Individuals who do not meet each of these tests would be disqualified from serving as an impartial hearing officer.

Administrative Hearings

Although due process hearings are not as formal as court cases, they are more formal than conferences or meetings held with school officials. Each side has the opportunity to present witnesses—school staff, evaluators, other professionals, neighbors, friends, family members who know the child—and each side is given the opportunity to cross-examine, that is, to ask questions of the other parties' witnesses. Parents and school officials can request that the hearing officer "subpoena" any witnesses that either party feels has information that is important to the case. All witnesses give their testimony under oath.

Parents are entitled to be represented by an attorney or accompanied and advised by individuals with special knowledge or training in the needs of children with disabilities. Both parents and school officials are entitled to a written transcript or verbatim recording of the hearing. Only parents have the right to request the child's presence at the hearing and to determine if the hearing will be open to the public.

The IDEA regulations require that a written decision, including findings of fact and conclusions, must be rendered no later than 45 days after the hearing is requested. In addition, in states that have chosen the two-tiered system of review, administrative appeal decisions must be made no later than 30 days after the request for the review is received. It is not unusual for hearing officials to extend these timelines at the request of either party for good cause.

Mediation

Neither the IDEA nor its regulations require mediation of special education disputes. However, many states have included mediation in their state scheme of dispute resolution prior to a due process hearing. Mediation is often very helpful in resolving disputes; however, it cannot be mandated or used to deny or delay the right to a formal due process hearing.

Appeals

The IDEA entitles any party who is aggrieved by a hearing decision (or a review decision in a two-tiered state) to bring a civil action in state or federal court. The court must receive the records of the administrative proceedings, hear additional evidence at the request of a party, and base its decision on the preponderance of the evidence. Courts are also required to give "due weight" to the administrative proceedings. If violations of the IDEA are found, courts may grant such relief as they deem appropriate, including ordering a new program or placement, the provision of related services, or such things as compensatory education and reimbursement for money spent for the provision of special education services pending resolution of the dispute.

Attorney's Fees

The Handicapped Children's Protection Act (HCPA) amended the IDEA in 1986 to empower courts to award attorney's fees to parents who prevail in IDEA disputes in court, through administrative due process hearings and, in some cases, for work done in settling IDEA disputes prior to administrative hearings. Parents who win all or some of what they sought in such disputes are entitled to "reasonable" attorneys' fees and costs, subject to certain conditions relating to settlement offers. (See 20 U.S.C. §1415(e)(4)(B) and (e)(4)(D) and (E).)

Exhaustion

Generally, the IDEA requires that, prior to the commencement of a civil action, a parent must use and complete (exhaust) the administrative procedures. If the use of these procedures can be shown to be "futile or inadequate," the Court may excuse the parent from the exhaustion requirement.

Time Lines

There is no expressed statute of limitation, or time period, within which a person must file an action in Court in the IDEA. As a result, courts have applied varying time lines depending on other analogous state law claims. Even within a particular state, the time lines that are applied are often different depending upon the particular issues raised by the case. Thus, it is very important to consult with an attorney as soon as possible after an unfavorable due process decision to determine the applicable time within which an appeal may be filed.

Status of Child's Program Pending Resolution

Once administrative procedures have been initiated, a child's program and placement cannot be changed without the consent of both the parent and the state or local school agency. The IDEA mandates that, while administrative proceedings, including any judicial proceedings, are pending, the child must remain in his or her then-current educational placement. This provision is often referred to as the "status quo" or "pendency" provision. This provision is applicable to all changes in placement, including graduation and disciplinary actions.

The "stay put" provision prohibits parents or school officials from unilaterally changing a child's classification, program, or placement while due process or judicial proceedings are pending. There are circumstances in which a parent can change a child's placement at their own expense, that is, provide educational services privately, and if they succeed in establishing their claim that such service is "appropriate," may be entitled to reimbursement from the school system. (See *Town of Burlington School Committee v. Department of Education*, 471 U.S. 359, 105 S.Ct. 1996 (1985).)

IN SUMMARY

The rights discussed in this chapter exist because parents, professionals, and others concerned about the needs of children with disabilities banded together and worked for the passage of state and federal laws. It will take the continued hard work of parents, advocates, and school officials to make sure these rights are not hollow promises, but instead result in quality programs for all children with disabilities.

While the special education system may seem complicated, its basic design is really quite simple. Parents and school officials must look at individual children, determine their learning needs, and develop a program that includes all of the services necessary to meet those needs. If parents and school officials stay focused on the needs of individual children, the rights of children with disabilities will be protected and appropriate programs will be provided to all children with disabilities.

SECTION 504 OF THE REHABILITATION ACT OF 1973

Overview

Section 504 of the Rehabilitation Act of 1973, 29 U.S.C. Section 794, prohibits discrimination against children and adults with disabilities, including those with spina bifida, by recipients of federal funds. All, or virtually all, state and local education agencies receive some federal money and are therefore bound by Section 504. Section 504 provides in pertinent part:

> No otherwise qualified handicapped individual in the United States, as defined in section 706(6) of this title, shall, solely by reason of his handicap, be excluded from participation in, be denied the benefits of, or be subjected to discrimination under any program or activity receiving Federal financial assistance or under any program or activity conducted by any Executive agency or by the United States Postal Service.

Federal regulations implementing Section 504 within the education area are found at 34 C.F.R. Part 104.

As previously mentioned, there is much overlap between the IDEA and Section 504 in the area of public education; however, there are some important distinctions. There are children protected by Section 504 who are not eligible for services under the IDEA. There are also rights provided under Section 504 that are not addressed by the IDEA.

Children Who Are Protected by Section 504

Like the IDEA, Section 504 has its own definition of who is considered *handicapped* and entitled to its protections. The definition of *handicapped* under Section 504 is much broader than that under the IDEA. A person is considered handicapped if he or she "has a physical or mental impairment, which substantially limits one or more major life activities;" has a record of such an impairment, even if the impairment is no longer significant; or, is regarded or treated as if he or she had an impairment (34 C.F.R. Section 104.3(j)). "Major life activities" include virtually all life skills, such as walking, speaking, learning, working, and care for one's self (see 34 C.F.R. Section 104.3(j)(2)(ii)).

Thus, the definition of who is a "handicapped" child entitled to the protections of Section 504 differs from that under the IDEA. While the IDEA requires the presence of an impairment *and* as a result a need for "special education," Section 504 looks only to the impairment. Youngsters with spina bifida are protected by Section 504 even if they do not need special education services, so long as their impairments limit one or more major life activities. Section 504 prohibits discrimination against individuals with disabilities who are "otherwise qualified" to participate in the program or activity in question. The regulations define all children as being "otherwise qualified" for public preschool, elementary, and secondary education if they are at an age at which services are provided to nondisabled children or are required to be provided to children with disabilities under the IDEA or state law (e.g., children in specialized early intervention programs).

The Protections of Section 504

For the child with spina bifida, Section 504 provides important protections. It broadly prohibits "discrimination" based on the youngster's impairment and mandates that children be given full access to public education. Section 504 also recognizes that to provide a student who has disabilities with "equal access" to public education, different or additional services from those provided nondisabled students are often necessary. Thus, Section 504 requires the provision of appropriate programs and special services where needed for a student to succeed in school.

Types of Discrimination Prohibited "Discrimination" can take many forms and can often be very subtle. The definition of discrimination under Section 504's regulations is therefore quite broad. Public school systems may not, on the basis of a disability:

(a) Deny a student with disabilities the opportunity to participate in or benefit from any aid, benefit, or service;

(b) Afford the student an opportunity to participate in or benefit from an aid, benefit, or service that is not equal to that afforded others;

(c) Provide that student with an aid, benefit, or service that is not as effective as that provided to others;

(d) Provide different or separate aids, benefits, or services to the student or any group or "class" of students unless such action is necessary to provide the students with aid, benefits, or services that are as effective as those provided to others;

(e) Aid or perpetuate discrimination against the student by providing significant assistance to an agency, organization, or person that discriminates;

(f) Deny the student the opportunity to participate as a member of a planning council or advisory board (e.g., the student union or student government);

(g) Otherwise limit the student's enjoyment of any right, privilege, advantage, or opportunity enjoyed by other students (34 C.F.R. Section 104.4(b)(1)).

To be considered "equally effective," the aids, benefits, and services provided by schools are not required to produce identical results, but must provide the student an *"equal opportunity to obtain the same result, to gain the same benefit, or to reach the same level of achievement, in the most integrated setting appropriate to the person's needs."* *Id.* at Section 104.4(b)(2).

Students with disabilities, including those with spina bifida, are thus entitled to more than just "access" to the school building. They are entitled to participate fully and equally in the entire school environment and in all aspects of student life.

The Right to Special Programs and Services   The regulations implementing Section 504 provide that public school systems which receive federal funds "shall provide a free appropriate public education" to each eligible student, regardless of the nature or severity of the youngster's impairment.

For purposes of Section 504, a "free appropriate public education" is "regular *or* special education" that is designed to meet the individual child's needs as adequately as the needs of nondisabled students are met. This can include a full special education program such as would be available under the IDEA. However, it may also be composed of a regular education curriculum, with or without adjustments or modifications, depending on the child's needs.

A student must also be provided the "related aids and services" needed to participate fully in school, whether in a regular education or special education program. Related aids or services can include physical or occupational therapy; assistance with mobility or self-care needs (including catheterization services); specialized equipment; lift-bus transportation, and so forth. These type of services also may be considered "related services" under the IDEA, and thus available under the IDEA to a child in a special education program (see definition of "related services" under the IDEA, 20 U.S.C. Section 1401(17)). As noted above, however, related aids and services must also be provided under Section 504 to the student with disabilities who attends regular education classes and activities, if the aid or service is needed for the youngster to have equal access to, and receive equal benefit from, the school program. Both the education program and all needed related aids and services must be provided without cost to the student or family.

Section 504 requires placement of the student in the regular education environment "to the maximum extent appropriate to the needs" of the student with disabilities. A youngster *must* be placed in a regular education class and school "unless it is demonstrated *by the recipient* [of federal funds] that the education of the student cannot be achieved satisfactorily in the regular education environment . . . even with the use of supplementary aids and services" (34 C.F.R. Section 104.34(a)).

Section 504 also protects students with disabilities in the area of a school's nonacademic services, such as counseling or placement services. The regulations expressly require schools to ensure that students with disabilities are not counseled toward more restrictive career or personal objectives than their nondisabled peers with similar interests and abilities. A school's extracurricular activities, such as field trips, clubs, or athletics, are also covered by Section 504, which guarantees that students with disabilities be provided the opportunity for full participation.

Physical barriers that prohibit a mobility-impaired or other student with disabilities from participating fully in the school program are not permitted under Section 504. School officials are required to remove such barriers or to adjust the program so that the barriers no longer pose a problem. While every section of every building within a district need not be fully accessible, a district must insure that, taken as a whole, all aspects of its program—from lunchrooms and libraries to vocational programs—are accessible to students with disabilities. These youngsters must also have access to classrooms and facilities that are comparable to those provided nondisabled students. (See *Hendricks v. Gilhool,* 709 F. Supp. 1362 (E.D. PA 1989), which held that the frequent movement of special education classes from one building to another "to make room" for regular education students and the placement of special classes in "out of the way" locations violate Section 504.)

Procedural Protections Section 504 requires that schools also provide students with disabilities and their parents certain "procedural safeguards." The program, services, and placement needed by the child must be determined through an evaluation and program planning process not dissimilar to that under the IDEA. In fact, the Section 504 regulations acknowledge that the implementation of an IEP for the student as required by IDEA is one way to meet the requirements of Section 504 (34 C.F.R. Section 104.33(b)(2)).

An impartial administrative hearing and appeal procedure must be made available to students and their families who disagree with any proposed school action or refusal to act concerning the student's identification, evaluation, or education program and placement. Written notice to parents of any proposed actions or refusals to act must also be given (34 C.F.R. Section 104.36).

Under a 1986 amendment to the IDEA, 20 U.S.C. Section 1415(f), children who are covered by both Section 504 and the IDEA generally must use and complete the IDEA's hearing and appeal system before bringing a court action, if the claim is one covered by the IDEA (e.g., the "appropriateness" of a special education program). However, if the student or the claim is not covered by the IDEA, an action can be filed directly in court without the need to go through the administrative hearing or complaint system. For example, a student with spina bifida who is excluded from a class trip because of the impairment may file a case in court and need not go first to an administrative hearing.

Parents and their youngsters who allege a violation of Section 504 may file a written administrative complaint with the Office for Civil Rights (OCR) of the U.S. Department of Education, the federal agency charged with enforcing civil rights laws within the education system. Finally, parents and children may file a civil rights complaint in federal court if they believe their Section 504 rights have been violated. Section 504, like the IDEA, provides that individuals who win their legal actions are entitled to reimbursement for their attorney's fees and costs (29 U.S.C. Section 794a).

EDUCATIONAL SERVICES AND RECOURSES FROM INFANCY TO GRADUATION[2]

OVERVIEW

Students who have spina bifida are a widely diverse group. The previous chapters have provided detailed information about specific access, cognitive, health, functional living skills, psychosocial, and vocational plan-

---

[2]This section on educational services is authored by Pamela Meyer Kunkle.

ning needs that unite this heterogeneous population along with recommendations for meeting those needs in a variety of settings. This section looks at some of the variables in those settings, notably appropriate personnel and type of service delivery system; how students gain access to appropriate services; and how recommendations made for specific students with spina bifida can be integrated into those systems by means of PL 101-476 (IDEA)–mandated procedures.

As education in the United States enters the 1990s, several trends have gathered sufficient momentum to seriously affect students with spina bifida in all three service delivery systems. Widespread calls for educational reform have triggered the proposals underlying those trends, which have been put forward by many influential individuals and groups. A small but representative sample of those groups include: President Bush and members of the task force of the National Governors' Association (e.g., America 2000, U.S. Dept. of Education 1991); business associations like the U.S. Chamber of Commerce; and national education groups like the National Council of Teachers of Mathematics (Cawley, Baker-Kroczynski, & Urban, 1992; Sindelar et al., 1992; Toch, 1991). Recommended changes to basic or "regular" education are beginning to influence state and local policy makers, causing them to reexamine the way they administer services in general, vocational (Cetron & Gayle, 1991), compensatory (e.g., Chapter 1 and special education), and preschool programs. As Anderson (1992) stated emphatically to members of the Council for Exceptional Children: ". . . school reform is here, it is serious, and it has major implications for the way schools will be doing business in the future" (p. 4).

Because virtually all students with spina bifida participate in one or more of these types of education programs, we will review the proposed changes and "promising practices" in each of them with particular focus on the philosophical and political movement called the "Regular Education Initiative" (REI). The REI has fueled tremendous debate among special education professionals because it implies a total restructuring of special, compensatory, and regular education systems to implement the "least restrictive environment" provision of the IDEA (Davis, 1989; Sailor, 1989; Smith, 1990). Although it is too early to assess the impact of specific REI-based programs on the education of specific students with spina bifida, we will examine and explain the implications of these service delivery configurations so that teachers and parents encountering one of the related models (e.g., "Inclusive Schooling," "Johnson City Model," "Rights without Labels") will be able to make informed decisions regarding appropriate adaptations for students with spina bifida.

Finally, the procedural rights and processes available to students in the current system will be outlined, and national, state, and local advocacy resources will be described.

INFANT/TODDLER SERVICES: BIRTH TO AGE 3

Infant stimulation is a program of therapies and developmental activities designed by a multidisciplinary team to assist infants "to actively explore, engage, and gain control over their environment" (Hanson, Ellis, & Deppe, 1989). It also includes support and information for families of those infants so that they can practice and develop new activities at home. Therapists, for example, "can also provide advice on techniques and materials that will encourage use of hands through manipulation of toys & objects" (National Information Center for Children and Youth with Disabilities, 1988, p.8).

The federal Departments of Education and Health and Human Services (1989) have provided a succinct overview of the benefits of early intervention:

> Congress anticipated that these services would enhance the development of infants and toddlers with handicaps, reduce the need for special education and related services after these infants and toddlers reach school age, maximize the likelihood that individuals with handicaps ultimately will live productive lives in the community, enhance the capacity of families to meet the needs of members who have handicaps, and reduce family stress. (p. 2)

This brief description points to three areas of benefit commonly believed by professionals in early intervention to provide the rationale for these services. These areas of benefit affect: 1) the child with special needs, 2) the family of such a child, and 3) society as a whole.

Researchers and practitioners describe observing such child benefits as: increased competence in cognition or thinking (Guaralnick, 1991; Peterson, 1989; Shonkoff & Meisels, 1990; Weiner & Koppelman, 1987; Williamson, 1987), development of social and communication skills (Hanson, 1984; Kleinberg, 1982; Ryan, Ploski, & Emans, 1991), and increased levels of functional independence (Carney, Brickenstein, Hollihan, et al., 1980; Fallen & Umansky, 1985; Lerner, 1987).

From studies of infant/environment interactions like that of Thurman and Widerstrom (1990), and an analysis of families and environments, early intervention professionals have described certain family benefits to those who participate in early intervention. These include: emotional support and facilitation of coping skills (Bailey et al., 1992; Bricker & Kaminski, 1986; Lerner, 1987; Myers & Millsap, 1985; Williamson, 1987), and the opportunity to learn how to facilitate the child's development (Connor, Williamson, & Siepp, 1978; Darling & Darling, 1982; Knutson & Clark, 1991; Meisels, 1992; Pueschel, Bernier, & Weiderman, 1988).

Finally, the benefits to society that accrue from providing early intervention to children with special needs and their families include reduction in number of children requiring extensive special education and services (Bricker & Kaminski, 1986; Thurman & Widerstrom, 1990) and increased public acceptance of individuals with disabilities (Fallen & Umansky, 1985).

All of the benefits described above are relevant to families and children living with spina bifida. These children are at high risk for impairments in cognitive, social, motor, and 'independent functioning skills. Meeting their complex needs can often result in high levels of family stress. When offered the opportunity to learn how to help facilitate their children's development, these families are, as Darling and Darling (1982) describe, "very receptive to infant stimulation programs because program involvement fulfills their need to 'do something' to help their child" (p. 133).

Appropriate infant and toddler programs for children with spina bifida and their families focus on promoting functional independence in mobility, high levels of social initiation with peers, and an increasing ability to focus on completing tasks independently. Families will contribute information about themselves and their children for a written plan with goals in the areas of motor, self-help, communication, cognition, and socialization skills (Tingey, Doret, & Rosenblum, 1989; Weisgerber, 1991). Program staff will assist families and children to meet these goals in a manner that will enable the family to gradually relinquish assistance and control over their child's daily activities and to develop effective methods for reducing stress. The use of goals in these areas is appropriate because they promote the development of what professionals in the field regard as "critical skills" (Weisgerber, 1991) for later school success.

Families living with infants who have spina bifida are just beginning to become effective partners with educators in designing appropriate educational services for their children. These families are currently living through the challenging medical situations described earlier in this volume (Reigel, chap. 1, this volume). Although they are afforded rights and protection in planning for and securing appropriate educational services for their infants and themselves, notably through their participation in and approval of family assessments and individualized family service plans (IFSPs), such things will not seem important to them at this stage. One way in which the educator or case manager named in the IFSP can support the family is by becoming a liaison to the clinic team at their regional spina bifida center. Parents' and agency staff questions at this stage can best be answered by the medical and allied health personnel familiar with the infant's current health status. This liaison function will also benefit early intervention staff who need health-related information to begin to select appropriate assessment instruments and to develop appropriate goals for the IFSP.

Educators and other program professionals can also support families of children with spina bifida by developing networks with community physicians unaffiliated with a spina bifida regional center; in this way *all* appropriate families will be referred for early intervention service. Physicians who encounter few infants with spina bifida may not readily identify them as being eligible for PL 99-457 services and will not encourage families to use these services. Early intervention staff will need to develop creative outreach techniques to inform these medical practitioners and families about benefits and to fulfill the Child Find mandate of PL 99-457. Local parent groups serving families living with spina bifida or other disabilities or the Spina Bifida Association of America may be helpful in getting information to families and may also provide information to community medical personnel about the advantages of early intervention.

Types of Infant and Toddler Services

Typical service delivery configurations for infants and toddlers fall into three patterns: home-based, center-based, and integrated daycare or toddler play groups (Morrison, 1988; Weiner & Koppelman, 1987).

Home-based services are generally delivered by a therapist or child development specialist who visits the child and family once or twice per week to demonstrate therapeutic routines and/or appropriate play activities. This professional may provide information on child development, behavior management, or other topics to the family during the regularly scheduled visits, and may also function as the IFSP case manager (Roberts & Wasik, 1990).

Center-based parent/child programs also provide therapies and developmental activities for children, but the variety, frequency, and intensity of related services may be greater with therapists on site and, therefore, more readily available (Meyen, 1988, pp. 27–29). Nursing and social work services are often on site also in a "multidimensional model" of intervention (Vincent, Salisbury, Strain, McCormick, & Tessier, 1990) which may include structured individual and group counseling or training sessions if the family's IFSP states a need.

A more recent service delivery option for this group is the integrated daycare or toddler play group program in which special education and allied health services are provided through contractual, consultative support to childcare workers. This type of service delivery may become increasingly important to employed single parents as well as to families where both parents are employed. It may also be the option chosen by families who want their children to spend as much time as possible with their nondisabled peers.

Parents electing this option should be alerted to a potential problem with eligibility for preschool services, however; successful performance in an integrated toddler program, especially one in which the child appears successful without any consultative therapy services, could jeopardize the child's eligibility for PL 99-457 preschool services. As Thiele and Hamilton (1991) point out, the flexibility states have in developing eligibility criteria under Part H of PL 99-457 (infant/toddler programs) allows them to interpret eligibility in a variety of ways that may differ from the eligibility criteria under the Part B (preschool) program. Thus an infant could be considered eligible up until age 3, then lose the right to services because of a different definition of eligibility. When families are choosing an infant/toddler program, they should be informed about the planning services for transition to preschool available in the program they're considering, as well as about other program options.

Personnel Delivering Infant and Toddler Services

In the evaluation and planning phases of these programs it is important that the family and child with spina bifida be assessed and monitored by the following personnel: physical, occupational, and speech therapists; nurses; special educators; and social workers. Each of their evaluations will contribute to the development of the individualized family service plan in collaboration with the clinical multidisciplinary team at the regional spina bifida center. For those children receiving care from several different medical specialists in the community, the 99-457 mandate for naming a case manager on the IFSP to coordinate medical, therapeutic, and education services is particularly apt. Fallen and Umansky (1985) point out that "the teacher becomes the resource for the parent, for education colleagues, and for community agency personnel." In most infant/toddler programs, it may make sense for an educator to be designated as case manager. This person will need to become familiar with the medical, health-related, psychosocial, and educational implications of spina bifida to provide accurate and ongoing communication between the regional medical center staff or community medical personnel and the infant/toddler program staff.

Technical details regarding medical test results and prescribed therapeutic or health-maintenance routines are essential pieces of information for successful implementation of the IFSP. The program nurse, for example, will need information about the child's status regarding clean intermittent catheterization (CIC) and the clinic staff's time line for teaching the procedure to the family. The infant program's physical and occupational therapists will need such details as dates of upcoming surgical procedures, information about new equipment, or contraindications to any of their current treatment plans. Finally, the program's social worker will need anecdotal information regarding the family's system for coping with repeated hospitalizations and the neighborhood or extended family supports available to them. Timely and comprehensive information such as the above is critical both to selecting appropriate assessment tools and to monitoring or revising goals on the IFSP.

Transition to Part B preschool programs must be planned with schedules and procedures documented on the IFSP (Filler & Olson, 1990; McGonigel, Kaufmann, & Johnson, 1991). As there may be questions regarding eligibility for some children with spina bifida (e.g., those with lower lumbar lesion levels and no hydrocephalus), providers would do well to follow Fowler, Hains, and Rosenkoetter's (1990) advice to "conduct timely assessments of the child's development so that eligibility can be determined before the child reaches 3 years of age" (p. 57). This will give parents and agency staff time to plan for alternate programs, or to investigate advocacy options.

PRESCHOOL PROGRAMS: AGES THREE TO FIVE

Many of the details regarding service delivery and personnel availability for infant/toddler programs also apply to the preschool population (Darling & Darling, 1982; White & Casto, 1987). The specific needs of students with spina bifida from age 3 through age 5 have been comprehensively described by Williamson (1987) and in the preceding chapters (see Baker & Rogosky-Grassi, chap. 2; Culatta, chaps. 5–7; & Rowley-Kelly, chaps. 9–12, 14, this volume). But eligibility and parent participation are significantly different in this system, and those differences will be examined.

Eligibility

Families may access the PL 99-457, Part B preschool system in one of the following ways: through recommendations and transition planning by infant program staff; by means of referral by clinic staff or other health care providers; or through local education agency developmental screenings held in various community locations. Unless the child enters this system through a planned transition from an infant program, there is a possibility that he or she will not meet local eligibility criteria for preschool services. Depending on the state's interpretation of PL 99-457, Part B definitions of "at risk" and "developmental delay" and on the type of assessments used to determine eligibility, the child's development may be judged too close to age-appropriate norms to qualify (Hausslein, Kaufmann, & Hurth, 1992; Weiner & Happelman, 1987).

Educators should be aware that preschoolers who have spina bifida require specialized testing by physical, occupational, and language therapists to determine whether or not they are showing subtle signs of delay in gross motor, fine motor, visual-motor, visual perception, cognitive, or receptive language skills. Educators should advise parents to seek specialized testing either through the clinic staff at their regional center, or through their local education system. Procedural safeguards apply to this age group, and parents need to be informed that they have the right to an independent evaluation.

If a child is deemed ineligible and a parent or educator feels the child needs the services to prepare for kindergarten because of developmental delays related to spina bifida, an educational advocate should be consulted to assist in securing services.

Types of Preschool Services

Traditionally, preschool programs were center-based "classrooms," many complete with mini-gyms or "gross motor/therapy areas" run by non-profit agencies exclusively for children with disabilities, to deliver a developmental package of therapy routines and pre-academic skills training (White & Casto, 1989). Parent participation was largely restricted to receiving education on how to train their children on the skills and methods used by the center, and was offered in a variety of ways: teacher or therapist conferences or phone calls to parents in between IEP meetings; formal therapeutic parent group counseling sessions on a regularly scheduled basis; or evening parent meetings featuring a speaker on some appropriate topic, to name a few. In many areas this is still the norm for preschool programs.

Two very strong, often contradictory, trends are gaining momentum in the field, however, and they have begun changing the nature of preschool programs. These trends, behavioral–ecologically based programming (Filler & Olson, 1990; Thurman & Widerstrom, 1990) and inclusive programming, draw their support from the early intervention research community and have strong legal support in the PL 99-457 mandates for family-focused intervention in the least restrictive settings. Vincent et al. (1990) offer a cogent description of the educational rationale for the behavioral–ecological approach to programming as follows:

> Strain (1987), Dunst et al. (1987), and others have pointed out that a change in the child is dependent, not just on professional skills or the child's disability, but also upon complex interrelationships among family values, intra- and extra-family supports, and the extent to which services offered match what families need and want. (p. 186)

This approach is appealing to practitioners interested in seeing a child's skills training carried over into the family's daily life. For families of young children with spina bifida, this approach shows promise in assisting the child and family with their often complex daily therapeutic routines (e.g., learning to walk in braces) and health care routines (e.g., mastering clean intermittent self-catheterization), and with learning to incorporate these routines into some semblance of a normal family life.

The other major trend affecting the preschool service systems, "inclusion," is an extension of the mainstreaming movement begun with the passage of PL 94-142 in 1975 with its mandate to educate students in the "least restrictive environment." This has traditionally been regarded by professionals in the field to mean an environment with nondisabled peers. Standard practice in preschool settings where mainstreaming is available consists of either a regular preschool or daycare center willing to accept children with disabling conditions (what Winton, Turnbull, & Blacher, 1984, refer to as "traditional mainstreaming"), or a preschool staffed by special education and therapy personnel in which children without disabilities attend the program, (i.e., "reverse mainstreaming") (Winton, Turnbull, & Blacher, 1984). If a child with spina bifida is found eligible for services in this type of setting, careful planning by the IEP team will be necessary so that any subtle deficits in the areas described previously will be identified and *compensatory strategy instruction* used for all appropriate IEP objectives.

One of the goals of successful inclusion programs is that students with special needs will learn independence and appropriate social skills through daily interactions with peers. Students with spina bifida may require structure and adult assistance in this area, as many of them will simply observe their peers interacting with each other rather than initiating interactions themselves. Unless the educator and aide are careful to monitor the interactions of students with spina bifida, inclusive programming will result in a less appropriate education than one in a preschool exclusively for children with disabilities.

Parent Participation

Unlike infant and toddler programs, preschools are not required to develop family goals or discuss family needs. Child goals and objectives and procedures for transition to kindergarten are the mandated focus of PL 99-457, Part H programs. Instead of an IFSP, the family will be included in writing an individualized education program (IEP) with child-related goals and objectives.

Parent education, counseling, or other support services, while alluded to in the listing of "related services" available to the preschool-age student, are not required. Many special education preschools have traditionally made such services available upon a family's request, but, with implementation of PL 99-457 still in the beginning stages, it is difficult to predict whether agencies will continue to provide them.

The types and levels of parent participation in regular preschool or daycare programs have always been highly individualistic to each program, and PL 99-457 guidelines in this area have not become widely available.

Personnel Delivering Preschool Services

Traditional, separate special education preschool centers may be staffed by a full complement of educational, therapy, and health care providers as described in the infant/toddler program.

This multidisciplinary approach is essential for most students with spina bifida as the preschool years are often the only time such children receive the intensive level of functional training they need to be mobile, dry, and as independent as possible in elementary and secondary schools and in later life. The description by Robertson, Alper, Schloss, and Wisniewski (1992) of clean intermittent catheterization (CIC) training gives a good account of the level of structure, staff time, and record-keeping required at this age in teaching functional skills to children with spina bifida.

Preschool personnel who have no training or who are inexperienced in working with children who have spina bifida may require, at a minimum, frequent contacts with therapy, nursing, and special education consultants to deliver appropriate services to such students.

A personal care aide or nurse's aide, for example, may be needed to assist the child with CIC and related hygiene procedures while the teacher is working with the rest of the class.

Another area where specialized related services are required for many students with spina bifida is in the area of mobility or gross motor skills. As Knutson and Clark (1991) point out, "the types of orthoses used by children with myelomeningocele (spina bifida) change with age. Changes are particularly common during the first 6 years of life and families should be assisted in planning for these changes" (pp. 958–959). As with learning self-catheterization, children learning to walk with or use braces need a specific IEP section on mobility with structured goals and objectives.

Finally, consultation in developing an adapted gross motor program may also be necessary for the child with spina bifida to participate with peers in games and activities to the fullest extent possible. Specific sections of the IEP should document appropriate goals, objectives, and activities in this area.

Transition planning for children who have spina bifida and are ready to enter kindergarten needs to be done far enough ahead to complete the following activities: a thorough evaluation of all functional skills and proposed IEP sections on access and mobility, self-care, and any other appropriate areas; and a planned sequence of events for parents, educators, and other appropriate personnel to develop a formal transition schedule and documented plan as mandated by 99-457.

Rule, Fiechtl, and Innocenti (1990) correctly summarize one of the pitfalls to be avoided by preschool staff in preparing young students with spina bifida for the transition to kindergarten entry:

> Despite the evidence that successful kindergartners must work independently (Hoier, McConnell, & Palley, 1987; Walter & Vincent, 1982; Carta et al., 1988; Cooper & Farren, 1988) there is little or no evidence to suggest that preschoolers with handicaps are taught or expected to function with minimal teacher assistance. (p. 79)

As young children who have spina bifida are often given moderate to extensive assistance while they work to master ambulation, dressing, and catheterization, preschool staff need to structure withdrawal of assistance throughout the year prior to kindergarten to prepare both the student and the student's family for a system where expectations for independence probably will be considerably higher. Here, as earlier, consultation with therapy, nursing, and possibly social work staff should be utilized to judge the level of independence that can reasonably be expected. One of several promising models in this area was developed by Conn-Powers, Ross-Allen, and Holburn (1990). Titled "The TEEM (Transitioning into the Elementary Education Mainstream) Model," this demonstration project includes preschool transition teaming methods, goals, time lines, and procedures for educators to adapt in working with young students with spina bifida and their families. Another promising practice in this area described by Sainato, Strain, Lefebvre, and Rapp (1990) deals with promoting the acquisition of independent work skills by strengthening preschoolers' ability to assess their own behaviors. This system might reduce the high frequency of requests for adult interaction attributed to students with spina bifida by some teachers.

KINDERGARTEN: THE ENTRY INTO LOCAL EDUCATION AGENCY PROGRAMS

Access to this system may bring the family of the student with spina bifida into contact with school district personnel for the first time. For families who have not been involved with early intervention special education services, it is best to make the first school district contact in April of the year before entry, to allow lead time for assessment and placement planning as well as to prepare for transportation, building, and classroom accessibility needs, health-related services, and any other services that may be required. The initial contact may be made with the school principal or the administrator referred to as either the "Special Education Director" or the "Pupil Personnel Director." This person will probably direct the activities of all school personnel whom families may encounter throughout the student's educational career. If the family was involved with any early intervention program, parents and preschool staff should meet and exchange information with this administrator before the formal multidisciplinary team or individualized education program meeting.

For children who have not attended a special needs preschool program, this contact provides the appropriate time for parents to present a written request for evaluation by a multidisciplinary team (MDT) to begin to plan for special education programming or related services.

It is very important that preschool educators acquaint these administrators with appropriate, timely, and accurate information about the special needs of children with spina bifida in general, as well as with detailed information about the particular child with whom they have worked. Ideally, preschool staff will already have a transition system and cooperative working arrangement with local school administrators. At the least the preschool educator should make sure parents and the school district staff receive therapy recommendations, nursing or health care plans, and detailed educational records to assist in multidisciplinary team decisions about kindergarten placement. This should all be done in conjunction with the local spina bifida center where the child receives care.

Types of Kindergarten Services

As kindergarten is not mandated in all states, length of day and types of services may vary. Some school districts may even offer an alternative program, sometimes called "pre-kindergarten" or "developmental kindergarten" for students who are not yet proficient in fine motor, paper and pencil activities, or in handling themselves in a structured academic setting (Oppenheim, 1989).

Special transportation and provision for teaching clean intermittent catheterization procedures are related services the student may need at this time. Districts accustomed to running half-day kindergarten programs where parents provide transportation and students are in school for fewer hours will need information about the social advantages to the student with spina bifida of riding on a school bus, even a modified one; and on the importance of maintaining the child's current CIC schedule by factoring in transportation times when developing the regular half-day schedule. Educators may need to support families who feel they are being coerced into providing either transportation or assistance with CIC.

Families of students who do not display significant gross motor, cognitive, or language deficits and who, therefore, are denied related services because the student is deemed not an "eligible student" under the IDEA should be given information about finding an advocate.

Kindergarten Personnel

Another new staff person families may meet is the paraprofessional assigned to the kindergarten class to assist the teacher. This instructional assistant or "teacher's aide" can be a positive support to the student with spina bifida. Under the supervision of the school nurse, for example, the aide could assist the student in performing CIC by handing supplies to the student, observing his or her techniques, or by teaching steps in the routine. The aide could also assist with any needed adaptations to the gross motor or physical education program. Other areas where a teacher's assistant could be useful are field trips or adapting outdoor activities.

Therapists may still need to be part of the school team for students with spina bifida. Physical or occupational therapists can provide suggestions to regular physical educators regarding appropriate adaptations to the general curriculum or to specific activities. They can also suggest ways to make classroom supplies more accessible or to assist the student to access books in the library. (See Baker & Rogosky-Grassi, chap. 2, this volume.) The therapist could also suggest appropriate ways for the staff to handle fire drills, slippery floors, and desk, work-space, locker, or coat closet modifications. Kindergarten teachers expect more independent work behaviors from children. They need to know that children with spina bifida can achieve comparable independence with appropriately modified environments and carefully structured assistance from adults. Kindergarten teachers can assist their students with spina bifida to prepare for a more academic, full-day first grade program by encouraging them to attempt all the same activities as the other students and then analyzing which parts of each activity should be modified. They can also assist students to understand that they can also analyze activities themselves and devise their own modifications.

Kindergarten may signal another important stage in the educational career of a student with spina bifida: access to one of the three existing education configurations in the United States today—"regular," "special," or "compensatory." As these three systems span both elementary and secondary school levels, and as all three may be radically restructured with the full implementation of the Regular Education Initiative, each is examined more closely.

THREE SYSTEMS OF EDUCATION

Regular or Basic Education

The most widely utilized system of education, this service delivery configuration presents academic and vocational curriculum to large groups of students, averaging 30 students per class, by teachers trained in child and adolescent development and specific academic subjects. Students assigned to this system are expected to progress through a K–12 sequence of information and skills in the area of "vocational," "general," or "college-prep."

Many students with spina bifida begin their public school careers in this system. Unless they display obvious motor, cognitive, or language difficulties, this is the system from which they emerge—successfully or not—at graduation. Teachers in this system are often the least prepared for recognizing subtle deficits in such students or for adapting instruction to meet individual needs. The IDEA rights are invoked in this system by identifying a student as "eligible" after a multi-step referral-assessment-referral process, which can be quite complex and time-consuming, as outlined in the first section of this chapter.

Compensatory Education

This service delivery configuration includes programs targeted at "disadvantaged," or, a term used more frequently of late, "at-risk" students. This system is funded separately from the other two, and has its own eligibility guidelines. Students being considered for this system usually come from lower socioeconomic backgrounds and have achievement test scores below the 40th percentile. The system may be accessed by students as young as 3 years through entry into the Head Start program. In elementary school, students may access the system by displaying academic difficulties but not economic disadvantage if the school they attend has a certain level of participation by students with economic disadvantage. Classes at the elementary level may be called "Chapter 1" or "Remedial" Reading and Math. In these classes, instructional aides and separate curriculum materials, books, and supplies may be provided to students. Teachers in all these classes may be itinerant or stay in the same building all the time. They are usually specialists in reading or math. Students attend all their other classes in a "regular education" classroom, and are considered no longer eligible for this program whenever achievement scores exceed eligibility criteria. Students with spina bifida may access this sytem if they encounter the academic difficulties described above and are considered not eligible for special education services.

Special Education

This system is considered by many administrators to be the most regulated, legalistic system of the three. From the student's standpoint it is the most flexible of all three since all decisions regarding participation in this program must, as mandated by the IDEA, be based solely on the specific needs of the individual student and not on only one measure of that student's needs (e.g., achievement test percentile ranking or economic background). Students may participate in this system on a part-time or full-time basis, again, based solely on their individual needs for adaptation of the "regular" system. Parents are much more closely involved in this system, and have rights unavailable to them in the other two.

The system's personnel include special education certified educators and licensed therapists, and may expand, based on the student's needs, to include psychologists, social workers, and paraprofessionals. The system is supported by separate clerical and transportation staff in many states. Most states also have regional special education systems parallel to the many regular education school districts. Some of the terms for this separate organization, as chosen by state governments, are: Intermediate Unit (IU) in Pennsylvania; Boards of Cooperative Education Services (BOCES) in New York; and Regional Education and Service Agency (RESA) in West Virginia.

Students may enter and leave this system as frequently, in theory at least, as their changing individual needs dictate (Sailor, 1989).

Students with spina bifida are found in all of these systems, some students participating in more than one at a time.

ELEMENTARY SCHOOL PROGRAMS

For the family experiencing full-day regular educational programming for the student with spina bifida, several school personnel will become increasingly important: the building principal; the subject matter, Remedial or Chapter 1, and resource or instructional support teachers; the school nurse; the guidance counselor; the school psychologist; the adaptive physical education teacher; the itinerant therapist(s); the librarian; and, finally, the paraprofessional staff—school secretary, food service staff, custodian, recess aides, and bus driver. The student's homeroom or primary teacher should arrange for successful interactions between these staff persons and families as early in the year as possible so that everyone can begin to build a strong communication system between the school and home of the student with spina bifida. Like the multidisciplinary clinical team caring for the student, school personnel have various professional and personal skills and strengths critical to assisting such students as they move through this system. Weekly or monthly staffings or frequent informal conversations among staff can promote the student's transfer and generalization of the skills taught by each professional.

Obtaining Services and Modifications

Most students who have spina bifida should be identified as "eligible" for the IDEA rights and services since they are at a higher-than-average risk for school problems in one or more of the following areas: health and physical access mobility, academics, perceptual-motor, language, and socialization. Some of the problems may occur as a result of lengthy or frequent absences from school after surgery; others result from subtle deficits caused by the neurological impairment itself. Regardless of the reason(s) for the occurrence, once students are deemed "eligible," a multidisciplinary team will provide background information and recommendations for solving current school problems as well as for preventing or ameliorating future ones. The recommendations can then be formalized by writing an individualized education program.

Many school personnel and parents find an appropriate IEP invaluable in facilitating communication among all the medical, therapy, and education personnel caring for the student with spina bifida. Clinical personnel can be provided with real-life information about the effects of their interventions as well as with an "early warning system" to alert them of progressive changes in functional status. Education personnel can utilize health and therapeutic information to plan for absences or declines in skill levels as well as to assist the student in understanding his or her own special needs.

State regulations vary in details surrounding the initial identification process, so educators and parents should get accurate, current information from their state's Department of Education or from a local advocacy agency. Some states, for example, have begun to use a "pre-referral intervention system" which gives school districts the opportunity to attempt to solve a student's school-related problems by modifications to the current program before or instead of consulting "outside experts" (Graden, Casey, & Christenson, 1985). Then, if the problem persists, the district may request evaluation by an MDT. In states where such a system is in place, parents should be advised to contact their spina bifida regional center or community medical personnel for written documentation about the effects of spina bifida on school-related performance as well as for specific details about their student's special needs. Parents should then draft a formal request for multidisciplinary evaluation to determine eligibility for the IDEA rights and services and include the appropriate medical and therapy documentation. If the school district disagrees with the need for such evaluation, the parents should be directed to an advocate for assistance in requesting a due process hearing.

Once the MDT evaluation is complete, an IEP team meets to determine the program and related services needed by the student.

Adaptations to the student's schedule and physical environment should be discussed by the IEP team and detailed on the student's IEP prior to school entry. A visit to the school by the student's family, followed by an informal meeting between the principal, other staff if appropriate, and the student's family to discuss potential trouble spots, or to discuss school policies and procedures, would be the first step to successful IEP implementation. Families made to feel welcome and whose contributions seem to be valued will become strong advocates for their child's school and will keep personnel up to date on all important medical or family information, such as planned hospital stays, medication side effects or changes, and contraindications for any programmatic activities.

Particular care is needed in planning the student's schedule. Consultation with the itinerant physical or occupational therapist(s) serving the student should also be arranged prior to school entry to assess adaptations to the physical space. Whenever appropriate, the student's classes should be in close physical proximity to each other as well as to the nurse's office since mobility skills may still be developing and the student may need more time than peers in changing classes and using the nurse's office restroom. Lieberman (1982) gives specific suggestions for ways of adapting students' schedules to ensure the fewest possible interruptions to actual learning time and efficiency. Lieberman suggests, for example, that school personnel consider carefully such things as building layout (e.g., how far does the student have to travel for classes, lunch and gym, and other activities; can the schedule be modified to group classes by both time and location?); establishing specific procedures for students to follow independently when they enter the classroom; and teaching the student to keep a daily log to record assignments.

Plans for adaptations to the cafeteria or lunch area should be made based on the goal of making the student as independent as possible. Therapy goals may need to be written specifically for this part of the student's educational program. Details such as width of food line, placement of personnel to collect lunch money, availability of paraprofessional support during lunch, and observing the student's skill in seeking a place at a table of nondisabled peers all need to be worked out for the student to experience success in this area. Analysis of the restroom facilities in the nurse's office should also be done during this early planning time. Suggestions about details in this area can be found in earlier chapters of this volume (Baker & Rogosky-Grassi, chap. 2; Leo, chap. 3; Rogosky-Grassi, chap. 8, this volume).

Other aspects of school organization that will affect students with spina bifida in either a positive or negative manner are: peer expectations, adult expectations, quality of communication among school staff, access to technology, and systems of monitoring student progress.

Peer Expectations

Educators cannot assume that simple proximity to appropriate peer models will result in the student's acquisition of essential peer relationship skills or in the spontaneous development of appropriate friendships between students with spina bifida and their nondisabled peers (Gural-nick, 1991; Rowley-Kelley, chaps. 9–12, 14, this volume). Positive social outcomes between such groups have been the focus of much recent research. Peck, Donaldson, and Pezzoli (1990), for example, cite research reviews by Gaylord-Ross and Peck (1985) that focus on the importance of adult-initiated structure and monitoring of interactions for success. Anecdotal information from Peck and his colleagues' research (1990) suggest that nondisabled students' social expectations regarding friendships do not carry over to peers with disabilities. Specifically, friends of nondisabled students will correct each others' inappropriate social behavior routinely as part of their ongoing relationships. Peers of students with disabilities, however, were found to be too uncomfortable with the idea of relating to their disabled peers in this way to perform that correction for them. Clearly, a real effort must be made by educators, counselors, and other appropriate staff to assist nondisabled peers in identifying, articulating, and understanding their own expectations about students with spina bifida. Educators should also explore with nondisabled peers their expectations and feelings about receiving help from peers with disabilities.

Access to organizational support for successful system-wide social integration could occur in any one of several ways. Educators could request, for example, consultative services from the school psychologist, school social worker, or other staff members in setting up a specific program with clearly structured goals for students both with and without spina bifida to facilitate their exploration and eventual modification of inappropriate expectations. Janney and Meyer (1990) present a consultation model that clearly addresses the organizational factors that support or impede successful implementation of a behavioral consultation program. Their findings indicate that specific attention and planning must focus on staff development, environmental variables in student programming (e.g., consistency of approach by all staff during contacts with target students), and resource utilization for "increasing the confidence and competence of individual staff to address student learning and behavioral needs" (p. 197).

Janney and Meyer (1990) found that staff needed support both while learning about and trying new promising practices, then while making the new skills and approaches standard practice. The authors suggest that "different levels of classroom support" rather than a standardized approach would assist educators and other building personnel to keep using the new approaches even under difficult circumstances. Administrators play an important role in maintaining support for staff in modifying interaction skills or in other areas for students with spina bifida. They can, for example, prearrange release time, purchase materials or pay in-service fees, and offer encouragement for new staff roles or activities. In spite of the program's positive outcomes for several students, the authors offer some cautionary advice applicable to all programs attempting to create new approaches to service delivery. If, they state, "neither the commitment nor the necessary resources exist to answer . . . needs in typical schools and the community, advancement in our knowledge about individualized interventions will continue to be associated with mixed outcomes that have more to do with systems needs than student needs" (p. 199).

Adult Expectations

The effect of teacher expectations on student performance has been so well documented for so long it will not be discussed here. Adult expectations for students with spina bifida, however, are frequently inaccurate. Usually adults expect less of such students than circumstances warrant, or expect too much in areas of subtle deficit. Either can have devastating effects on the students' entire educational careers.

Underestimating the student's potential for growth and learning tells the student he or she is incapable of achieving an independent and productive lifestyle. Overestimating the level of strength in deficit areas and refusing to supply modifications or support tells the student that his or her own assessment of strengths and weaknesses is hopelessly inaccurate, and can also result in frustrating the student's drive for independent adulthood.

Educators should collect all available information about such students from parents, clinic staff, qualified school or neuropsychologists, and any other appropriate sources. Educators should then meet with school staff to discuss the implications of that information on academic performance or routines as well as on those aspects of daily school life such as keeping to a schedule, remembering books and supplies, and following classroom procedures that are often referred to as "the hidden curriculum" (Baksh, 1990).

Staff Communication

The IDEA mandates only two meetings during the average entry and first programming year: the multidisciplinary team (MDT) meeting to determine eligibility for services (if the student has not previously attended special preschool education) and the IEP meeting for detailed planning of service delivery. School staff working with a student who has spina bifida should meet more frequently, however. Some health-related aspects of spina bifida are dynamic processes (see Reigel, chap. 1, and Leo, chap. 3, this volume). Staff need to plan for sudden absences or changes in routine in a frequent and timely manner. Also, ongoing and updated information from therapists, parents, or clinic staff may be needed for certain times during the student's school career (e.g., a change in mobility status from assisted walking to wheelchair use) when school staff all have roles to play in managing the change appropriately. Teachers may need to meet, for example, for short wrap-up sessions with instructional aides or the school nurse (Bos & Vaughn, 1991; Langone, 1990; Shea & Bauer, 1991). Regular and special or remedial teachers should meet formally every month, at a minimum, to review the student's progress in managing classroom organizational skills, changing classrooms, managing materials and books during those changes, and managing transport of messages and materials to and from home. These meetings could also be used for the exchange of information regarding nursing or therapy updates. Paraprofessionals and support staff should be encouraged to participate at these meetings, whenever appropriate, to contribute observations from lunchroom, recess, transportation, or custodial domains regarding the student's behavior and peer interactions (Rosenfield, 1987). Only through such free and full information exchange will the overall IEP planning and implementation processes contribute to increasing the independent functioning of the student with spina bifida (Vandercook & York, 1990).

Access to Technology

Educators should consult with the student's occupational therapist regarding the need for intensive use of computer-assisted instruction (CAI) to compensate for visual-motor, fine motor, or visual perception deficits. If necessary, access to technology should be included as a related service on the student's IEP.

Research done by Withrow, Withrow, and Withrow as well as by Kerchner and Kistinger (cited by Galloway, 1990) describes some of the psychosocial benefits of CAI in increasing students' tolerance for repetition and increasing academic performance (Trifiletti, Frith, & Armstrong, 1984). Educators interested in modifying current building priorities for computer access and instructional modifications appropriate for students with spina bifida should begin by consulting the Council for Exceptional Children (CEC) publication, *Beyond Drill and Practice: Expanding the Computer Mainstream* (Russell, Corwin, Mokros, & Kapisovsky, 1989). Majsterek and Wilson (1989), however, caution that "even the best software is inappropriate unless it fulfills a specific instructional need." Educators should contact their state departments of education for information regarding assistive device centers in their states, and how such centers could assist in providing materials or instructional support to their students. They should also find out how their state intends to implement the federal Technology-Related Assistance for Individuals with Disabilities Act (PL 100-407).

Monitoring Student Progress

Many students with spina bifida have difficulty in monitoring their own performance of academic and adaptive activities. Some have unrealistic expectations about the type of activities they will be able to perform successfully in later life without assistance or without improvement in their present performance. Educators can provide support in these areas by teaching self-monitoring skills and procedures for requesting appropriate assistance from adults or peers.

To help such students become aware of the areas of their lives in which they currently receive and expect adult assistance, educators and other building staff need detailed progress monitoring systems to present students with specific examples of their current performance levels and the current results of their efforts. Educators counseling such students and teaching them more socially appropriate or efficient skills can use specific examples of current performance as starting points for discussions of new skills, adaptations to tasks, or language patterns. Educators could investigate the Precision Teaching model, for example (Koorland, Keel, & Uberhorst, 1990; Lovitt et al., 1990; West, Young, & Spooner, 1990), and adapt it for use in areas of greatest need. Like many other students with disabilities, students with spina bifida profit from consistency of approach across classrooms, therapy sessions, and home. With their documented organizational deficits, many such students simply won't assimilate new behavior or academic skills unless practice and consistent cuing are part of their daily experience.

Accurate monitoring of student progress is critical for planning the transition to middle school.

MIDDLE SCHOOL: GRADES 6–8

Much of the information presented above regarding elementary school systems, personnel, and practices applies as well to the middle school or junior high school educational program.

Educators should be aware that students with spina bifida who reach their 14th year during attendance at middle or junior high may be legally entitled to another kind of planning: the transition to post-high school life. This planning should occur in consultation with the state Office of Vocational Rehabilitation. These federally funded agencies assist individuals with disabilities in beginning or resuming gainful employment. Although the IDEA states that transition planning must occur no later than age 16, many states are moving toward a model of delivery starting at age 14 (Clark, Carlson, Fisher, Cook, & D'Alonzo, 1991, p. 110). Administrators should find out their state's department of education requirement, then provide appropriate inservice information to their regular, compensatory, and special education staff.

Frequent staff communication and ongoing progress monitoring are particularly pertinent to this part of the educational delivery system. Students with spina bifida in the middle or junior high school setting are at very high risk of academic and social failure because of the environmental complexity in which they find themselves. New teachers and higher adult expectations regarding independence (e.g., in organizing academic activities and managing time and travel between classes efficiently) may cause considerable stress. Educators at this level need detailed information about the student's past performance in these areas so they can convey appropriate expectations to the student. One staff person, possibly the school counselor, should be designated as a support or resource person to the student and the student's family. One of the major tasks of the IEP team at this level is to continue a progress monitoring system until such time as the student has demonstrated consistently efficient and effective performance in self-monitoring of all academic and nonacademic activities.

Experiences of young adults with spina bifida after high school as reported to agency staff indicate that opportunities to develop good work habits, an effective work personality, and skills in time management, organization, and problem-solving are critical to future success in vocational training, higher education, and employment (Rowley-Kelly, chaps. 9–12, 14, this volume). Planning by the IEP or ITP (individualized transition plan) team should therefore focus on structuring occupational education programs, extracurricular activities, and field trips to assist the student in developing those skills. Ongoing exposure to and instruction in computer skills is another area to be developed by the team.

A final, potentially more complex area requiring team planning and appropriate modification is health education, particularly the curriculum dealing with sexuality. Because of the effects of neurological impairment on this part of the student's life, students with spina bifida may need independent study in this area, with an adult knowledgable about dimensions of sexuality and reproduction related to spina bifida. Parents should be part of all planning activities, and, in this area especially, their opinions will be crucial. Clinic staff from the regional center where the student receives medical care or the student's urologist or gynecologist should also be consulted about this curriculum area to make sure the student is not discriminated against by receiving inaccurate or emotionally damaging information. The student should also be provided with exposure to the mainstream curriculum to ensure an understanding of the sexual and reproductive functions of potential future partners.

Finally, students with spina bifida may require independent living and community skills training by a physical or occupational therapist beginning at this stage of the student's educational career. Mobility status should be reevaluated with particular emphasis on how well the student can utilize community transportation, public restrooms, community service agency and health providers' offices, cultural and sports facilities, and any other buildings or systems the student will need. This "transition" therapy evaluation should also assess the student's safe and efficient use of school facilities such as fire exits, auditorium and gym seating, cafeteria facilities, school store, school stage area, pool, and even parking lot. Therapists and educators should also assess the student's ability in community problem-solving (e.g., where to find a phone in an emergency, where to carry money and personal effects, and how to manage personal safety).

HIGH SCHOOL

As the student with spina bifida prepares to enter high school, educators should consult with counselors from the state vocational rehabilitation agency about scheduling a complete neuropsychological and vocational evaluation to assist the ITP team with educational planning. At the ITP planning meeting, families should be encouraged to articulate their expectations for the student's future. These can then be discussed in relation to assessment results. Appropriate decisions about vocational, general, functional or college-prep curricula and related services can then be made. Many students at this age will have much to contribute and should, therefore, be included.

Opportunities for high school extracurricular activities must be available to the student with spina bifida to ensure compliance with both the IDEA and with Section 504. If the student is otherwise qualified to participate, details about such things as accessible transportation to off-site tournaments, or modifications to marching band formations, must be worked out to allow full participation. Community isolation, especially in rural areas, may be a problem for the high school student with spina bifida, so opportunities for social, job-related, and language skill generalization available during school activities assume critical effect on future career success. Off-site vocational education transportation schedules should accommodate the daily health care routine needs of students with spina bifida. Although the student may no longer require assistance in these routines, vocational program personnel must participate in planning for potential problems associated with them. Students should be instructed in accessing available support personnel and supplies in the event they are needed. Travel times between programs must be managed in such a way that the student does not miss essential learning support or computer access time, or social-skill practice opportunities. No schedule will ever be perfect; but with special care and creativity, as well as administrative support for changes in staff role obligations, a reasonable level of student needs can be met.

By the time the student with spina bifida is 16 years old, all community agencies such as the local mental health/mental retardation office and the state vocational rehabilitation agency that provide services to adults with disabilities should be invited to participate in the student's transition plan. Support personnel such as therapists, adapted physical education teachers, school nurses, and team members from the regional spina bifida center where the student receives medical care could lend expertise to this planning in the following topics: community survival, independent living, work behavior, and functional or academic reading, communication, and mathematics; and should, therefore, also be asked to participate.

If the student is preparing to go on to college, the guidance counselor should provide the student and student's family with information about accessibility, independent living systems, funding, and learning support services available at several different colleges.

Promising practices in this area include summer orientation programs for students like the one at Edinboro University in Pennsylvania. Its focus is on teaching academic survival and independent living skills prior to the student's acceptance into the university. The program also includes extensive assessment and observation of the student's current level of functioning in these areas, and recommendations for academic or career programs based on that data. Another promising practice in western Pennsylvania is the Gatehouse Independent Living Rehabilitation and Training Program. This program provides assessment and training in a variety of areas designed to prepare the individual with spina bifida for success in higher education, vocational training, employment, and independent living. The 3-month residential program focuses on self-care and health care skills, organization and time management, problem-solving, initiative and other interpersonal skills, task completion, community access, and vocational exploration. Developmental delays in any or all of these areas have been identified as providing obstacles to an effective transition from high school to training and employment for persons with spina bifida.

For students interested in an academic alternative to university life, community college information should be given early in the transition plan year, and the student encouraged to attend adapted Home Economics and Industrial Arts class. Goals and objectives should focus on independent living skills, menu planning, cooking, wardrobe planning and clothing maintenance, and basic home repair. Consultation with the student's occupational therapist will be useful here, as will information and suggestions from the student's parents and vocational rehabilitation counselor.

STUDENTS WITH MODERATE OR MULTIPLE DISABILITIES

The preceding description details the educational systems, personnel, and adaptations necessary for implementing the rights of students with spina bifida who have traditionally received appropriate services through the regular education system. There are other students with spina bifida, however, whose special needs require a more intense level of support. Although these students' needs could also be met through some combination of regular and special education services, many local school districts prefer to refer them to the special education system.

Many interventionists (administrators, teachers, therapists, health care personnel) and parents see this population moving out of the segregated, special education system that traditionally served them and moving into settings with their nondisabled peers (Laski, 1991; Lipsky & Gartner, 1989; Sailor, 1989). In fact, these people are among the growing numbers of researchers and practitioners in favor of moving toward a system of schooling where *all* students learn together in individualized classrooms. We will explore the details of this rapidly growing movement in our discussion of the regular education initiative (REI).

Advocacy for Students with Spina Bifida

> All systems tend to resist change: otherwise P.L. 94-142 (now IDEA) would be fully implemented because it is the law of the land . . . and you would not be reading books on how to get services. (Cutler, 1981, p. 56)

The systems and services described in the previous sections of this chapter represent ideal situations for students who have spina bifida. The reality of many students may be different. The National Council on Disability in its 1989 report entitled *The Education of Students with Disabilities: Where do we stand?* described a variety of problems still facing students with special needs seventeen years after passage of PL 94-142. The following comprise a representative sample of its findings:

Parent–professional relationships too often are strained and difficult, and parents and professionals frequently view one another as adversaries rather than as partners.

Some parents (Harris & Associates [1989] say 56%) have difficulty finding appropriate services for their children.

Services are often not available to meet the needs of disadvantaged, minority, and rural families who have children with disabilities.

Clearly, parents and professionals working with students who have spina bifida will need to take an active role in encouraging their local school system to move current services toward the IDEA. One way of taking that role is by learning to employ advocacy skills.

Advocacy skills include the "knowledge, assertiveness, and persistence" (Darling & Darling, 1982; Espinosa & Shearer, 1986) needed for decision making, self-determination (Markel & Greenbaum, 1979), obtaining services, and "supporting innovative programs and encouraging change" (Pueschel et al., 1988). Parents and professionals can acquire and use these skills in a variety of ways to assist students with spina bifida.

Professionals as Advocates

Professionals can advance their own advocacy skills, for example, by becoming familiar with federal and state regulations pertaining to the education of students with disabilities and then assisting families to learn about the rights afforded them by those regulations. As Espinosa and Shearer (1986) point out, "parents who have developed advocacy skills . . . are likely to be more effective in acting on behalf of their children" (p. 260).

Parent and Professional Advocates

Professionals and parents working in collaboration can develop detailed background information regarding the specific health, academic, social, and access needs of individual students with spina bifida for use by multidisciplinary evaluation and IEP planning teams.

After the development, and during the implementation of the IEP, professionals "should monitor programs to make sure that they are adequate. Parents who are not always aware of programming alternatives trust professionals educators to meet their children's needs, and professionals must honor that trust" (Darling & Darling, 1982).

Parents should be informed of the following rights mandated throughout the referral, evaluation, placement, and review process: the right to:

- Request screening or evaluation for service eligibility.
- Receive notification and give consent for initial evaluation.
- Receive notification of results of and access to information in evaluation.
- Be assured of confidentiality for all of the student's educational records.
- Independent evaluation, if appropriate.
- Be notified of multidisciplinary team decision regarding eligibility.
- Participate in preparation of IFSP, IEP, or ITP.
- Accept or refuse IEP recommendation for placement and related services.

- Request revision of IEP, IFSP, or ITP.
- Be notified of and consent to a change in eligibility, placement, or services from the current IFSP, IEP, or ITP.
- Request a due process hearing and appeal to resolve disputes about eligibility, placement, or related service evaluation.

Professionals who are unable to provide information and training to parents in this area should be prepared to refer them to a local advocacy agency, professional organization, or parent support group (Dickman & Gordon, 1985; Shore, 1986) or to the closest office of the state's Protection and Advocacy system. They should assist the parent to learn the names and titles of personnel in the local school system with whom they'll be working. An especially helpful tool to give parents would be a diagram similar to the "Key People Chart" developed by Anderson, Chitwood, and Hayden (1990), pages 1–2.

Parents should be informed of the evaluation planning process used by the district to determine eligibility and to provide and monitor services. They should know, for example: how to request an evaluation for determining eligibility and be given a sample letter as a model, what kinds of medical and therapy information from their regional spina bifida center or local providers would be helpful in determining eligibility, what kinds of assessments the school district is likely to request from district personnel, how to understand frequently encountered educational terminology, what types of classroom placements and regular education supports are currently available in the district, and, finally, what the time line is from initial request for evaluation to an IEP meeting.

Parents who may need to become the advocate for their child will need to consult the following resources in preparation for acting in that capacity:

National Information Center for Children and Youth with Disabilities (NICHCY)
P.O. Box 1492
Washington, DC 20013
1-800-999-5599

A Reader's Guide for Parents of Children with Mental, Physical, or Emotional Disabilities (3rd edition), by Cory Moore, 1990
Published by Woodbine House
5615 Fishers Lane
Rockville, MD 20852
1-800-843-7323

Other general strategies parents will find useful in serving as their child's advocate include:

1. Asking medical and therapy providers familiar with the student to thoroughly document all needs and recommendations frequently and to serve as consultants to the school district
2. Taking someone—a friend, relative, or professional—to all meetings with the school, both for moral support and for collaboration, if needed
3. Keeping a very detailed file of all contacts with school and clinic staff with notes on phone conversations, copies of evaluations, and report cards (Fowler, 1990)
4. Taking accurate notes during all meetings with the school and asking for clarification or repetition of any information as needed (Markel & Greenbaum, 1979)

Working with a Community Advocate

Parents who live in a community that has one or more agencies providing advocacy services to students with spina bifida or any other disability (Hazel et al., 1988) or with a parents' group organized to do educational advocacy may wish to discuss their child's situation with a specific person (Fowler, 1990) who can then sort through documents with them, assist them in prioritizing their child's needs, attend meetings (Dickman & Gordon, 1985), and, if the volunteer functions as a "legal advocate," provide an attorney or paralegal (Pueschel et al., 1988).

Bloom (1990) has compiled a list of topics parents may wish to discuss with the person who may serve as their advocate. Such topics as the cost for advocacy services if any, necessary preparations the parent will need to make before contact is made with the school, possible repercussions the child may face during adversarial proceedings, and alternatives, if any, to a due process hearing are critical areas where parents and their advocate must be in complete agreement before meeting with school personnel.

Parents and their advocate may disagree with the school district as early in the process as the evaluation stage. As Bloom (1990) describes it, "advocates often encourage clients to get an independent evaluation . . . since the school evaluators are often . . . under personal pressure to keep services to a minimum."

Dane (1990) provides another reason for outside evaluation, as she warns that "multidisciplinary teams may be inclined to select goals they know can be achieved with the use of their school's resources, rather than goals that would require additional staff expenditures." Medical and therapy personnel familiar with the student's ongoing development should be consulted, and asked to provide evaluations, therapy progress notes, and anything else that will clearly describe the child's special needs.

At the IEP meeting, parents may find the advocate's services invaluable in analyzing proposed goals and objectives, program details, related services, and placement (Dickman & Gordon, 1985) in relation to the documented needs of their child. If consultation with the regional center or community therapists has resulted in concrete suggestions for educationally related goals and services, the advocate can lobby strongly for specific IEP sections addressing functional skills areas. Perhaps the most helpful support the advocate can give parents at this time, especially if the IEP fails to address the communication between regular and special education personnel (Dane, 1990; Darling & Darling, 1982), is in reminding parents that they may take the proposed IEP home to study before signing (Dickman & Gordon, 1985).

After the IEP is signed, an advocate can assist parents in making sure the IEP is actually being carried out and in notifying the appropriate state level education agency personnel if it is not.

At any point along the way where negotiations break down irrevocably, the advocate can assist the parents in deciding whether to pursue mediation or an administrative hearing. Such a decision must not be made emotionally nor without extensive reevaluation of resources available both to support the parent's legal position and to provide emotional support. According to the 1989 report by the National Council on Disability, parents must be made aware of the drawbacks to pursuing due process, among them:

- There is a perception that the outcomes of due process hearings are biased in favor of the schools.
- Due process hearings are costly.
- There is a paucity of attorneys with expertise in special education law to represent parents.
- There are no standard qualifications or training requirements for hearing officers.

Goldberg and Kuriloff (1991) echo the warning of the Council. Their research and review of past research suggests that parent outcomes are rarely positive. An advocate can help parents decide whether they and the district have truly exhausted all other remedies and can prepare the family and student for the future.

New developments in the American education system will profoundly affect students, parents, and advocates in the years to come. The effects of these developments on the futures of specific students with spina bifida are impossible to predict. Advocates, parents, and professionals will all need to monitor these developments as well as any subsequent revisions to federal, state, or local mandates extremely carefully to preserve the rights afforded by the IDEA and Section 504.

CURRENT EDUCATION TRENDS

In the early 1980s, some special educators began advocating a change in the nature of what they saw as two parallel systems: special education and regular education. Compensatory and regular education were considered as one system. These researchers believed that two systems represented a duplication of effort and overprotection of students considered eligible for the "least restrictive environment" clause of the IDEA. Such students, they stated, might succeed better if they spent more time with their nondisabled peers. In 1986 the Assistant Secretary of the Office for Special Education and Rehabilitative Services (OSERS), Madeleine Will, published a policy paper in support of the concept of including students with special education needs in as many of the activities of the regular school as possible. Titled "The Regular Education Initiative," the concept became a highly controversial political movement within the special education community. It is strongly supported and roundly denounced still, but it is a very powerful movement. Semmel, Abernathy, Butera, and Lesar (1991) who provide a summary of the REI research, state the major arguments for the merger, as expounded by its proponents. Those who favor adoption of the REI maintain that:

- "instructional services for children with disabilities be delivered within the regular classroom environment" (p. 9)
- there is a "lack of data supporting the efficacy of special education 'pullout' programs" (Semmel, Gottlieb, & Robinson, 1979, quoted in Semmel et al., 1991, p. 9)
- "the dual system separates special education and, therefore, minimizes communication between special and regular classroom teachers" (Semmel et al., 1991, p. 9)
- "implementation of the REI is a means for reducing the need for assessment of students with lower levels of functioning, thereby eliminating harmful labeling practices" (Semmel et al., 1991, p. 10)

Educators, parents, and advocates must be aware of this growing movement because it is consistent with the mandate of the IDEA for "least restrictive environment" placement and because much of the research spawned by this movement is extremely important for students in all three education systems. Lipsky and Gartner (1989) discuss some of the methods considered effective in promoting successful integration by the regular education movement and used by state funded "model" or "pilot" programs:

- Cooperative learning
- Peer learning
- Mastery learning
- Adaptive learning environments

Researchers have not as yet been able to examine what effects, if any, REI-based programs will have on the provision of related services. Parents of students with spina bifida who require related services such as adapted physical education therapies or adapted restroom facilities and support for CIC, need to be particularly careful to safeguard their student's rights in this area as related services are most vulnerable to cutbacks during budget tightening (Hobbs, Perrin, & Ireys, 1985). With appropriate functional skills assessment by physical and occupational therapists from the spina bifida regional center or local community, parents may be able to convince reluctant school district personnel to identify and provide related services for students with spina bifida in the educational setting because skills in mobility, self-care, and prevocational areas are an integral part of the student's safe and efficient movement around the school, as well as of the student's successful transition to adult life.

Because students who have spina bifida make up such a small segment of the population of students with special needs, parents, educators, and advocates must work together to articulate their unique needs to the educational community. A knowledge of current promising practices and political trends must be combined with detailed information about the specific student and the local supports available to enable educational, medical, and therapy personnel to provide truly appropriate services. Families who spend years preparing their children and young adults for independent community living must be encouraged and supported during all planning/implementation stages of their students' education careers. They alone fully share their children's successes and failures as they move through the education system; they are, therefore, truly the "experts" on these students.

GLOSSARY

Adaptive learning environment An educational model developed by Margaret Wang that combines regular and special education techniques to provide individualized instruction in a regular education classroom.

Allied health services Testing and/or treatment provided by persons trained in physical, occupational, or speech therapy.

At-risk Refers to any student who may experience academic and/or social failure in school because of biological, social, or economic factors.

Behavioral consultation An educational model for the regular classroom which includes assessment, a structured plan and monitoring carried out by a classroom teacher and one or more of the following: special educator, social worker, or school psychologist. The plan usually addresses changing the behavior of a particular student, or teaching a student a particular social skill.

Behavioral–ecological model A service delivery system based on two philosophical approaches: one, that the goal of education or intervention is to produce a change or changes that are apparent and measurable; and second, that
all members of the family and social network (neighbors and friends) affect and
are affected by the goals of a particular intervention.

Child Find The local system for identifying, serving, and keeping a census of all
young children or students thought to be in need of special education or related services; mandated by the IDEA.

Cooperative learning A group of educational techniques developed by
Robert Slavin and David and Roger Johnson to assist students in developing
positive social relationships with their peers and to strengthen students' self-
esteem. The techniques of group work are carefully structured so that each
member of the group attempts to assist all the other members to understand a
concept or complete a task.

Environmental complexity The sum of a number of variables in a student's
daily school life which may impact on the student's success in school, among
them: number of room changes and travel time, number of different adults and
their expectations for that student, variety of teaching styles encountered, and
variety of classroom or school "rules" encountered.

Generalization The cognitive ability—also referred to as "transfer of learning"—to use information from one particular learning situation in a variety of
situations outside the classroom.

Inclusive schooling The philosophical position which states that all students,
regardless of their individual differences or severity of disabilities, should
spend most, if not all, of their educational time together with appropriate
supports.

Integrated schooling The philosophical position which states that students
with varying degrees of disability should participate in the educational and
social activities of their nondisabled peers to the fullest extent possible; and
should receive services away from their nondisabled peers when appropriate.

Johnson City Model (also referred to as the **Outcomes-Driven Developmental Model**) The educational project developed by the Johnson City Central School District in New York to combine both regular and special education
personnel in providing appropriate, measurable academic and social skill development for all students in a regular neighborhood school.

Mastery learning The structured teaching technique that utilizes clear goals
for each student with appropriate assessment of the student's progress in
reaching them and reteaching and retesting any material not understood by
the student rather than moving on to new material.

Mediation A system for resolving educational disputes which is not legally
binding and rests on the good will of each party in implementing its decisions.
It is used as an alternative to legal administrative hearings whenever there is a
chance that a school district and family may be able to work out an agreement
with the assistance of an objective third party.

Multidisciplinary A delivery system that utilizes the expertise of several different professions to assess, plan, provide and monitor services to individual

students and/or families. Each profession contributes a slightly different approach and all are combined to provide services that address more than one particular area of the student's or family's life.

Peer learning   A group of classroom management and instructional techniques based on the cooperative learning philosophy (i.e., that many students' motivation, self-esteem, and academic success is positively influenced by the elimination of competition from the classroom and the substitution of a structured system of sharing and encouraging each others' growth).

Pre-academic skills   A term used until recently by early intervention practitioners to describe goals and activities thought to be necessary for kindergarten and elementary school success. Usually included were such things as: using scissors correctly, naming primary and secondary colors, and recognizing common shapes.

Precision Teaching Model   A system for individualizing instruction through the use of precise behavioral goals and daily or frequent measurement of a student's progress toward each goal. More detailed than the Mastery Learning Model.

Pre-referral intervention   The group of activities planned and carried out by local school district staff to attempt to remediate a student's academic or social problems without the use of special education services or personnel. It may include behavioral consultation.

Rights without labels   The belief that appropriate educational services should be available to all who need them without the need for documenting specific disabilities in order to secure or provide those services. Initially described by Maynard Reynolds, Margaret Wang, and Herbert Wahlberg as a way to combine regular and special education for students with mild disabilities.

Self-monitoring skills   The ability of students to control or change their own behavior after identifying and monitoring a particular behavior then rewarding themselves for increasing or decreasing that behavior, and for monitoring themselves successfully. Using these skills is believed by many practitioners to increase student independence.

Social initiation   The social skills involved in activities such as the following: beginning a conversation; introducing oneself to a group of strangers; requesting permission to join a group in an activity already in progress; or convincing a group to join one in beginning an activity.

Technology Assistance for Individuals with Disabilities Act   (PL 100-407) Passed in 1988, encourages states, through federal grants, to establish programs to match consumers with "any item, piece of equipment, or products system . . . that is used to increase, maintain, or improve functional capabilities of individuals with disabilities."

Transition   The planning and activities which take place whenever a family and student with special needs prepare for moving from one service delivery system to another. Typical transition times include: changing from an Infant Simulation program to a preschool; moving from preschool to kindergarten; and graduating from high school.

REFERENCES

Anderson, J. (1992, Winter). Educational reform: Does it all add up? *Teaching Exceptional Children, 24*(2), 4.

Anderson, W., Chitwood, S., & Hayden, D. (1990). *Negotiating the special education maze: A guide for parents and teachers* (2nd ed.). Rockville, MD: Woodbine House.

Bailey, D.B., Jr., Buysse, V., Edmondson, R., & Smith, T.M. (1992). Creating family-centered services in early intervention: Perceptions of professionals in four states. *Exceptional Children, 58*(4), 298–309.

Baksh, I.J. (1990). The hidden curriculum. In E.O. Miranda & R.F. Magsino (Eds.), *Teaching, schools and society* (pp. 170–189). New York: The Falmer Press.

Bloom, J. (1990). *Help me to help my child: A sourcebook for parents of learning disabled children.* Boston: Little, Brown.

Board of Education of the Hendrick Hudson Central School District v. Rowley, 458 U.S. 176, 102 S.Ct. 3034 (1982).

Bos, C.S., & Vaughn, S. (1991). *Strategies for teaching students with learning and behavioral problems* (2nd ed.). Boston: Allyn & Bacon.

Bricker, O., & Kaminski, R. (1986). Intervention programs for severely handicapped infants and children. In L. Bickman & D.L. Weatherford (Eds.), *Evaluating early intervention programs for severely handicapped children* (p. 57). Austin, TX: PRO-ED.

Carl D. Perkins Act. Public Law 98-524, 20 U.S.C., §§ 2301 et seq. (1984).

Carney, G., Brickenstein, M., Hollihan, J., & Allegheny County Local Children's Team (1980, May 15). *Position paper on pre-school special education placement: Discrimination in eligibility for educational assignment to approved private pre-school programs.* Testimony presented to Pennsylvania Department of Education.

Carta, G., Sainato, D.M., & Greenwood, C.R. (1988). Advances in the ecological assessment of classroom instruction of young children with handicaps. In S.L. Odem & M.V. Karnes (Eds.), *Early intervention for infants and children with handicaps: An empirical base* (pp. 217–239). Baltimore: Paul H. Brookes Publishing Co.

Cawley, J.F., Baker-Kroczynski, S., & Urban, A. (1992). Seeking excellence in mathematics education for students with mild disabilities. *Teaching Exceptional Children, 24*(2), 40–43.

Cetron, M., & Gayle, M. (1991). *Educational renaissance: Our schools at the turn of the century.* New York: St. Martin's Press.

Clark, G.M., Carlson, B.C., Fisher, S., Cook, I.D., & D'Alonzo, B.J. (1991). Career development for students with disabilities in elementary schools: A position statement of the division of career development. *Career Development for Exceptional Individuals, 14*(2), 109–120.

Conn-Powers, M.C., Ross-Allen, J., & Holburn, S. (1990). Transition of young children into the elementary mainstream. *Topics in Early Childhood Special Education, 9*(4), 91–105.

Connor, F.P., Williamson, G.G., & Siepp, J.M. (1978). *Program guide for infants and toddlers with neuromotor and other developmental disabilities.* New York: Teacher's College Press.

Cooper, D.H., & Farran, D.C. (1988). Behavioral risk factors in kindergarten. *Early Childhood Research Quarterly, 3,* 1–19.

Cutler, B.C. (1981). *Unraveling the special education maze: An action guide for parents.* Champaign, IL: Research Press.

Dane, E. (1990). *Painful passages: Working with children with learning disabilities.* Silver Spring, MD: National Association of Social Workers, Inc.

Darling, R.B., & Darling, J. (1982). *Children who are different: Meeting the challenges of birth defects in society.* St. Louis: C.V. Mosby Company.

Davis, W.E. (1989). The regular education initiative debate: Its promises and problems. *Exceptional Children, 55,* 440–446.

Department of Education and the Department of Health and Human Services. (1989). *Meeting the needs of infants and toddlers with handicaps: Federal resources, services, and coordination efforts in the Departments of Education and Health and Human Services: A report to Congress.* Washington, DC: Author.

Dickman, I., & Gordon, S. (1985). *One miracle at a time: A guide for parents of disabled children.* New York: Simon & Schuster.

Dunst, C.J. (1986). Overview of the efficacy of early intervention programs. In L. Bickman & D.L. Weatherford (Eds.), *Evaluating early intervention programs for severely handicapped children and their families* (pp. 79–147). Austin, TX: PRO-ED.

Dunst, C.J., Lesko, J.J., Holbert, K.A., Wilson, L.L., Sharpe, K.L., & Lies, R.F. (1987). A systematic approach to infant intervention. *Topics in Early Childhood Special Education, 7,* 19–37.

Espinosa, L., & Shearer, M. (1986). Family support in public school programs. In R.R. Fewell & P.F. Vasasy (Eds.), *Families of handicapped children: Needs and supports across the life span* (pp. 253–277). Austin, TX: PRO-ED.

Fallen, N.H., & Umansky, W. (1985). *Young children with special needs* (2nd ed.). Columbus, OH: Charles E. Merrill.

Family Education Rights and Privacy Act of 1974 (34 C.F.R. Part 99), 20 U.S.C. §1232G (1982).

Filler, J., & Olson, J. (1990). Early intervention for disabled infants, toddlers, and preschool age children. In R. Gaylord-Ross (Ed.), *Issues and research in special education, I* (pp. 82–109). New York: Teacher's College Press.

Fowler, M.C. (1990). *Maybe you know my kid: A parents' guide to identifying, understanding and helping your child with attention deficit hyperactivity disorder.* New York: Carol Publishing Group.

Fowler, S.A., Hains, A.H., & Rosenkoetter, S.E. (1990). The transition between early intervention services and preschool services: Administrative and policy issues. *Topics in Early Childhood Special Education, 9*(4), 55–65.

Galloway, J.P. (1990). Policy issues for learning disability computer integration. *Journal of Learning Disabilities, 23*(6), 331–334, 348.

Gaylord-Ross, R., & Peck, C.A. (1985). Integration efforts for students with severe mental retardation. In D. Bricker & J. Filler (Eds.), *Severe retardation: From theory to practice* (pp. 185–207). Reston, VA: Council for Exceptional Children.

Goldberg, S.S., & Kuriloff, P.J. (1991). Evaluating the fairness of special education hearings. *Exceptional Children, 57*(6), 546–555.

Graden, J.L., Casey, A., & Christenson, S.L. (1985). Implementing a preferral intervention system: Part I, the model. *Exceptional Children, 51*(5), 377–384.

Guralnick, M.J. (1991). The next decade of research on the effectiveness of early intervention. *Exceptional Children, 58*(2), 174–183.

Hanson, M.J. (1984). *Atypical infant development.* Baltimore: University Park Press.

Hanson, M.J., Ellis, L., & Deppe, J. (1989). Support for families during infancy. In G.H.S. Singer & L.K. Irvin (Eds.), *Support for caregiving families: Enabling posi-*

tive adaptation to disability (pp. 207–219). Baltimore: Paul H. Brookes Publishing Co.

Harris, L., & Associates. (1989). *International center for the disabled survey III: A report card on special education.* New York: Author.

Hausslein, E.B., Kaufmann, R.K., & Hurth, J. (1992). From case managment to service coordination: Families, policymaking, and Part H. *Zero to Three, XII* (3), 10–12.

Hazel, R., Barber, P.A., Roberts, S., Behr, S.K., Helmstetter, E., & Guess, D. (1988). *A community approach to an integrated service system for children with special needs.* Baltimore: Paul H. Brookes Publishing Co.

Hobbs, N., Perrin, J.M., & Ireys, H.T. (1985). *Chronically ill children and their families.* San Francisco: Jossey-Bass.

Hoier, T.S., McConnell, S., & Palley, A.G. (1987). Observational assessment for planning and evaluating education transitions: An initial analysis of template matching. *Behavioral Assessment, 9,* 8–19.

Individuals with Disabilities Education Act, 20 U.S.C. Section 1400 et seq.

Irving Independent School District v. Tatro, 468 U.S. 883, 104 S.Ct. 3371 (1984).

Janney, R.E., & Meyer, L.H. (1990). A consultation model to support integrated educational services for students with severe disabilities and challenging behaviors. *Journal of The Association for Persons with Severe Handicaps, 15*(3), 186–199.

Kerchner, L.B., & Kistinger, B.J. (1984). Language processing/word processing: Written expression, computers, and learning disabled students. *Learning Disability Quarterly, 7,* 328–335.

Kleinberg, S.B. (1982). *Educating the chronically ill child.* Rockville, MD: Aspen Systems.

Knutson, L.M., & Clark, D.E. (1991). Orthotic devices for ambulation in children with cerebral palsy and myelomeningocele. *Physical Therapy, 71*(12), 947–960.

Koorland, M.A., Keel, M.C., & Ueberhorst, P. (1990). Setting aims for precision learning. *Teaching Exceptional Children, 22*(3), 64–66.

Langone, J. (1990). *Teaching students with mild and moderate learning problems.* Boston: Allyn & Bacon.

Laski, F.J. (1991). Achieving integration during the second revolution. In L. Meyer, C. Peck, & L. Brown (Eds.), *Critical issues in the lives of people with severe disabilities* (pp. 409–421). Baltimore: Paul H. Brookes Publishing Co.

Lerner, J. (1987). *Special education for the early childhood years.* Englewood Cliffs, NJ: Prentice Hall.

Lieberman, L.M. (1982). The nightmare of scheduling. *Journal of Learning Disabilities, 15*(1), 57–58.

Lipsky, D., & Gartner, A. (Eds.). (1989). *Beyond separate education: Quality education for all.* Baltimore: Paul H. Brookes Publishing Co.

Lovitt, T.C., Fister, S., Freston, J.L., Kemp, K., Moore, R.C., Schroeder, B., & Bauernschmidt, M. (1990). Translating research: Using precision teaching techniques. *Teaching Exceptional Children, 22*(2), 16–19.

Majsterek, D.J., & Wilson, R. (1989). Computer-assisted instruction for students with learning disabilities: Considerations for practitioners. *Learning Disabilities Focus, 5*(1), 18–27.

Mancuso, E., Rieser, L., & Stotland, J. (1991). *The right to special education in Pennsylvania: A guide for parents.* Philadelphia: The Education Law Center.

Markel, G.P., & Greenbaum, J. (1979). *Parents are to be seen and heard: Assertiveness in educational planning for handicapped children.* San Luis Obispo, CA: Impact Publishers.

McGonigel, M.J., Kaufmann, R.K., & Johnson, B.H. (1991). A family-centered process for the individualized family service plan. *Journal of Early Intervention,* *15*(1), 46–56.

Meisels, S.J. (1992). Early intervention: A matter of context. *Zero to Three, XII* (3), 1–6.

Meyen, E.L. (1988). A commentary on special education. In E.L. Meyen & T.M. Skrtic (Eds.), *Exceptional children and youth: An introduction* (pp. 3–48). Denver: Love Publishing.

Morrison, G.M. (1988). Mentally retarded. In E.L. Meyen & T.M. Skrtic (Eds.), *Exceptional children and youth: An introduction* (pp. 139–181). Denver: Love Publishing.

Myers, G.J., & Millsap, M. (1985). Spina bifida. In N. Hobbs & J.M. Perrin (Eds.), *Issues in the care of children with chronic illness* (pp. 214–255). San Francisco: Jossey-Bass.

National Council on Disability. (1989). *The education of students with disabilities: Where do we stand?* Washington, DC: Author.

National Information Center for Children and Youth with Disabilities. (1988). Early intervention for children birth through 2 years. *NICHCY News Digest, 10,* 1–12.

Oppenheim, J. (1989). *The elementary school handbook: Making the most of your child's education.* New York: Pantheon Books.

Ordover, E., & Boundy, K. (1991). *Educational rights of children with disabilities.* Cambridge: Center for Law and Education.

Peck, C.A., Donaldson, J., & Pezzoli, M. (1990). Some benefits nonhandicapped adolescents perceive for themselves from their social relationships with peers who have severe handicaps. *Journal of The Association for Persons with Severe Handicaps, 15*(4), 241–249.

Peterson, N.L. (1987). *Early intervention for handicapped and at-risk children: An introduction to early childhood special education.* Denver: Love Publishing.

Pueschel, S.M., Bernier, J.C., & Weiderman, L.E. (1988). *The special child: A source book for parents of children with developmental disabilities.* Baltimore: Paul H. Brookes Publishing Co.

Rehabilitation Act of 1973, Section 504, 29 U.S.C. §794, as amended.

Reynolds, M.C., & Birch, J.W. (1988). *Adaptive mainstreaming: A primer for teachers and principals* (3rd ed.). New York: Longman.

Roberts, R.N., & Wasik, B.H. (1990). Home visiting programs for families with children birth to three: Results of a national survey. *Journal of Early Intervention, 14*(3), 272–284.

Robertson, J., Alper, S., Schloss, P., & Wisniewski, L. (1992). Teaching self catheterization skills to a child with myelomeningocele in a preschool setting. *Journal of Early Intervention, 16*(1), 20–30.

Rosenfield, S.A. (1987). *Instructional consultation.* Hillsdale, NJ: Lawrence Erlbaum Associates.

Rule, S., Fiechtl, B., & Innocenti, M.S. (1990). Preparation for transition to mainstreamed post-preschool environments: Development of a survival skills curriculum. *Topics in Early Childhood Special Education, 9*(47), 78–90.

Russell, S.J., Corwin, R., Mokros, J.R., & Kapisovsky, P.M. (1989). *Beyond drill and practice: Expanding the computer mainstream.* Reston, VA: The Council for Exceptional Children.

Ryan, K.D., Ploski, C., & Emans, J.B. (1991). Myelodysplasia—the musculoskeletal problem: Habilitation from infancy to adulthood. *Physical Therapy, 71*(1), 935–946.

Sailor, W. (1989). Preface. In W. Sailor, J.L. Anderson, A.T. Halvorsen, K. Doering, J. Filler, & L. Goetz, *The comprehensive local school: Regular education for all students with disabilities.* Baltimore: Paul H. Brookes Publishing Co.

Sainato, D.M., Strain, P.S., Lefebvre, D., & Rapp, N. (1990). Effects of self-evaluation on the independent work skills of preschool children with disabilities. *Exceptional Children, 56*(6), 540–549.

Semmell, M.I., Gottlieb, J., & Robinson, H. (1979). Mainstreaming: Perspectives on educating handicapped children in the public schools. In D. Berliner (Ed.), *Review of research in education* (pp. 223–279). Washington, DC: American Educational Research Association.

Semmel, M.J., Abernathy, T.V., Butera, G., & Lesar, S. (1991). Teacher perceptions of the regular education initiative. *Exceptional Children, 58*(1), 9–23.

Shea, T.M., & Bauer, A.N. (1991). *Parents and teachers of children with exceptionalities: A handbook for collaboration* (2nd ed.). Boston: Allyn & Bacon.

Shonkoff, J.P., & Meisels, S.J. (1990). Early childhood intervention: The evolution of a concept. In S.J. Meisels, & J.P. Shonkoff (Eds.), *Handbook of early childhood intervention* (pp. 3–31). New York: Cambridge University.

Shore, K. (1986). *The special education handbook: How to get the best education possible for your learning disabled child.* New York: Warner Books.

Smith, S.W. (1990). Individualized education programs (IEPs) in special education—from intent to acquiescence. *Exceptional Children, 57*(1), 6–14.

Strain, P. (1987). Comprehensive evaluation of intervention for young autistic children. *Topics in Early Childhood Special Education, 7,* 97–110.

Strain, P.S. (1991). Ensuring quality of early intervention for children with severe disabilities. In L. Meyer, C. Peck, & L. Brown (Eds.), *Critical issues in the lives of people with severe disabilities* (pp. 479–483). Baltimore: Paul H. Brookes Publishing Co.

Thiele, J.E., & Hamilton, J.L. (1991). Implementing the early childhood formula: Programs under P.L. 99-457. *Journal of Early Intervention, 15*(1), 5–12.

Thurman, S.K., & Widerstrom, A.H. (1990). *Infants and young children with special needs: A developmental and ecological approach* (2nd ed.). Baltimore: Paul H. Brookes Publishing Co.

Timothy W. v. Rochester School District, 875 F2d 954 (1st Cir. 1989) cert denied, 110 S.Ct. 519.

Tingey, C., Doret, W.B., & Rosenblum, R. (1989). Individual goals for children and their families. In C. Tingey (Ed.), *Implementing early intervention* (pp. 139–165). Baltimore: Paul H. Brookes Publishing Co.

Trifiletti, J.J., Frith, G.H., & Armstrong, S. (1984). Microcomputers versus resource rooms for LD students: A preliminary investigation of the effects of math skills. *Learning Disability Quarterly, 7,* 69–76.

Vandercook, T., & York, J. (1990). A team approach to program development and support. In W. Stainback & S. Stainback (Eds.), *Support networks for inclusive schooling: Interdependent integrated education* (pp. 95–121). Baltimore: Paul H. Brookes Publishing Co.

Vincent, L.J., Salisbury, C.L., Strain, P., McCormick, C., & Tessier. (1990). A behavioral-ecological approach to early intervention: Focus on cultural diversity. In S.J. Meisels & J.P. Shonkoff (Eds.), *Handbook of early childhood intervention* (pp. 173–195). New York: Cambridge University Press.

Walter, G., & Vincent, L. (1982). The handicapped child in the regular kindergarten classroom. *Journal of the Division for Early Childhood, 6,* 84–95.

Weiner, R., & Koppelman, J. (1987). *From birth to five: Serving the youngest handi-*

capped children. Alexandria, VA: Capital Publications.

Weisgerber, R.A. (1991). *Quality of life for persons with disabilities: Skill development and transitions across life stages.* Gaithersburg, MD: Aspen Systems.

West, R.P., Young, K.R., & Spooner, F. (1990). Precision teaching: An introduction. *Teaching Exceptional Children, 22*(3), 4–9.

White, K.R., & Casto, G. (1989). What is known about early intervention. In C. Tingey (Ed.), *Implementing early intervention* (pp. 3–20). Baltimore: Paul H. Brookes Publishing Co.

Williamson, G.G. (Ed.). (1987). *Children with spina bifida: Early intervention and preschool programming.* Baltimore: Paul H. Brookes Publishing Co.

Winton, P.J., Turnbull, A.P., & Blacher, J. (1984). *Selecting a preschool: A guide for parents of handicapped children.* Baltimore: University Park Press.

Withrow, F.B., Withrow, M.S., & Withrow, D.F. (1986). Technology and the handicapped. *Technological Horizons in Education Journal, 13*(6), 65–67.

Individuals with Disabilities
Education Act (IDEA)
34 C.F.R. Part 300
Reg. 300.5   Handicapped Children

(a) As used in this part, the term "handicapped children" means those children evaluated in accordance with Regs. 300.530–300.534 as being mentally retarded, hard of hearing, deaf, speech impaired, visually handicapped, seriously emotionally disturbed, orthopedically impaired, other health impaired, deaf-blind, multihandicapped, or as having specific learning disabilities, who because of those impairments need special education and related services.

(b) The terms used in this definition are defined as follows:

(1) "Deaf" means a hearing impairment which is so severe that the child is impaired in processing linguistic information through hearing, with or without amplification, which adversely affects educational performance.

(2) "Deaf-blind" means concomitant hearing and visual impairments, the combination of which causes such severe communication and other developmental and educational problems that they cannot be accommodated in special education programs solely for deaf or blind children.

(3) "Hard of Hearing" means a hearing impairment, whether permanent or fluctuating, which adversely affects a child's educational performance but which is not included under the definition of "deaf" in this section.

(4) "Mentally retarded" means significantly subaverage general intellectual functioning existing concurrently with deficits in adaptive behavior and manifested during the developmental period, which adversely affects a child's educational performance.

(5) "Multihandicapped" means concomitant impairments (such as mentally retarded-blind, mentally retarded-orthopedically impaired, etc.), the combination of which causes such severe educational problems that they cannot be accommodated in special education programs solely for one of the impairments. The term does not include deaf-blind children.

(6) "Orthopedically impaired" means a severe orthopedic impairment which adversely affects a child's educational performance. The term includes impairments caused by congenital anomaly (e.g., clubfoot,

absence of some member, etc.), impairments caused by disease (e.g., poliomyelitis, bone tuberculosis, etc.), and impairments from other causes (e.g., cerebral palsy, amputations, and fractures or burns which cause contractures).

(7) "Other health impaired" means

(i) having an autistic condition which is manifested by severe communication and other developmental and educational problems; or

(ii) having limited strength, vitality, or alertness, due to chronic or acute health problems such as a heart condition, tuberculosis, rheumatic fever, nephritis, asthma, sickle cell anemia, hemophilia, epilepsy, lead poisoning, leukemia, or diabetes, which adversely affects a child's educational performance.

(8) "Seriously emotionally disturbed" is defined as follows:

(i) The terms means a condition exhibiting one or more of the following characteristics over a long period of time and to a marked degree, which adversely affects educational performance:

(A) An inability to learn which cannot be explained by intellectual, sensory, or health factors;

(B) An inability to build or maintain satisfactory interpersonal relationships with peers and teachers;

(C) Inappropriate types of behavior or feelings under normal circumstances;

(D) A general pervasive mood of unhappiness or depression; or

(E) A tendency to develop physical symptoms or fears associated with personal or school problems.

(ii) The term includes children who are schizophrenic. The term does not include children who are socially maladjusted, unless it is determined that they are seriously emotionally disturbed.

(9) "Specific learning disability" means a disorder in one or more of the basic psychological processes involved in understanding or in using language, spoken or written, which may manifest itself in an imperfect ability to listen, think, speak, read, write, spell, or to do mathematical calculations. The term includes such conditions as perceptual handicaps, brain injury, minimal brain disfunction, dyslexia, and developmental aphasia. The term does not include children who have learning problems which are primarily the result of visual, hearing, or motor handicaps, of mental retardation, of emotional disturbance, or of environmental, cultural, or economic disadvantage.

(10) "Speech impaired" means a communication disorder such as stuttering, impaired articulation, a language impairment, or a voice impairment, which adversely affects a child's educational performance.

(11) "Visually handicapped" means a visual impairment which, even with correction, adversely affects a child's educational performance. The term includes both partially seeing and blind children.

(20 U.S.C. 1401(1), (15))
[42 FR 42476, Aug. 23, 1977, as amended at 42 FR 65083, Dec. 29, 1977. Redesignated at 45 FR 77368, Nov. 21, 1980, and further amended at 46 FR 3866, Jan. 16, 1981]

Individuals with Disabilities Education Act (IDEA)
34 C.F.R. Part 300
Reg. 300.13   Related Services

(a) As used in this part, the term "related services" means transportation and such developmental, corrective, and other supportive services as are required to assist a handicapped child to benefit from special education, and includes speech pathology and audiology, psychological services, physical and occupational therapy, recreation, early identification and assessment of disabilities in children, counseling services, and medical services for diagnostic or evaluation purposes. The term also includes school health services, social work services in schools, and parent counseling and training.

(b) The terms used in this definition are defined as follows:

(1) "Audiology" includes:

(i) Identification of children with hearing loss;

(ii) Determination of the range, nature, and degree of hearing loss, including referral for medical or other professional attention for the habilitation of hearing;

(iii) Provision of habilitative activities, such as language habilitation, auditory training, speech reading (lipreading), hearing evaluation, and speech conversation;

(iv) Creation and administration of programs for prevention of hearing loss;

(v) Counseling and guidance of pupils, parents, and teachers regarding hearing loss; and

(vi) Determination of the child's need for group and individual amplification, selecting and fitting an appropriate aid, and evaluating the effectiveness of amplification.

(2) "Counseling services" means services provided by qualified social workers, psychologists, guidance counselors, or other qualified personnel.

(3) "Early identification" means the implementation of a formal plan for identifying a disability as early as possible in a child's life.

(4) "Medical services" means services provided by a licensed physician to determine a child's medically related handicapping condition which results in the child's need for special education and related services.

(5) "Occupational therapy" includes:

(i) Improving, developing or restoring functions impaired or lost through illness, injury, or deprivation;

(ii) Improving ability to perform tasks for independent functioning when functions are impaired or lost; and

(iii) Preventing, through early intervention, initial or further impairment or loss of function.

(6) "Parent counseling and training" means assisting parents in understanding the special needs of their child and providing parents with information about child development.

(7) "Physical therapy" means services provided by a qualified physical therapist.

(8) "Psychological services" include:

(i) Administering psychological and educational tests, and other assessment procedures;

(ii) Interpreting assessment results;

(iii) Obtaining, integrating, and interpreting information about child behavior and conditions relating to learning.

(iv) Consulting with other staff members in planning school programs to meet the special needs of children as indicated by psychological tests, interviews, and behavioral evaluations; and

(v) Planning and managing a program of psychological services, including psychological counseling for children and parents.

(9) "Recreation" includes:

(i) Assessment of leisure function;

(ii) Therapeutic recreation services;

(iii) Recreation programs in schools and community, agencies; and

(iv) Leisure education.

(10) "School health services" means services provided by a qualified school nurse or other qualified person.

(11) "Social work services in schools" include:

(i) Preparing a social or developmental history on a handicapped child;

(ii) Group and individual counseling with the child and family;

(iii) Working with those problems in a child's living situation (home, school, and community) that affect the child's adjustment in school; and

(iv) Mobilizing school and community resources to enable the child to receive maximum benefit from his or her educational program.

(12) "Speech pathology" includes:

(i) Identification of children with speech or language disorders;

(ii) Diagnosis and appraisal of specific speech or language disorders;

(iii) Referral for medical or other professional attention necessary for the habilitation of speech or language disorders;

(iv) Provisions of speech and language services for the habilitation or prevention of communicative disorders; and

(v) Counseling and guidance of parents, children, and teachers regarding speech and language disorders.

(13) "Transportation" includes:

(i) Travel to and from school and between schools,

(ii) Travel in and around school buildings, and

(iii) Specialized equipment (such as special or adapted buses, lifts, and ramps), if required to provide special transportation for a handicapped child.

(20 U.S.C. 1401(17))

Comment. With respect to related services, the Senate Report states:

The Committee bill provides a definition of "related services," making clear that all such related services may not be required for each individual child and that such term includes early identification and assessment of handicapping conditions and the provision of services to minimize the effects of such conditions.

(Senate Report No. 94-168, p. 12 (1975))

The list of related services is not exhaustive and may include other developmental, corrective, or supportive services (such as artistic and cultural programs, and art, music, and dance therapy), if they are required to assist a handicapped child to benefit from special education.

There are certain kinds of services which might be provided by persons from varying professional backgrounds and with a variety of operational titles, depending upon requirements in individual States. For example, counseling services might be provided by social workers, psychologists, or guidance counselors; and psychological testing might be done by qualified psychological examiners, psychometrists, or psychologists, depending upon State standards.

Each related service defined under this part may include appropriate administrative and supervisory activities that are necessary for program planning, management, and evaluation.

Supporting
Effective Education

Developing a School Outreach Program

Fern L. Rowley-Kelly and Pamela Meyer Kunkle

A school outreach program serves to assure optimum educational opportunity for students with spina bifida. The greater purpose is to provide a maximum degree of functional independence in all spheres after graduation, including the practical, economic, and social spheres. The central strategy in achieving an optimum education is to obtain and distribute relevant and accurate information to all parties involved in the student's education.

DISCOVERING THE NEED

The need for a school outreach program becomes evident as dissatisfaction with school performance and vocational outcomes emerges. Parents articulate dissatisfaction with their child's academic performance or the extent of their socialization with classmates. Teachers continue to question why the student is not learning or performing at expected rates. People who deal with the graduated student in pursuing job placements, vocational training, or further education notice a lack of preparation in academic skills and personal traits, or observe failures that cannot be readily explained or overcome. In some cases, medical personnel notice dependent or noncompliant behavior with regard to the treatment regimen, particularly at a time when the patient should be approaching emancipation.

The information provided in this chapter is based on the School Consultation and Personnel Training Program of the Spina Bifida Association of Western Pennsylvania. Now in the third year of operation, the program was developed by the Association and operates in conjunction with the Spina Bifida Center at Allegheny General Hospital in Pittsburgh. Although the procedures described herein are derived from the School Consultation and Personnel Training Program, references to specific regional circumstances have been avoided where possible to allow for duplication of the concept in other regions.

Any of these signs may indicate that the student's education has not been planned or undertaken with a full knowledge of the educational aspects of spina bifida. As policy makers continue to opt in favor of mainstreaming students with disabilities in classrooms with the nondisabled, increasing numbers of students, parents, teachers, and others have begun to suspect that something is amiss, and that the information needed to educate these students properly is missing or unavailable.

PROVING THE NEED

The mere suspicion that something is not working as it should is not in itself enough to establish the need for an educational outreach program, to obtain funding and support for such a program, or to plan what specific needs should be met by the program. It is critical at this juncture to conduct a formal survey of teachers and parents to determine the extent of their knowledge of the educational aspects of spina bifida, and the depth of their desire for further information. The process that led to the preparation of this manual and the accompanying videotape as well as the development of the School Consultation and Personnel Training Program began with a formal needs assessment that established the absence of current and comprehensive information about these students. The needs assessment surveyed 200 parents and teachers, all of whom currently had a child in mainstream education or were currently teaching one or more students with spina bifida in a mainstream setting. Appendix A is the needs assessment survey questionnaire. The survey found that the majority of teachers had not been given the information they needed about the unique academic, social, and vocational needs of students with spina bifida.

Completion of this type of assessment is effective in identifying the scope of the problem and can be a key tool in mobilizing resources, obtaining funding, and engaging key persons and agencies in a collaborative endeavor. The development of this manual and the video tape and the initiation of the School Consultation and Training Program were both direct responses to the information obtained through the needs assessment.

PERSONNEL: THE MULTIDISCIPLINARY TEAM

Although an educational outreach program may be centered around one person primarily responsible for the operation of the program, a full multidisciplinary team must be available to provide specific information about the unique needs of any of the program's clients, in any dimension of life where a need may exist. The multidisciplinary team need not be assembled from scratch, as major elements of such a team are often already in place and functioning as a team, and may already be addressing educational needs. The outreach program enlists, coordinates, organizes, and targets these efforts, while identifying areas where more needs to be done. The team ultimately includes professionals working under medical funding, other professionals funded through one or more private nonprofit organizations, consultants, parents and other volunteers, and members of cooperating agencies and organizations.

The Regional Medical Center and Staff

Mission   In most sections of the United States, comprehensive care for persons with spina bifida is provided by the staff of a regional center or clinic, assembling the talents of a full range of professionals and serving the population of an entire state or a major portion of a state. The original mission of the regional centers has been to provide life-long coordinated health care. Along with success in meeting this primary mission has come a growing awareness of the needs of persons with spina bifida that go beyond the medical to the educational, vocational, social, economic, and emotional.

As these needs have become obvious and resources have become available, some regional centers have expanded their mission to address the total needs of persons with spina bifida in all of the systems in which they must function. In some cases, these additional needs are addressed through an expansion of the regional team, and in others through the creation of a collateral nonprofit consumer advocacy agency, usually a spina bifida association. Regional centers and their associated agencies are best equipped to move effectively into educational outreach if they have a history of strong community involvement and have had a focus on training professionals through medical and educational conferences.

Medically Funded Personnel   Within the medical funding stream of the regional centers will be found a variety of physicians, nurses, and allied health care professionals. Physicians on staff may include specialists in neurosurgery, neurology, orthopedics, urology, endocrinology, plastic surgery, and neuropsychology. Generally, one of these also serves as the medical director of the regional clinic, and may have additional executive or directive functions in an associated advocacy agency. The primary role of the physicians in the educational outreach program is to provide information and documentation as needed of the client's medical condition and its impact on education.

Nurses will serve in a variety of capacities including pediatric coordinator, clinic coordinator, pediatric nurse, or adolescent and adult medicine specialist. Allied professionals may include a physical therapist, occupational therapist, nutritionist, social worker, and financial coordinator. Any of these people may be needed to address a particular educational need. If, for example, a student's primary need is for an adapted work space and other adaptations in the school environment, the occupational or physical therapist may be the key person involved in the school outreach program for this student, and would serve as case manager for this case, coordinating other outreach services for the student. Similarly, if bladder training were the key need, a pediatric nurse educator might be the chief interventionist, and would serve as case manager, with informational support from the urologist as needed, and family and school information from the social worker.

Consumer Advocacy Agency Staff

Although a range of professional support for an educational outreach program can be provided through a regional clinic or center, some functions may only be properly funded through a private nonprofit consumer advocacy agency, such as a regional spina bifida association. These include specific advocacy functions including testimony before legislative committees, school boards, and other government bodies. It may also be necessary that the coordinator for the educational outreach program be provided through the advocacy agency. Specific personnel assigned to the outreach program include a program director or executive director as supervisor and a full-time school program coordinator. The school program coordinator should have an educational background and a full understanding of the unique educational needs of students with spina bifida.

Consultants may be required to work with the advocacy association. Consultants are usually funded by the organization that provides them. In Pennsylvania, an attorney from the Education Law Center may be contacted regarding particular cases, especially as those cases may serve as precedents for assuring educational rights for large numbers of students. A neuropsychologist can be very valuable in providing neuropsychological assessments of the educational needs and potential of given students, especially as such an assessment can prove a connection between a particular behavior or disability and the underlying neurological condition. Besides being of value in advocating for adapted programs, these assessments are useful in giving specific directions to concerned educators.

Funding sources for particular projects and for the overall budget of an advocacy agency vary from region to region. Funds have been provided through United Way, memberships, various fund-raising campaigns, and other techniques. Specific projects such as the informational videotape that accompanies this manual can be funded through state and local foundations.

Cooperating Agencies and Organizations

In addition to the personnel and expertise available through the regional medical center and the local advocacy association, the school outreach program and its coordinator need to have recourse to a local network of cooperating agencies and organizations. In most cases these agencies and their key personnel are already known to the local advocacy association from prior collaborative efforts in behalf of the same population.

In western Pennsylvania, these agencies and organizations include the Instructional Support Center, funded by the state and providing instructional materials to the special education community, and the Office of Vocational Rehabilitation, also funded by the state and commissioned to provide an optimum degree of vocational preparation for persons with disabilities. Private agencies include the Visiting Nurse Association and the Learning Disabilities Association of Pennsylvania. The latter provides advocacy and education about the learning disabled. Of course, the specific constellation of collateral agencies will vary from state to state and region to region.

Community Consultation Network

In addition to a trained staff and a system for information management, the educational outreach program benefits from a network of community consultants. This network can be drawn from both lay persons and professionals and from local and national sources. Advocacy associations that have sponsored or attended educational conferences can draw network members from conference presenters as well as participants. Parents involved with the association can serve in the consultation network and can refer other persons to the school program coordinator. Educators and other professionals who have been involved in prior missions of the association may also be available, or may be able to recommend additional resource persons. All of the above should of course be recruited in advance of any specific task, identified with their skills in an accessible file, and called on specifically as needed to assist with specific tasks. Appropriate recognition after a task has been completed, including a note of thanks from the director of the association, can be invaluable in maintaining and expanding the network.

Team Organization Overview

Figure 14.1 provides a visual model of the relationship between the components of the school outreach program. It shows how resources that already exist are organized around the task of contributing support and expertise to the student's education. The final outcome of the system is a higher quality of education and greater degrees of independence.

Team Organizational Overview

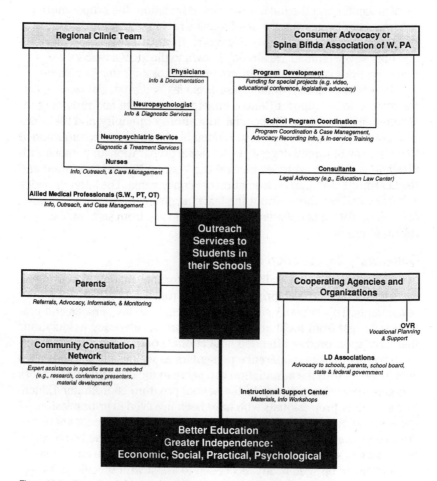

Figure 14.1.   Team organizational overview.

GETTING STARTED

Referrals

A new school outreach program begins with both solicited and unsolicited referrals. The outreach program itself begins because school problems that have not been successfully resolved by anyone else have been referred to the advocacy association. It is through this type of unsolicited referral that the need for a school outreach program is discovered. Active solicitation for referrals begin when the association has decided to address itself to this need in a systematic manner.

Active solicitation for referrals can be undertaken in a number of ways. Some referrals will be generated in response to articles in the advocacy association's newsletter, especially if referrals are explicitly solicited and the name of the contact person given. Referrals are also generated by presentations before community and parent groups throughout the area served by the association, and by presentations made to parents during their regularly scheduled clinic visits.

A comprehensive screening for referrals can be conducted during the regularly scheduled clinic visits by filling out the School Needs Identification Form (Appendix A) with the parents. This instrument provides for thorough identification of needs in fifteen different areas. Each identified need can then be described on a School Needs Action Form (Appendix B) and referred to a particular specialist for service. The referral and action process will be described more fully below.

Staff Development

Staff development for an educational outreach program begins with the medical and clinical orientation of the school program coordinator. During this phase, the coordinator is introduced to key personnel, briefed on standard procedures, and introduced to the procedures developed for educational case management.

Ongoing staff development then becomes the responsibility of the school program director or coordinator. All personnel involved in educational outreach are to be kept informed of changes in regulations and current issues through handouts, presentations, and speakers. Ongoing training also occurs through the regular operation of the program through team staffings, weekly case conferences, and case management reviews by the supervisor.

Information Management and Recording

The School Needs Identification Form (Appendix A) is completed with the parents by the school program coordinator during the regularly scheduled clinic visits at the regional center or during other contact opportunities. This form can also be completed with the clinic social worker, nurse, or any other person familiar with the form. This is a comprehensive eight-page survey designed to identify any school needs of which the client family may be aware. Although some school needs may well be identified through the normal course of contacts during clinic visits, parents are not always aware of what their child's educational rights allow or what situations can be changed. This process also allows a regional clinic to stay current on educational needs of the hundreds of clients who may be served. Upon completion, the School Needs Identification Form is reviewed by the school program coordinator and brought to the next team staffing.

The School Needs Action Form (Appendix B) is used to assign a particular problem from the School Needs Identification Form to the appropriate specialist. These forms are generally completed during or after the team staffing in which the School Needs Identification Form is reviewed and an action plan developed. The assigned specialist records the plan and keeps one copy of the form until closure, at which time the outcome and date of closure are recorded. A second copy is kept in the student's file and updated as the work is performed.

The School Needs Progress Report (Appendix C) provides for more detailed ongoing recordkeeping by each assigned specialist. This form documents any phone calls, letters, or other contacts between regional center staff and persons in the student's home, school, or community. As many pages as are needed are completed and placed in the student's file as the work progresses.

The School Needs Outreach Program Visit Form (Appendix D) provides for the recording of field visits to the home or school, along with the findings or recommendations that result. Note that one or more staff members may be involved in the visit, depending on the needs identified previously and the specialists assigned. One copy is kept in the student's chart and another is centrally filed to record all of the outreach work done.

The School Needs Release Form (Appendix E) is completed by the parent or guardian and authorizes access to school records for those involved in the educational outreach program. It should be completed along with the School Needs Identification Form at the time of the clinic visit, or as early as possible in the service delivery process.

New referrals and current "Priority" cases are reviewed by the entire treatment team at a weekly team staffing. The School Needs Team Staffing notice (Appendix F) form is used to announce which students will be presented at team staffing. The School Needs Summary of School Staffings form (Appendix G) is kept by the school program coordinator to maintain an overview of all of the cases reviewed at a given weekly staffing. This is also used as a case management tool for the school program coordinator.

The School Needs Case Load Management form (Appendix H) provides a method to prioritize service delivery while keeping track of all clients in the service area. Because some regional centers serve hundreds of students, a system such as this is necessary to make the most effective use of personnel without allowing important needs to be over-looked. This form places each student in one of five service categories depending on the status of the student's current needs. The service categories are described below under the heading "Overall Case Management." This form also provides for supervision of the program coordinator.

The School Needs Service Record (Appendix I) provides for tracking and reporting of the types and numbers of problems identified and the types and numbers of services provided by each team member. These records are valuable for the identification of recurrent problems that may require research or new approaches. They are also used for oversight of program operations, and serve as the basis for reports to the board of directors and to funding sources about the ongoing need for the program and the quantity of services provided.

PROGRAM OPERATION

The description of the information management system given above has provided a rough outline of the program operation. The following are additional details of specific areas.

Screening and Case Assignments

Screening of referrals is conducted primarily by the school program coordinator, under the supervision of a program director or the association director. Case assignments are made at the team staffing immediately subsequent to the completion of the School Needs Identification Form. An Action Form is completed for each identified need and given to the appropriate professional. Generally, the management of each case is assigned to the professional who will be most involved with that case. Required input from other team members is solicited and organized by the assigned case manager. Action plans and results are forwarded to the school program coordinator and filed and recorded in accordance with the information management system described above.

Although most cases are identified at the regional clinic, all referrals are not made in this way. The regional advocacy association may serve clients who do not attend the regional clinic. They may also obtain referrals through newsletters to members and through presentations to the general public. Whatever the referral source, service delivery begins with completion of the School Needs Identification Form and proceeds with some variation of the case assignment process described above. Personnel of the regional clinic are of course not assigned to work for clients who are not active with the clinic. When possible, educational advocacy is coordinated with the student's medical service providers, with the bulk of the outreach work being performed by the school program coordinator.

A Sample Case

Screening Donny S. and his parents came to the Allegheny General Hospital Regional Spina Bifida Center for Donny's regular quarterly visit. The clinic social worker talked to the family about how they're all doing in their jobs, including Donny's oldest brother who was recently unemployed. She then asked the family how Donny was doing in school and asked them to fill out a survey with her regarding his educaiton. She explained the purpose of the survey and talked about the School Outreach and Personnel Training Program. As they answered questions about Donny's regular education fourth-grade class, Donny's mother reported a slight problem with gym class. She said that Donny spends most of his gym time in his wheelchair, lifting weights or keeping score. The social worker asked if the fmaily would like someone to look into the situation and see if the school would like some help in developing ways to increase Donny's participation. They completed the School Needs Identification Form and signed a Release of Records form.

Team School Staffing The social worker gave the completed forms to the school program coordinator, who sent the Release of Records to Donny's principal along with a brief letter of introduction to the school program. The coordinator then added Donny's name to two lists: the weekly Case Management Form and the weekly School Staffing announcement. The name was listed under "new referrals" on both forms. The team assembled and began with cases identified as "Priority" cases because of some urgent problem or upcoming deadline. Each team member had previously discussed his or her activities in each case with the acting case manager. The case manager provided a brief summary of this activity and requested suggestions regarding a plan of action. The coordinator then asked if the case should retain "Priority" status and asked how soon the team should evaluate progress at an upcoming staffing.

Donny's Needs Identification information was then summarized by the coordinator and the social worker. Other team members provided pertinent information about Donny's medical, social, or educational history. The physical therapist reported that Donny had just recently gone from walking with crutches and long leg braces to using his wheelchair full-time. The coordinator then asked the physical therapist to act as case manager for as long as the "Priority" status was related to physical education. The team agreed to consider this case appropriate for action by the school outreach program until the physical therapist had spoken to the physical education teacher and brought back further information to the team. The physical therapist began filling out the Action form by noting how the referral was made, briefly describing the problem, and stating the treatment plan formulated by the team. As the work continued, the physical therapist would record what was done and the outcome of the intervention on the Action Form. During the staffing she stated that she would call Donny's mother after talking to the teacher. Both calls would be reported on a Progress Report form. The coordinator then logged the problem and plan on the Staffing Summary form and the team proceeded to other business.

Follow-Up Team Staffings   Two weeks later the physical therapist reported at team staffing that she had been unable to reach the physical education teacher but had left several messages. (Had she made the contact and obtained the information, this would have been reported at the first staffing following the contact.) The team agreed to keep Donny's name on the "Priority" list until some progress was made and scheduled the case for the following week. The coordinator noted these developments on the Staffing Summary Form and placed Donny's name in the "Priority" section of the new weekly Case Management form.

At the third weekly staffing concerning Donny, the physical therapist reported that she had talked to the physical education teacher and that the teacher had requested a school visit and written information about spina bifida and adaptation to the physical education program. She had also called to update Donny's mother and discuss the plans. The physical therapist had documented these two phone conversations on a Progress Report form and had scheduled a school visit. The team then moved Donny's name to the "Active" list and set a staffing date for a few weeks after the school visit to allow time for the school to incorporate the recommendations into Donny's physical education program. The physical therapist planned to tell Donny's mother what was accomplished at the school visit and to ask that she report any information she was given by the school. The physical therapist would also complete the School Visit Report form. After the staffing, the coordinator filed all of the documents on the case including a copy of the written recommendations that would be presented to the physical education teacher.

At the next staffing at which Donny's case was discussed, the physical therapist reported that she had talked to the teacher, who was very pleased with the changes in his class. The team moved Donny's name to the "Monitor" list and noted the date of his next clinic visit. Before that visit, a member of the clinic team would make the usual pre-clinic phone call to ask if there are any problems that need to be addressed at clinic.

Donny's name remained on the "Monitor" list for 1 year to make sure everything at school went smoothly. His parents were reminded at each clinic visit to inform any team member of any school situation. Since no new problems surfaced and the adaptations to the physical education class continued to be appropriate, Donny's name no longer appeared on the case management form after 1 year. His file would remain with the other current files until he finished high school and higher education. A detailed illustration of the school referral and action process is provided by Figure 14.2.

Team Staffings

The weekly team staffing reviews and updates the record of each client who is currently in service "priority" and/or "active" status. New referrals are also discussed, and students who are in "Monitor" status are presented prior to their clinic visits, occurring every 3–4 months. Available team members from all disciplines should be present. Action plans are developed in common and priorities for casework are established. Personnel resources are allocated by revising and finalizing decisions about which tasks will be managed by the various team members.

Team staffings are also used to select clients for educational assessment on the next weekly clinic day. In this way a regional clinic that serves hundreds of clients can ensure that a School Needs Identification Form is completed for each client at least once each year.

School Visits

School visits may include any or all of the following services. In-service training may be provided in cases where there is no specific problem or when a new student is entering the school. The videotape "Teaching the Student with Spina Bifida" may be presented to all of the student's teachers and other relevant personnel. This presentation can be made prior to the student's entry or while the student is attending school. It provides an effective overview of the needs the student may have and will serve as a starting point for discussion. The videotape may also be presented at the beginning of a case conference to serve as a starting point for discussion.

In some cases when referral information is inadequate, the primary purpose of the visit is to perform direct observation, gather information, and report back to the team. The observer should note the adequacy of the physical environment including characteristics of the workspace and proximity to the teacher and the blackboard. Speed and ease of written work should be observed, as well as attentiveness and general involvement in the subject matter. Opportunities should be found to observe the student's social position in the class peer group, including observation of informal times such as lunch, class changes, or work breaks. In addition to classroom observation, a tour of the school can be conducted to determine accessibility of all programs. Direct observation should be performed during other school visits when possible.

Informal case conferences can be held with the classroom teachers, school nurse, guidance counselor, and administrator. These sessions

Referral Protocol

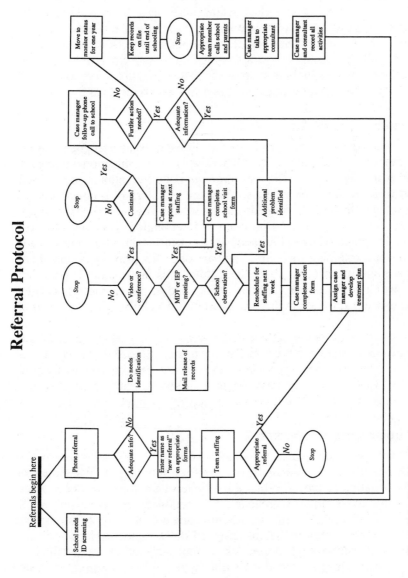

Figure 14.2.   Referral protocol.

provide for information sharing, cooperative planning, and the building of productive relationships. More formal meetings also occur, including Multidisciplinary Team meetings, individualized education program conferences, pre-hearing conferences, and Due Process Hearings. These formal meetings include the presentation of the results of independent evaluations by the team members attending. Sections to be included in the IEP are also presented by team members in these formal meetings. The selection of team members to attend school visits and conferences varies with the subject matter of the visit and the requirements of the case.

Parental Involvement

The importance of parents in an educational outreach program cannot be overstated. Parents are often key drivers of the educational outreach and advocacy process. They are providers of information to the school and to advocacy professionals. They are monitors of progress and of compliance by both the student and the school. They are the first to judge the success or failure of a program or intervention. They are also frequently appointed by either medical or educational professionals to administer a training procedure. They are often the primary recipients of advice and information about their child. This information is provided during clinic, by phone, in home visits, and at parent meetings. They are also and at the same time the most direct advocates for the needs of their child.

There are several very specific areas where parents must be included in the outreach process. Parents must authorize the release of records in writing. (See Appendix E.) Parents are also required to approve school visits. Whenever possible, parents should participate in school meetings, and they should be present for IEP conferences.

Ongoing Case Management

Overall case management is designed to ensure that all cases receive the level of attention they currently require. (See Appendix H.) The system of categorization employed is based on the level and frequency of contact. "Priority" cases require a great deal of attention during the current week. "Active" cases require ongoing attention and are currently being served. "Monitor" cases require that the assigned staff keep themselves informed of current status and developments. "Completed" cases have had the prescribed services performed with satisfactory results. Completed cases will become active again when new needs are identified. "New Referrals" require Needs Identification (Appendix A) and one or more Action Forms (Appendix B).

Individual case management is designed to ensure effective service delivery. Many informal contacts can be followed by correspondence to document the contact. Correspondence serves as a courtesy that maintains relationships. It provides information in a retrievable form and makes decisions, suggestions, acknowledgements of progress, and reports of further need accessible to persons not involved in the original contact. It also provides a safeguard against future dispute about what was stated and decided. The simple act of putting communication in writing is also an important form of assertiveness.

It is likewise important to follow a contact with a subsequent visit or phone conference. This provides an opportunity to learn what has worked and what difficulties have been encountered. It also lets all parties know that the outreach program remains involved with the student's needs.

Recording

Recording forms (Appendices A, B, C, D, E, F, G, H, and I) have been described above (Information Management and Recording). An education file is maintained by the school program coordinator who should ensure that all relevant forms are completed and forwarded. Upon completion of the release form, access to the medical files of the regional clinic should be provided. When students are not active with the regional clinic, medical information is secured from the medical service provider as needed and with a release form. This information can then be stored in the student's education file.

SUPPORTIVE MATERIALS AND SERVICES

The materials and services in the educational outreach program are all designed to meet needs in the areas of health and access issues, cognitive issues, social and emotional issues, and vocational issues. Materials and services include this manual, the accompanying videotape, informational handouts, and educational conferences.

Using the Videotape

The videotape, "Teaching the Student with Spina Bifida," runs for 30 minutes. It provides an overview of the major topics treated in the manual and is an excellent brief introduction into the medical history and educational needs of students with spina bifida. It is directed to a general audience and is well suited for in-service training, parent meetings, and educational conferences. The videotape was developed to support the Educational Consultation and Personnel Training Program and is currently being used for in-service training and prior to case conferences. It is best presented by an educational advocate or outreach coordinator who is familiar with the contents of the manual and prepared to accurately answer questions raised by the audience after the videotape has been presented.

Using the Book

This book, *Teaching the Student with Spina Bifida*, is designed as a reference guide, with sections covering most of the major areas that may be encountered in the education of a student with spina bifida. As supportive material in an educational outreach program, it can be used in two ways. The entire book can be provided to classroom teachers, administrators, school psychologists, and any other professional who serves this population. It may also be used in sections to provide selected information to personnel who are grappling with a particular need or issue. Both forms of use require that the educational outreach coordinator and other members of the outreach team be thoroughly familiar with the contents of the book.

Using Informational Handouts

A wide variety of fact sheets, brochures, and other informational handouts are available from a variety of sources. The outreach coordinator can obtain and maintain a supply of these materials and provide them to parents and educators as needed. Appendix J is a partial list of current sources of these materials.

Providing Educational Conferences

Educational conferences can be held on an annual basis at a site near the regional clinic or center. Parents and educational professionals can be invited to a program of presentations and workshops designed by the local spina bifida association. A faculty of presenters and discussion leaders can be drawn from the local support network, the clinic team, and the association. This faculty can be supplemented and enriched by the addition of speakers who are more nationally known. Besides disseminating information, conferences can serve to identify resource persons for future tasks and can provide opportunities for groups of experienced people to seek new solutions to difficult problems.

ADDITIONAL PROGRAM COMPONENTS

Although case management and direct client service are the most critical responsibilities of an educational outreach program, additional services and functions can and should be performed.

Research

Research into all aspects of education for students with spina bifida is ongoing and needs to be pursued, promoted, and followed. In addition to obtaining recent research findings and incorporating them into the information being provided, the educational outreach program should encourage and promote ongoing research into the needs of this new population.

Policy Advocacy

Policy advocacy is an ongoing need as federal, state, and local policies and regulations governing education are repeatedly revised. Outreach personnel must be alert to proposed changes and opportunities for improvement. The impact of such changes on students with spina bifida should be thoroughly evaluated, position statements developed, and members of the support network mobilized to give testimony, contact decision makers, and draft concrete and specific amendments to proposed regulations.

Parent Education

Parent education workshops are vital for bringing new parents into the full information stream as early as possible. They also provide updated information to parents of older students as new information and research findings become available. A final function of these workshops is to keep parents informed about changes in regulations governing their children's educational rights, to inform them of new programs that are available, and to enlist them as appropriate in current advocacy campaigns.

Program Coordination

Program coordination with local rehabilitation or camping programs can ensure that full knowledge of the students educational needs and abilities is made available to other professionals who will be working with the student.

CONCLUSION

The best possible education for students with spina bifida may be ensured by developing and operating an effective school outreach program. Although additional resources may require the full- or part-time services of a school program coordinator, the bulk of the program and personnel resources mobilized by the program are already in place at many regional centers. Through organization, coordination, and monitoring of these resources, an effective school outreach program supports both the school and the student by intervening with needed information and services at critical points in the student's career. The more effective education that develops will result in higher levels of academic, vocational, and social competence and will promote a greater degree of independence for the young adult with spina bifida.

GLOSSARY

Action plan Written description of the short-term activities (e.g., phone contacts, correspondence, meetings) to be performed by specific school program team members on behalf of particular student.

Active status Case management category to describe school situations that require frequent but not crisis-oriented activity to carry out the specific action plans.

Case conference Any meeting between two or more individuals involved in the education of a particular student (e.g., parent[s] or guardian[s], school program team member, location educational or allied health professional) to identify a school problem or to implement/update the student's action plan.

Case management Organization of all of the activities and documentation required for obtaining and monitoring services needed by an individual student throughout the student's educational career. It often includes long-range planning and interpreting information with the student and the student's family.

Case manager Specific member of the school program team assigned to coordinate all the information and activities described in a specific student's action plan. Assignment is based on matching the member's specialty (e.g., physical or occupational therapy, social work, health, nutrition, or education) with the nature of the specific problem.

Completed status Case management category to describe school situations in which the initially-reported problems as well as any/all subsequently discovered problems have been satisfactorily resolved. Also used whenever a parent/guardian or student refuses any further assistance.

Consumer advocacy agency (also referred to as a volunteer association) Any organized group whose mission is the advancement of knowledge and services for individuals with a common interest (e.g., disability). It may also refer to a direct services provider agency whose consumer population shares specific needs.

Endocrinology The medical specialty dealing with the systems of glands, hormones, and organs that affect growth, metabolism, and other internal body states.

Functional independence Often referred to as the most crucial goal of education, related services, and vocational preparation, the term refers to mastery of the skills necessary for successful adulthood; such skills include those used to live, work, and enjoy a social life in one's community with minimal assistance from parents or professionals.

Individualized family service plan Individualized, written description of the goal, activities, and services which will enable the family of a child with a disability to assist the child in his/her development. It is prepared by early intervention (infant and toddler) program staff and the specific family and is based on meeting needs which the family has identified. It cannot be implemented without the consent of the family.

Mission Overall philosophy and purpose of an organization which directs its choices of services to provider, and guides its long-range planning activities.

Monitor status Case management category that describes school situations requiring only quarterly activity. Information-gathering from parents is done preceding the quarterly visit to the regional center clinic.

Multidisciplinary team Group of specialists representing various professional disciplines (e.g., nursing, therapies, nutrition, social work, and education) who exchange information and make recommendations for action plans to assist students in obtaining appropriate educational services.

Neurology Medical specialty dealing with the organs and network of the central nervous system.

Neuropsychological assessment Collection of tests designed to measure and describe brain functioning for the purposes of educational or vocational planning as well as for medical diagnosis.

Neuropsychology Branch of psychology concerned with the relationship between the brain and behavior.

Neurosurgery Medical specialty dealing with operations involving the central nervous system (brain and spinal cord).

Orthopedics Medical specialty dealing with bones, joints, and muscles.

Outreach All the activities of a regional center that focus on building a collaborative relationship with local education and allied health personnel in a student's community.

Plastic surgery Medical specialty dealing with operations involving the skin and underlying structures.

Policy advocacy All of the activities (e.g., presenting testimony, writing position papers) undertaken to educate administrators or politicians about the impact of new systems, eligibility requirements, or service quantity on the persons they serve.

Position statement Formal document written to describe the philosophy, recommendations, new technical knowledge, or important background data related to a specific social concern or proposed social change (e.g., inclusion of students with spina bifida in their neighborhood, schools, or provision of aggressive medical treatment to all newborns with spina bifida). It is distributed by a consumer advocacy agency to educate the community at large about the needs of the consumers it serves.

Priority status Case management category to describe school situations that are either in crisis, or that have an upcoming deadline requiring immediate activity (e.g., an IEP conference, or a surgical procedure). Cases in this category receive daily or weekly activities and weekly team staffing.

Regional center Medical facility specializing in the care and treatment of a particular health condition or disability by means of high-level technology, expertise, and multidisciplinary team management. It is usually affiliated with a medical school or university research center.

School team staffing Weekly meeting of the clinical and education specialists who staff the School Consultation and Personnel Training Program. Each case is reviewed to update the Action Plan by adding outcome information or other data and by revising the Plan if necessary. Cases where activities are no longer required are closed or moved to a monitoring level of activity for one year. New cases may be added at this meeting also.

Treatment plan Written description of particular medical or therapeutic activities and services provided to a specific student. It is usually kept in the student's medical chart, and may be reviewed if appropriate, at a school team staffing.

Urology Medical specialty dealing with bladder and urinary tract. For males, this specialty may also deal with matters of sexuality and reproduction.

School Needs
Identification Form

Student's name _____

_____ A cooperative program of _____

Spina Bifida
Association of
W. Pennsylvania

ALLEGHENY GENERAL HOSPITAL
320 East North Avenue
Pittsburgh, Pennsylvania 15212-7986

Spina Bifida Center

School Needs
Identification Form

Student's name _____ Date of Birth _____
Parents' names _____ Phone (h) _____ *month day year*
Address _____ (w) _____
_____ zip _____ County_____

Name of school _____ I.U. _____
Supervisor of Special Services _____

School program _____ Current grade _____
Primary teacher _____ School principal _____

Referred by _____ Interview date_____
Name of interviewer _____

Area(s) of Reported Need

1 ☐ Health related services

2 ☐ Physical management instructions

3 ☐ Accessibility

4 ☐ Safety and fire drills

5 ☐ Preparation for school entry

6 ☐ Educational rights and related services

7 ☐ Academic difficulties

8 ☐ Psychological assessment

9 ☐ Perceptual motor deficits

10 ☐ Visual perception deficits

11 ☐ Self help skills

12 ☐ Social acceptance

13 ☐ Social and emotional issues

14 ☐ Parent and school relationships

15 ☐ Transitional services

16 ☐ Other needs _____

_____

_____

School Needs Identification Form   Name _____

Please check each area where services are needed.
Check the name of the problem or needs and provide a brief description.

☐ 1 Health Related Services

☐ Bladder program   ☐ Orthopedic management

☐ Bowel program   ☐ Diet

☐ Seizures   ☐ Food and nutrition

☐ Hydrocephalus   ☐ Other (please specify) _____

☐ Skin care   _____
                            _____

Description _____
_____
_____

☐ 2 Physical Management Instruction

☐ Bracing and body mechanics   ☐ Handling of a child who is braced or
                                        unbraced
☐ Entering doorways
                                    ☐ Providing opportunities for
☐ Ascending steps   position change

☐ Descending steps   ☐ Care of adaptive equipment
                                        ☐ Braces
☐ Getting down to floor   ☐ Crutches
                                        ☐ Wheelchair
☐ Transfer from wheelchair to standing position

☐ Transfer from wheelchair to sitting position   ☐ Other (please specify) _____
                                    _____
☐ Classroom position   _____

Description _____

School Needs Identification Form

Name _____

page 3

☐ 3 Accessibility

☐ Access to classroom   ☐ Access to all school activities

☐ Access to cafeteria   ☐ Appropriate seating, desk, locker

☐ Access to field trips   ☐ Other (please specify) _____

☐ Access to library   _____

☐ Provisions for special bathroom   _____

Description _____

_____

☐ 4 Safety and Fire Drills

Description _____

_____

_____

☐ 5 Preparation for School Entry (preschool & school age)

☐ Preparing the parents   ☐ Other (please specify) _____

☐ Notifying the school   _____

☐ Testing   _____

Description _____

_____

_____

School Needs Identification Form   Name _____

☐ 6 Educational Rights and Related Services

☐ Individualized Education Program   ☐ Occupational therapy

☐ Clean intermittent catheterization   ☐ Speech and language therapy

☐ Transportation   ☐ Classroom aide

☐ Psychological assessment   ☐ Other (please specify) _____

☐ Adaptive physical education   _____

☐ Physical therapy   _____

Description _____

_____

_____

☐ 7 Academic Difficulties

☐ Mathematics   ☐ Abstract conceptualization

☐ Reading   ☐ Attention span deficits

☐ Reading comprehension   ☐ Selective attention

☐ Writing   ☐ Organizational problems

☐ Perceptual and language difficulties   ☐ Other (please specify) _____

                                          _____

                                          _____

Description _____

_____

_____

School Needs Identification Form   Name _____

☐ 8 Psychological Assessment

Description _____
_____
_____

☐ 9 Perceptual Motor Deficits

☐ Eye-hand coordination   ☐ Other (please specify) _____

☐ Hand dominance   _____

☐ Crossing midline   _____

Description _____
_____
_____

☐ 10 Visual Perception Deficits

☐ Visual memory   ☐ Other (please specify) _____

☐ Figure ground   _____

☐ Spatial relations   _____

Description _____
_____
_____